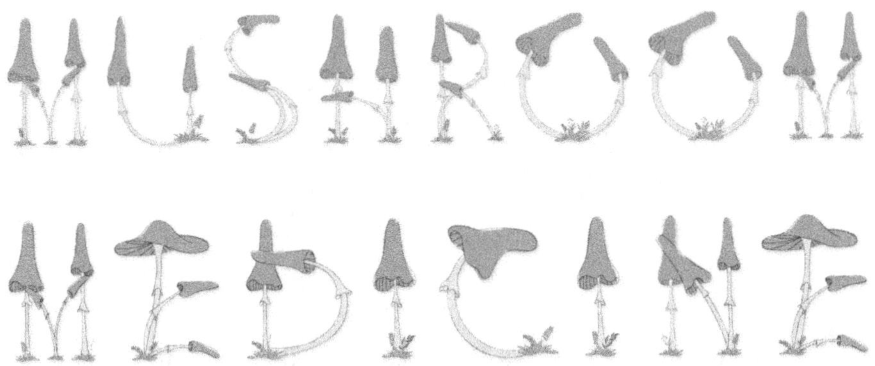

The Future of Functional Fungi

ROBERT DALE ROGERS (RH) AHG

ISBN: 979-8-3627-8793-6

CONTENTS

INTRODUCTION

Over a decade has passed since the latest edition of *The Fungal Pharmacy*.

Interest in the potential of Medicinal Mushrooms has rapidly increased, with new discoveries and research published nearly every week.

I published *Medicinal Mushrooms: The Human Clinical Trials* several years ago, to help fill the gap of misinformation regarding the benefits associated with double-blind, placebo-controlled trials. Oncologists who continue advising their patients undergoing chemotherapy and/or radiation, to avoid all supplements, are either misinformed or repeating un-scientific dogma, resulting from their medical training. Mushrooms not only alleviate side-effects, associated with these toxic invasions, but show significant clinical efficacy in extending survival rates.

This book, with complete citations present information on numerous medicinal mushrooms, and their distinct, and unique compounds. A few chapters are updated from articles previously printed in *Fung*i magazine.

This book includes information on various *in vitro*, *in vivo* and human clinical trials that may lead to novel, safer, and less invasive natural approaches to restoring health and wellness.

This book examines the health-related potential of 64 genera and 159 species of mushrooms. Enjoy the journey!

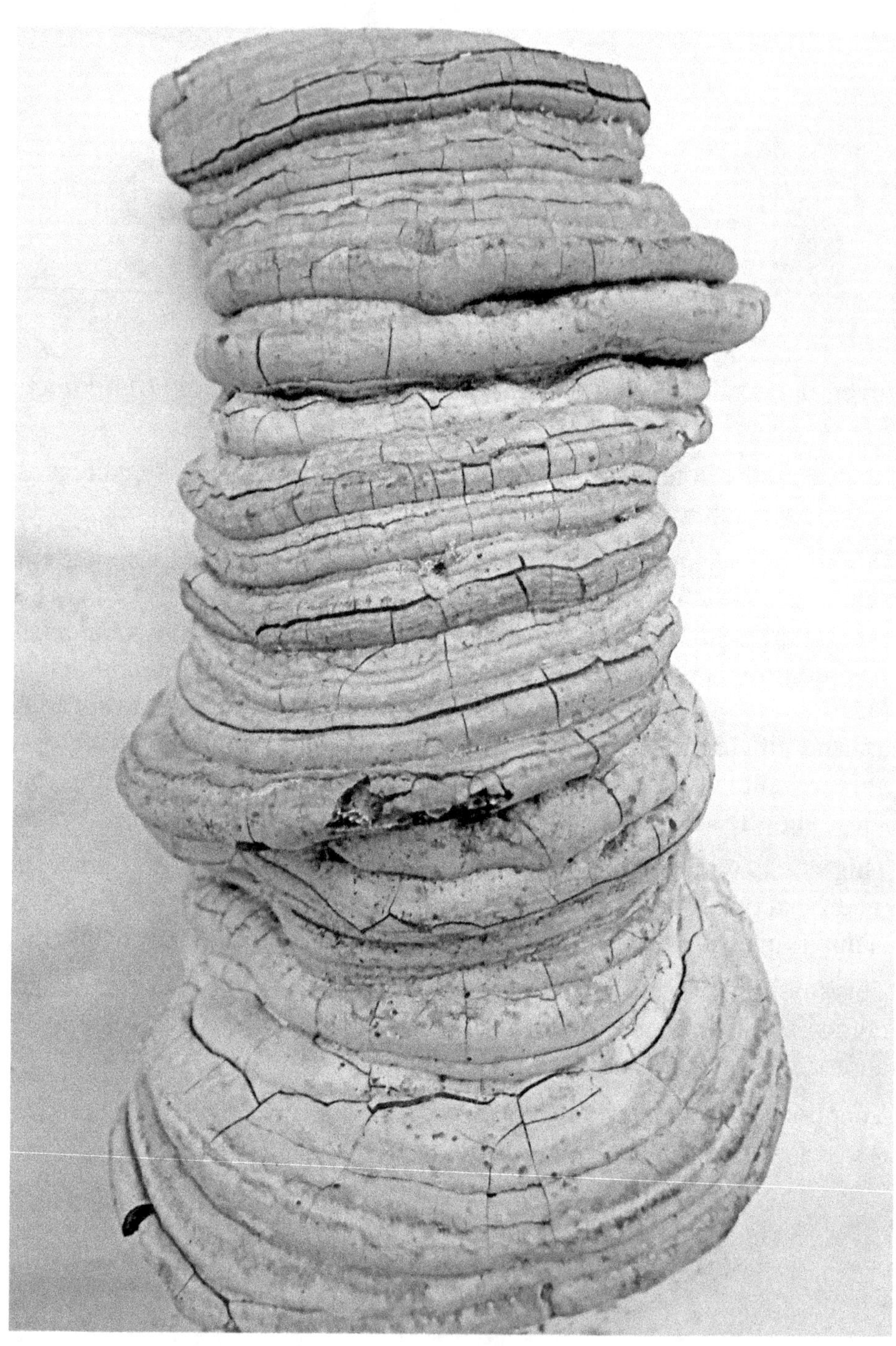

Stacked Artist's Conk, often mistaken for Agarikon

AGARIKON
(Fomitopsis officinalis)
(Laricifomes officinalis)

Larche tre…giueth also…ye famous medicine called Agarick.
TURNER

One dramme of Agaryke and a half dramme of fine Rheubarbe.
ELYOT 1533

Quinine Conk or Agarikon is occasionally found in the Pacific Northwest mainly on Douglas Fir, but also on Englemann spruce, white and black spruce, and occasionally on pine or larch. It has a roasted, tea-like odour, when fresh.

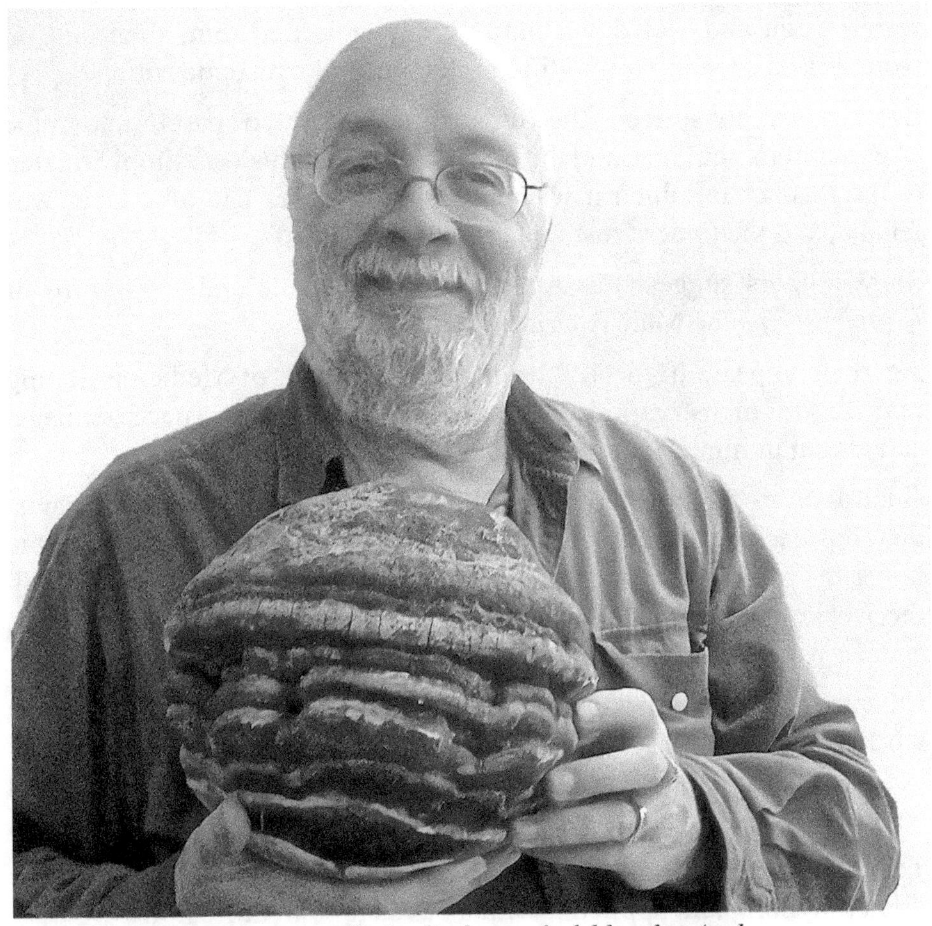

Fomitopsis officinalis being held by the Author

Dioscorides used the name Agarikon. "Its properties are styptic and heat-producing, efficacious against colic and sores, fractured limbs and bruises from falls...it is given in liver complaints, asthma, jaundice, dysentery, kidney diseases and cases of hysteria. In cases of phthisis it is administered in raisin wine, in affections of the spleen with honey and vinegar. By persons troubled with pains in the stomach and by those who suffer from acrid eructations the root is chewed and swallowed without any liquid."

The Roman writer Pliny, who copied anything, named it Agaricum.

The powdered dry fungus was used for hemostatic application like the powder of puffballs. Thin strips were cut from younger specimens after the hard pellicle and undersurface tubes were removed. These strips were beaten and wet down until soft, pliable and thin; then laid on wounds as a dressing, providing protection and antiseptic action.

Dioscorides considered the fungus to have two parts, one male (Agaricum masculum), and the other female, but this was simply related to the manner in which it was cut for commerce. The tube layer was female, and the upper crust male (no pun intended).

Some authors suggest this Agaric was the Female and *F. ignarius* or *F. fomentarius* the Male Agaric.

Agaricon appears in the 12th century Syriac Book of Medicines, citing remedies for menstruation, excessive urination, repairing nerve damage, and aiding in immortality.

Gerard, in his famous herbal of 1597 recommended, "it is good against the shortnesse of breath, called Asthma, the inveterate cough of the lungs, the ptysicke, consumption and those that spet blood: it comforteth the weake and feeble stomacke, causeth good digestion, and is good against wormes."

Ethnomycology of the Pacific Northwest is somewhat scarce. Early work by Newcombe (1897 & 1898-1913) remains unpublished, but has been "re-discovered" by Nancy Turner (1979, 1990, 1998, 2004) and colleagues.

The Alberta Cree know it as **WAH PAH TOOS**. They powdered the dried polypore, and applied it with a bandage to treat frostbite.

Spirit figures placed on shaman graves of the British Columbia coast, were carved from the large, perennial polypores. They often include mouth and/or stomach orifices, which gave them spirit-catching capability.

Paul Stamets suggests that some of the 50 year-old conks resemble women, like Venus of Willendorf, in form. The Native tribes considered the conks as objects with supernatural powers and were used by shaman in various rituals.

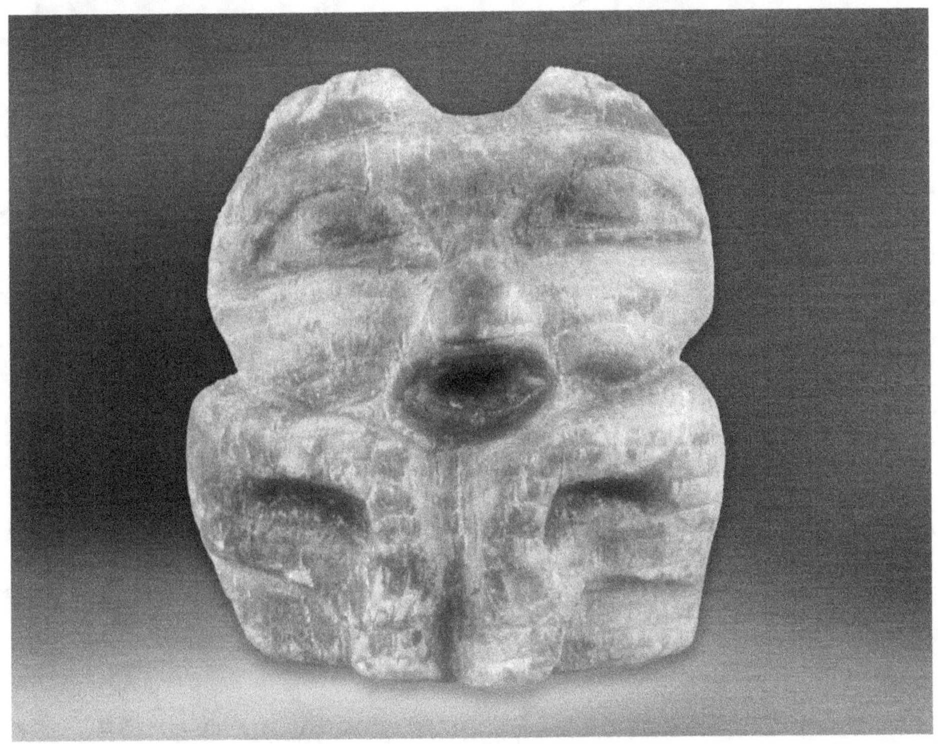
Agarikon carving picture courtesy of Robert Blanchette

After the death of a shaman, the carved conks were placed, as guardians at the head of their grave, letting others know spirits occupied the site.

It was known as **'ADAGAN** or "Bread of Ghosts", by the Coast Tsimshian, with important medicinal and spiritual use. The Tlingit call it **TAK'A DI**, meaning, "tree biscuit". They formerly used it as a poultice for swollen and inflamed areas.

The Bella Coola created effigy figures used in a special "fungus dance" of their Kusiut ceremonies (Turner 1979).

Paul Kroeger (2012), noted west coast mycologist, adds to the mushroom mythology and its relationship to totem poles in his excellent book.

"The origin of the Back-pack or fungus described as having been obtained from Nelli, a Nitcaoten man of the Gitemdanyu clan, by the Hagwelget Gitemdanyu, in acknowledgment of their cooperation in a potlatch, in the Nicaoten country, Nelli had granted to his helpers the right to use his crest (*nettse*) the Fungus."

"Wutarhayaets of Gitwinlkul, a Gitksan, was the carver…When the pole was erected, a wooden imitation of a huge lump of fungus or punk, resembling a hollow ball; was made out of wood by Teelee, a Larhsaelyu, of what is now Moricetown; and it was fastened to the pole; at the back of the human figure below the two ravens. It disappeared many years ago." (Barbeau 1929)

The Haida word for bracket fungus is **GYAALGAS NAAN-GHA**, which translates as "sea biscuit's grandmother". They also used it for carving shaman's effigies and/or to mark graves. The fungi were used to move fire, in the form of hot coals, much like the false tinder conk, *Fomes fomentarius*.

The Haida personified the bracket fungi as Fungus Man, and due to his strength was used by Raven (Yaahl) to steer his canoe. According to legend, they went to find female genital associated with the origin of women and, of course, the female archetype. It is considered a protector of women's sexuality.

The Haida narrative about the origin of women (if that is really what it is about) was drawn on the white, underside of the Tree Fungus (*Ganoderma applanatum*). Nancy Turner, who has helped preserve Pacific Northwest ethnomycology, writes. "This story is pictorially represented in an argillate plate carving (slate dish No. 17952, Field Museum of Natural History, Chicago) designed and made by Charlie Edenshaw…in 1894.

The supernatural powers were increased through the shaman's art forms. Various carved "wooden" objects in many museums are actually the carved sporophores of *F. officinalis*. They were often in animalistic form meant to protect from evil spirits.

G. Emmons collected large numbers of these carved objects in the late 1800s, sailing up and down the coast of British Columbia and Alaska. He shipped them to the American Museum of Natural History in New York.

Notes by Emmons suggest the grave guardians were made from wood and placed on graves to protect the shaman during his long death sleep. They appear to have been oiled or greased, to increase their dark colour. Others were painted and one was ornamented with copper.

During society rituals, the conks were displayed in the ceiling timbers of special dance houses of the shaman for ritual protective purposes. The Squamish hung them in their homes to protect the inhabitants from evil thoughts. The carved fungi were also believed to re-direct evil or malicious thoughts directed their way, back to the person who sent them.

Their role as spirit catchers and objects helping the shaman séance may be interpreted from various shape orifices of the mouth and stomach region.

These forms are significant, and when the shaman died, were placed to guard his grave. The grave guardians let other people know the area was sacred and not to be disturbed.

Enrico (1995) re-translated, Tree Fungus, Xuya's [Raven's] Steerman, a story told to Swanton (1905) by John Sky:

Xuya [Raven] wanted to go on a journey to a certain reef to fetch "certain short objects," which were female genitalia: "Then they say he left there. While he was going along, they say he managed to pick up his sister. He let her off at his wife's place. Then they say he left. He asked Junco to be crew for him and took him with him. He also took a spear. The female genitalia were climbing on each other on the reef there [like chitons]. When the canoe got near it, Junco became deranged. Then Raven went back with him, they say. He asked Steller's Jay [**kl'aay kl'aay**] to be crew for him and set out with him, too. When they got near it, Stellar's Jay too just flapped his wings around. Raven failed with everything [that he asked to go with him] and he drew a design on a bracket fungus and sat it in the stern. Then, 'Keep your eyes open and backpaddle every once in a while,' he said to him. Then he left with him. When the canoe got near the roof, the fungus just shook its head.

He [**Xuya**] speared a big and a little one [female genitalia] and put them aboard and went back with them. He landed and summoned his wife and stuck one on her. Then he put one on his sister too. **Siwaas** [his sister] cried. Then he said to her, 'But your little one will be safe [from me]!

John Enrico elaborates on this translated passage. "Raven here refers to lineage exogamy. Nevertheless, he soon tricks his sister into having sex. Swanton noted here that women of the Raven moiety, to which Raven and his sister belonged, were said to behave less promiscuously than Eagle women, hence the description of **siwaas**'s genitals as "little".

The Hanaksiala of Pacific Northwest decocted the ground polypore gathered from spruce to treat tuberculosis (Compton 1991).

Work by Blanchette et al, (2021) suggest mycelial fabric mats, in two museums, may have been produced from the fungi, by indigenous people of North America.

European strains of this polypore are rapidly in decline, and in many areas are close to extinction. It grows best at temperatures between 20° to 24° Celsius.

Today, medicinal mushroom companies are importing fruiting bodies from larch trees growing in the Altai Mountains of western Siberia. Sustainability issues are of concern.

In Japan, the polypore is known as **EBURIKO**, and used as a general tonic and natural anti-oxidant and bactericide. The belt of waxes and oils around the mushroom margin are used sparingly in the seasoning of foods. This oil, upon extraction is used to treat slow healing skin wounds, to smooth dry, coarse and chapped skin and to repair skin tissue, and treat phlebitis, psoriasis and eczema.

It is a novel source of gamma linoleic acid, fungal omega 3 polyunsaturated fatty acids, and other lipids including trans-retinoic acid.

Super critical CO_2 extracted oil is used for sensitive skin products, facial tonics, hair shampoos, liquid soaps and rinse off skin and hair products.

Cosmetic companies utilize this polypore in natural products to effectively refine pores and make the skin look smoother and easy to apply color make up. One extract is marketed as Astrindyl LS-8865.

MEDICINAL

CONSTITUENTS - fruiting body - agaricic, agaricolic and agaricinic acid, agaricin (containing 97% agaric acid and 3% agaricol), ergosterol, eburical, cetyl alcohol, ricinolic, eburicoic, dehydro-eburicolic, ricinoleic, agaric and dehydro-buriconic acids, fomefficinic acid A-G, fomefficinol !-B, fomlactone A-C, versisponic acid D, agaricol, phytosterin, dehydromatricaria ester, octadien-(1,7)-diin-(3,5)-diol-(1,2)-carbonic acid-1, ergosta-4,6,8(14),22-tetraenon-(3), beta glucans, triterpenoids, dehydrotrametenolic, dehyrdroburicoic, 3-ketodehydrosulfurenic and sulfurenic.acid, various gums, resins and carbohydrates.

mycelium - various indole compounds (L-tryptophan, 6-methyl-D,L-tryptophan, melatonin, 5-hydroxy-L-tryptophan [518mg/100g d.w.), p-hydroxybenzoic and gallic acid, catechin, phenylamine, ergosterol, ergosterol peroxide.

Argarikon has slightly sweet, bitter and cooling energetics, reducing intermittent fevers; night sweats in tuberculosis, and is a mild laxative.

It was included in the famous Warburg's Tincture, also known as *Antiperiodica Tinctura*, of the late 1800s. This compound was used mainly for relief of night sweats associated with tuberculosis.

It tones the lungs, removes lumps from the abdomen, soothes vital energy, allays asthmatic wheezing, reduces edema and promotes diuresis.

Grzywnowicz (2004) has reported traditional Polish use of Agarikon to treat coughing illness, asthma, rheumatoid arthritis, and infections.

The Ainu of Northern Japan have long used the peeled and dried fruiting body for stomachache, body pain and reducing sweat.

Gerard, the famous English herbalist of the 17th century, used agaric for cleansing the intestine, jaundice, menstrual problems, asthma, chronic and recurring fevers, and edema.

Quinine fungus from larch has been used traditionally for hemorrhoids, water motions, and vomiting. It helped to cure coughing, asthma, nephritis, urinary calculii, nosebleed, swollen sore throats, and peritonitis.

It possesses a distinct quinine, bitter taste that helps distinguish it from other polypores.

It is not much used today, as it has a slight irritating effect on the bowel. Because it arrested sweating slowly, it was often mixed with ground wild carrot seed.

It dries up breast milk, and in the past was used for cases of chorea or epilepsy.

It was official in the Pharmacopoeias of Switzerland, Austria and Portugal until recent times. It is rarely found in Europe and Asia at the present time.

The fungus is used in Unani medicine for coughs and colds, as well as asthma, and as an expectorant. It is known as **GHAARIQOON** in this medical system that moved from Greece to Arabia and then to India. One compound medicine called *Habb-e-Iyarij* contains Agaric and is use for facial paralysis, epilepsy, a brain tonic and melancholia. The fungus is given with honey to promote the eruption of measles, chicken pox and other childhood infections. Recent work by Paul Stamets identified anti-pox properties in the polypore, confirming an ancient folkloric use (2005).

More recent work by the National Institute of Health, the National Institute of Allergy and Infectious Disease and the US Army Medical Research Institute screened various mushroom extracts against a number of viruses.

Agarikon showed very strong activity against cowpox, mentioned above, and vaccinia. The mycelium shows promise against smallpox.

Other viruses including influenza B, the H1N1 (swine flu), H3N2 and H5N1 (avian flu) strains, yellow fever, West Nile, arenaviruses such as Tacaribe and Pichinde, and Punta Toro a hemorrhagic virus similar to Rift Valley Fever Virus, all showed inhibition by extracts of this polypore (Rogers 2011).

Recent work by Teplyakova (2012) found strong anti-viral activity against H5N1 flu virus. It may prove useful in drug-resistant tuberculosis strains. (Hwang et al, 2012).

Both fruiting bodies and mycelium possess medicinal benefit.

Work by Fijalkowska et al, (2020) found anti-proliferative effects of mycelium and fruiting bodies on A549 lung cancer, DU145 prostate, and A375 melanoma cancer cell lines.

The following year, Fijalkowska et al, (2021) supplemented zinc and magnesium salts in the culture medium, helping increase various active substances.

The mycelia extract and purified cytokinin fractions reduce HepG2 cell growth in vitro (Vedenicheva et al, 2021).

Practitioners believe it exerts a potent synergistic activity in neurological and inflammatory conditions. Work by Graf and colleagues investigated the transformation of hydroxytriterpene acids in the polypore to 11-keto-corticosteroids (1960).

The extraction of the fruiting body with Fo3-chloroformic acid, promoted apoptosis, activated G2/M-phase cell cycle and induced NF-kappaB proteins against HepG2 cancer cell lines (Altannavch et al, 2022).

Sauer, an 18th century German American wrote in his *Compendious Herbal*, translated by Weaver (2001). "Agaric operates through its divers earthy salts, as well as through a caustic, soft resinous component. It is thus endowed with rather bitter after tasting compounds with the capacity to purge both by stool and urine, and to expectorate phlegm from the chest...for persons afflicted by the falling evil (epilepsy), an agaric decoction ... should be used to scrub the head. Agaric is employed with great favour in laxatives made with wine. But it is also possible to achieve an excellent extraction of agaric's properties by infusing it in brandy and then boiling it to a soft extract that can then be rolled into balls and administered in the amount of 20-24 grains as laxative pills."

The main indication for use, however, is alternating chills and flushes of heat, with bearing down pain in the back.

Alcohol extracts of the mushroom resemble atropine, with relaxation of intestinal spasms, smooth muscles, and drying up of nasal secretions.

It shows inhibition against sarcoma 180 cancer cell lines of 80%.

Early work by Robbins found this polypore inhibits *Staphylococcus aureus and E. coli* (1945).

(Sato et al, 2002) found dehydrotrametenolic acid acts as an insulin sensitizer in glucose tolerance tests and reduces hyperglycemia in non-insulin dependent diabetes.

Work by Chen et al, (2005) looked at the aromatase and 5alpha reductase inhibition properties of button (*A. bisporus)* mushrooms. Several strains of *F. officinalis* were found to contain compounds with similar activity, suggesting possible benefit in the prevention of breast, prostate and other hormone sensitive cancers.

Decoctions are best, one teaspoon every two hours. Prepare with 0.3-0.9 grams in one pint of water as slow simmer (<75°C) for at least one hour.

Tincture 10-15 drops as needed. The official medicine is made from the inner portions of the freshly picked polypore. Prepare at 1:5 and 90% alcohol. Let sit two weeks. Press and remove the marc. Decoct at 1:20 until reduced to half, cool, strain and combine two liquids.

NOTE - It should be noted that extraction with boiling water does not isolated active Beta-glucan. Active B-glucan can be obtained in individual state by cold alkali extraction after dehydration of the fruit bodies and removal of components extractable by boiling water (Golovchenko et al, 2020).

HOMEOPATHY

Boletus laricis is made from the triturated dried fungus *Fomitopsis officinalis*.

The main indications are night sweats, pancreatic and hepatic inflammation. The eyes may be glued shut in morning with dull pain in the eyeballs, painful gums, and a thick yellow coating on tongue.

There may be a metallic taste in mouth, with nausea and vomiting, burning pains in area of gall bladder. Stools may be yellow and thin, or bloody with a high fever, dull pain in the back and legs, and shivering up and down the back, hot flushes and profuse sweats at night.

Burt and Lord identified some peculiar symptoms including the sensation of teeth pressed out of their sockets and frightful dreams of water.

Other symptoms include coppery taste in mouth, dry, dark lumpy stools, great weakness and prostration, great restlessness at night.

DOSE - 1st-3rd potency as needed. Burt and Lord did a proving on 6 males in 1868.

Laricifomes officinalis e mycelio is used for night sweats, asthma, coughs, chronic polyarthritis and as a laxative. It is produced from the mycelium according to a process developed by Dr. G Enderlein.

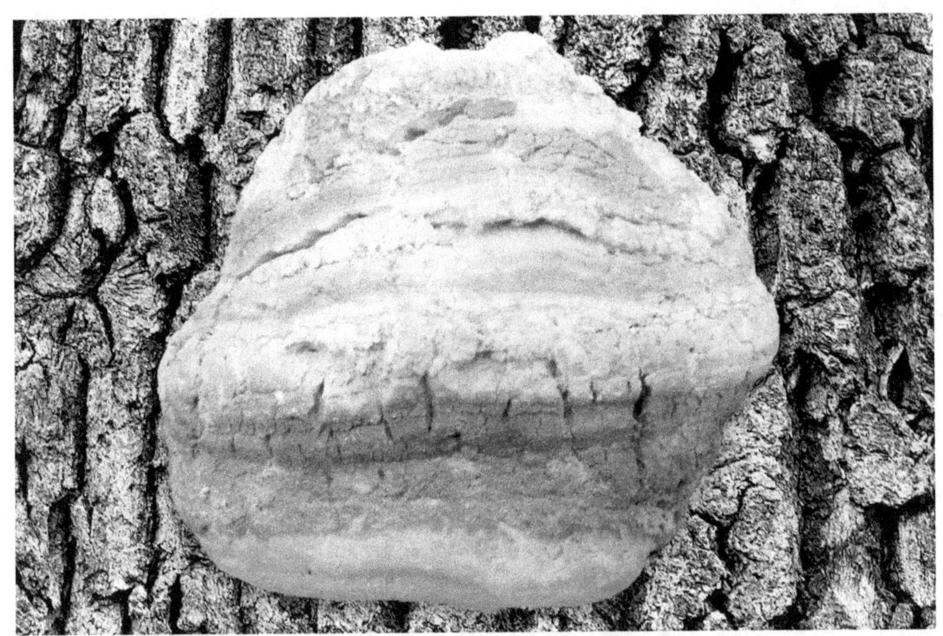

Laricifomes officinalis

DOSE - 4X-5X. Take 5-10 drops under tongue before meals. For polyarthritis, it can be rubbed into affected area. A commercial product Larifikehl is available as drops, ampoules, capsules or suppositories.

Agaracin is a substance isolated from *F. officinalis*, and then attenuated for medicine. It is valued for conditions like Sydenham's chorea. This is mainly a childhood condition affecting more girls than boys, and associated with rheumatic fever.

It is recommended for night sweats in doses of one quarter to one half gram, by Boerike.

It is used for chorea associated with dilation of the heart and pulmonary emphysema, fatty degeneration and erythema.

Anxiety, impaired memory and speech are present, as well as contraction of the muscles of the body and extremities. May be helpful in erythema.

Agaracin may help those prone to epileptic seizure or parasethesia.

In King's American Dispensatory, agaritin in doses of 1/16 to 1/6th grain is reported to show great benefit in excessive sweating, especially in phthisis, where it allays thirst and controls cough and diarrhea.

Blackwood says that "this remedy is of special service in those patients who have nervous dyspepsia…In those patients who have been addicted to the excessive use of tea, coffee or tobacco, are recovering from some debilitating disease that has greatly weakened the heart; the pulse is weak and irregular, while the heart's action is weak and attended at times by violent palpitations. There is profuse sweating with twitching of muscles and dilatation of the heart".

DOSE - Third to sixth potency as needed.

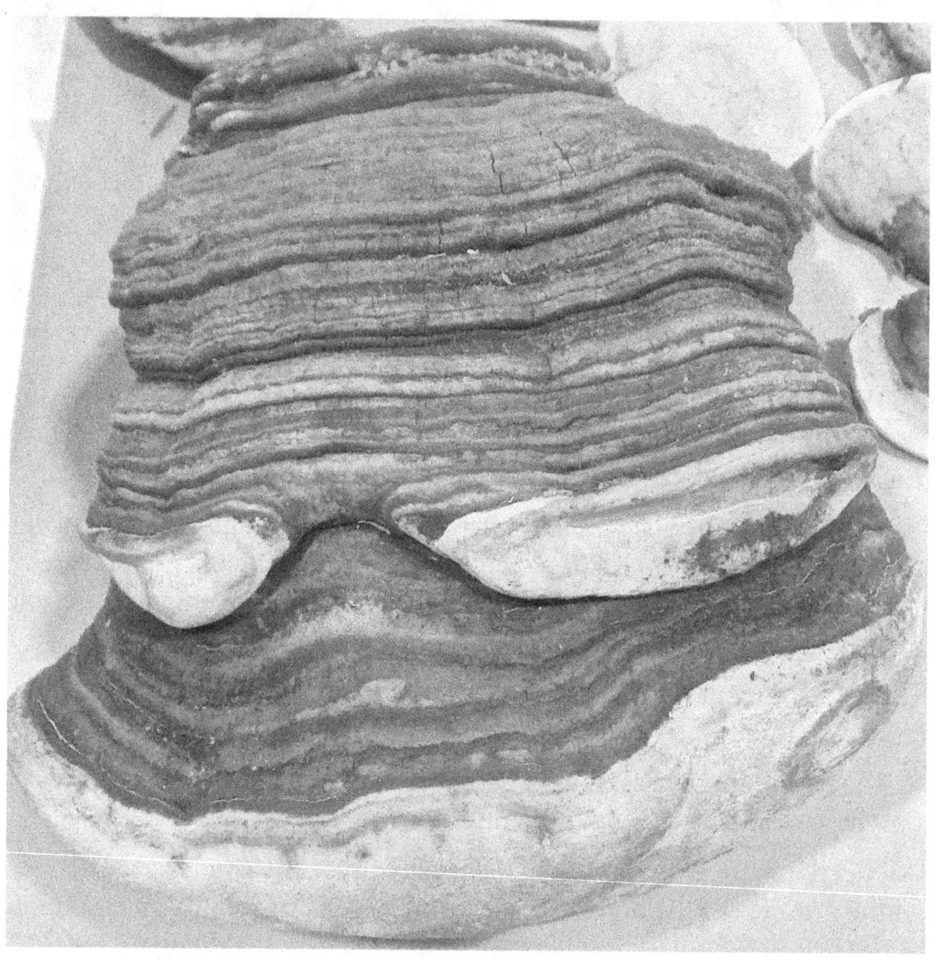

Agarikon

ALBATRELLUS
Sheep Polypore
Forest Lamb
(*Albatrellus ovinus*) (Scaeff.) Kotl. & Pouzar
Goat's Foot
(*Scutiger pes-caprae*) (Pers.) Bondartsev & Singer
(*A. pes-caprae*) (Pers.) Pouzar
Confluent Polypore
(*A. confluens*) (Alb. & Schwein.) Kotl. & Pouz.
Blue Capped Polypore
(*A. flettii*) Morse ex Pouz.
Crested Polypore
(*A. cristatus*) (Schaeff.) Kotl. & Pouz.
Greening Goat's Foot
(*Scutiger ellisii*) (Berk.) Murrill
(*A. ellisii*) (Berk.) Pouzar
Blue-Pored Polypore
(*Neoalbatrellus subcaeruleoporus*) Audet & B.S. Luther

CONSTITUENTS - *A. ovinus*- neogrifolin, methyl-neogrifolin, grifolin, scutigeral, acetyl-scutigeral, ilicicolin B, ovinal, ovinol, albatrellins A-F, confluentin, meroterpenoid pigments. *A. confluens*- albaconol (prenylated resorcinol), neoalbaconol, (+)-(R)-grifolinone, albatrellin, grifolin, neogrifolin, grifolinone A-B, conflamides A-I. Mycelial culture contains aurovertin B and E. *A. fletti*- confluentin, grifolin, neogrifolin. *A. cristatus*- grifolic and cristatic acid, cristatomentin. *N. subcaeruleoporus*- various farnesylpenols, including 8 neogrifolin derivatives, grifolin, neogrifolin, albatrelin G-H, albatrellin.

Albatrellus is a pored member of Russulales family, found growing on the ground. They are firm of texture and quite edible, when well cooked.

Ovinus refers to sheep, and confluens means, "running together." The entire genus could benefit from further DNA analysis. *Scutiger*, *Albatrellopsis*, and *Neoalbatrellus* are legitimate species variations, at the present moment.

Many of the 12 NA species exhibit blue or green coloring, and are associated with either hardwood or conifer species. Spore prints are white.

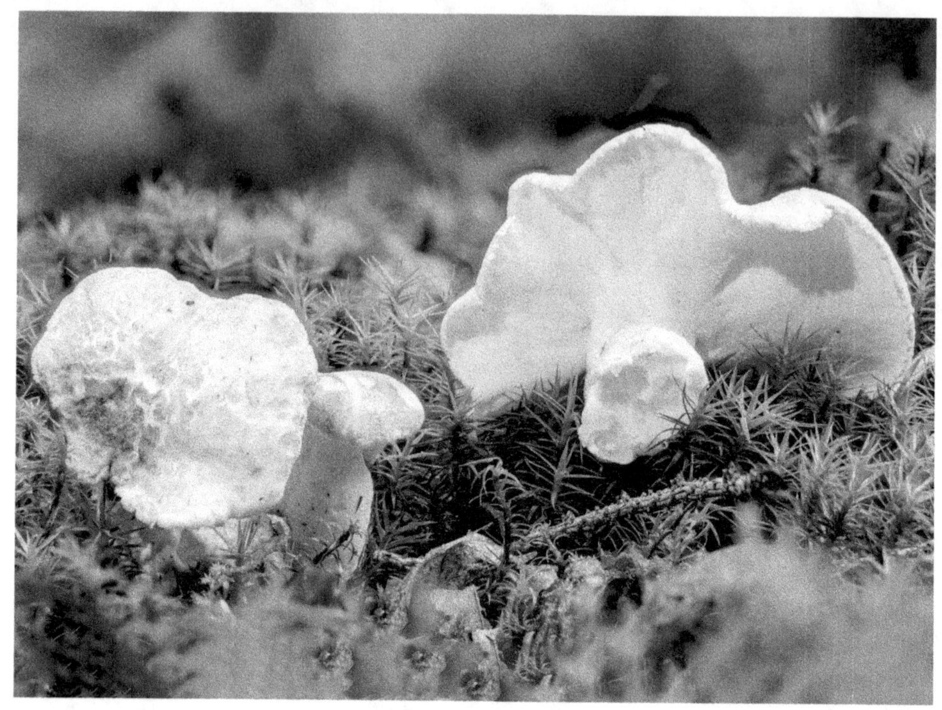

Albatrellus ovinus

The highly edible Goat's Foot (*A. pes-caprae*) is brown to reddish-brown, and further north under conifers, is found the equally delicious Greening Goat's foot, with its yellow-green to yellow-brown cap. Both spore surfaces stain green.

Sheep polypore is harvested commercially, and found under conifers in the Pacific Northwest. In Japan, the mushroom is known as *Ningyoutakemodoki*.

Grifolin, also present in Maitake (*Grifola frondosa*) fruiting body, is common to several Albatrellus species, and shows significant activity against a wide range of cancer cells, via various pathways.

Early studies suggested anti-bacterial activity, reduced cholesterol levels, anti-oxidant properties and inhibited histamine release from mast cells, all based on *in vitro* and *in vivo* animal studies. Grifolin, it should be noted, is insoluble in water.

Grifolin targets DAPK1 (death-associated protein kinase 1) signaling to induce cell cycle G1 phase arrest of nasopharyngeal carcinoma cells (Luo, X.J. et al. 2011).

It directly targets and binds to ERK1/2 protein kinases; supressing adhesion, migration and invasion of high-metastatic cancer cells, in a mouse model (Luo, et al, 2015).

A mouse study found grifolin induced apoptosis (cell death) in various human osteosarcoma xenografts. It induced cell death by inhibiting NADH generation and ATP production, without obvious toxicity (Zhao, et al, 2018a).

Earlier work by Chen et al. (2015) found neogrifolin induced apoptosis in human osteosarcoma cells, including U2OS and MG63 cell lines.

Grifolin has been investigated for potential treatment of sensitive skin conditions, by blocking TRPV1 receptors. A cosmetic formulation containing 3% *A. ovinus* extract, including grifolin, significantly reduced stinging and burning sensations from capsaicin or thermal stress, in a randomized, controlled trial. (Hettwer et al, 2017). A neurocosmetic on the market, Defensil®Soft, contains the mushroom extract, propanediol and citric acid.

Grifolin, derived from *A. confluens*, induces apoptosis and promotes cancer cell cycle arrest in A2780 human ovarian cancer cell lines. The pathway is via AKT and ERK1/2 signaling, to some extent (Yan et al, 2017).

The latter pathway, in a study by Wu and Li (2017) suggests inhibition of gastric cancer cell lines by the compound.

Early work by Ye et al. (2005) found grifolin strongly inhibited CNE1 (nasopharyngeal), HeLa (cervical), MCF-7 (breast), SW480 (colorectal), K562 (chronic myelogenous leukemia), and Raji (human Burkitt's lymphoma). The first four cell lines exhibited induced apoptosis.

Grifolic acid is a derivative of grifolin, and induces GH3 (anterior pituitary adenoma rat cells) toward apoptosis (programmed death) through inhibition of NADH production. The study by Zhao et al. (2018b) found grifolic acid significantly reduced the mitochondrial membrane potential, decreased cellular ATP, and increased the intracellular NAD/NADH ratio.

Scutigeral, derived from Sheep Polypore, interacts with vanilloid receptors, suggesting an orally active pain-reducing compound, that unlike capsaicin, is not pungent on the human tongue (Szallasi, A. et al., 1999).

Scutigeral, grifolin, neogrifolin, albaconol and confluentin were studied by Hellwig et al, (2003) and were found weak antagonists, as opposed to agonists, on human and rat vanilloid receptors.

Confluentin is weakly cytotoxic against human HL-60 (myeloid leukemia), SMMC-7712 (hepatic), A549 (lung), and MCF-7 (breast) cancer cell lines, *in vitro* (Liu et al, 2013). Liu et al. (2014) found albatrelin G and H, derived from *N. subcaeruleoporus*, weakly cytotoxic to the same cell lines.

Conflamides D and E, derived from *A. confluens*, exhibit potent inhibition against lipopolysaccharide-induced B lymphocyte cell proliferation. The human implication is unclear, as B cells can be both pro- and anti-inflammatory and tumor activating and apoptosis-inducing in various types of cancer cells (Zhang, S. et al, 2018). Because medicinal mushrooms possess immune modulating benefit, the potential benefit, or aggravation, in auto-immune conditions is unknown.

Albaconol, at doses higher than 1.0 microgram/ml inhibited production of macrophages, and induced apoptosis at 7.5 mcg/ml. At lower doses, without apoptosis, it significantly inhibited LPS-induced TNF-alpha, IL-6, IL-1beta and NO production. This suggests potential for immunosuppressive and anti-inflammatory applications (Liu et al., 2008). Suppression of dendritic cell function may be due to impairment of NF-kappaB activation.

Albatrellin exhibits *in vitro* activity against HepG2 human lung carcinoma cell lines (Yang, X.L. et al, 2008).

Grifolin and neogrifolin, derived from *A. confluens*, is cytotoxic to human prostate adenocarcinoma (PC-3), and colorectal adenocarcinoma (HT-29) cell lines (Dube et al, 2022).

Neoalbaconol induces energy depletion and induces apoptosis in various cancer cell lines by targeting the PDK1-PI3-K/Akt signaling pathway (Deng et al, 2013).

Neoalbaconol also induces apoptosis in human cholangiocarcinoma (bile duct) cell lines both *in vitro* and *in vivo*. It appears to work via the AKT pathway by targeting phospharate and tension homolog detected on chromosome 10 (Zhou, G.Y. et al, 2016).

Work by Yu et al, (2017) found neoalbaconol inhibits angiogenesis (the formation of blood vessels) and tumor growth in a breast cancer xenograft model, *in vivo*.

The cultured mycelia contain aurovertins, very unusual for basidiomycetes. Aurovertin B is an ATP synthase inhibitor that halts proliferation of breast cancer cell lines, but does not affect normal MCF-10A cell lines (Huang, I.C. et al, 2008).

Recent work by Wu et al, (2020) found aurovertin B exhibits potent anti-proliferative activity against triple negative breast cancer cells (MDA-MB-231). The authors suggest the compound could possibly induce more apoptosis than taxol (tamoxifen) treatment.

Aurovertin B stimulates the expression of the natural killer group 2D receptor on natural killer cells. It appears to sensitize colorectal cancer cells to recognition and targeting these cells to death (Zhu, H.F. et al, 2018).

Cristatic acid, present in Crested Polypore, is cytotoxic and anti-bacterial against various Bacillus species (Bycroft, 1987).

Work by Akiba et al, (2020) identified several new and seven known compounds in the related A. yasudae. Grifolic acid and neogrifolin, showed inhibition of amyloid-beta aggregation, suggestive of potential benefit in Alzheimer's disease (AD). Maybe. One study of amyloid-beta plaquing associated with AD, found that when cut open, 70% of them contained the human herpes simplex virus 1. This suggests the leaky brain, often associated with leaky gut, acted to protect itself from viral invasion and formed the plaques in defense. As one author noted, it may be amyloid-beta is the fireman, not the fire. Surely something to think about as ongoing research into prevention and potential cures are explored. My recommendation is that individuals prone to cold sores, regularly take lysine, and avoid high arginine-rich foods, especially nuts.

Medicinal mushroom research at the University of Northern British Columbia continues to discover possible health benefits from regional fungi.

Confluentin, isolated from *A. flettii* ethanol extracts, suppressed KRAS expression in SW480 human colon cancer cells, inducing apoptosis and arresting cell cycle at the G2/M phase (Yaqoob et al, 2020).

Blue Albatrellus (*A. flettii*) mushroom essence is associated with behaviors and mental patterns of optimism and pessimism. Thomas Friedman writes, "Pessimists are usually right, and optimists are usually wrong, but all the great changes have been accomplished by optimists." Rogers (2016).

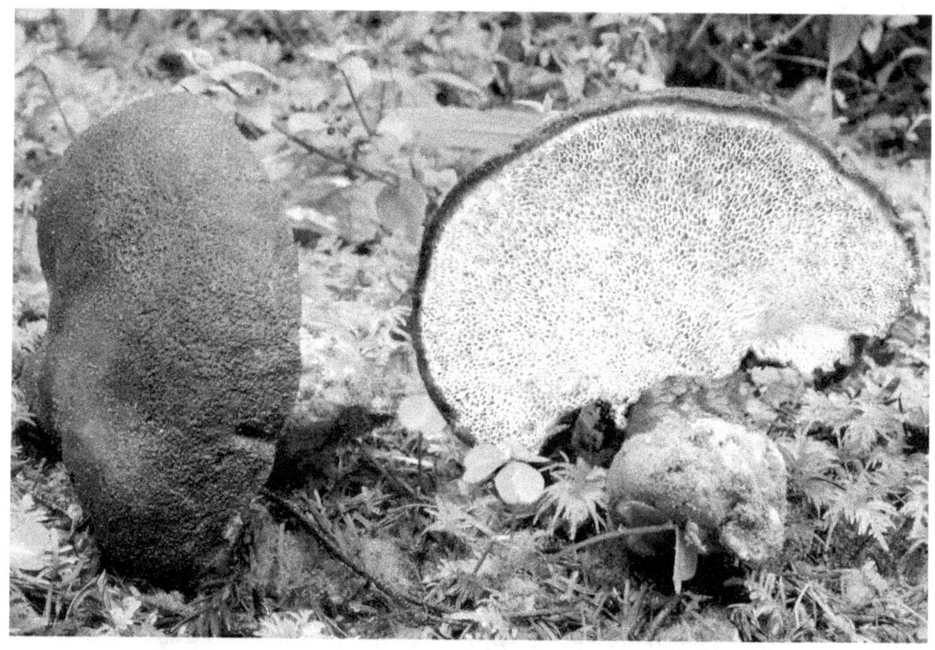

Scutiger pes-caprae courtesy of Daniel Winkler

ARMILLARIA
HONEY MUSHROOM
(Armillaria mellea group)

Honey mushroom is one of my favorite fall collectibles, in the rarer, wetter years it fruits in my part of the world.

Its distinct tawny color and massive fruiting gives rise to excessive gathering. The fresh, cooked mushroom is not my favorite, so it means lots of drying for winter meals. The stalks are tough, and best used for broth in soups and stews.

Honey mushroom is not just one species, with at least ten distinct North American variations (Ross-Davis et al, 2012).

The Honey mushroom (*A. solidipes*/*A. ostoyae*) growing on 2400 acres in the Blue Mountains of eastern Oregon, is considered the largest living organism in the world. Some scientists suggest it may be over 2400 years old.

It is tenacious and develops these "shoe string" rhizomorphs which robustly invade over 600 different species of trees and herbaceous perennials.

Douglas Fir is a favorite. Suzanne Simard (2022) in her intriguing book Finding the Mother Tree, notes a unique relationship between the conifer and birch. It appears that the latter roots contain *Pseudomonas fluorescens*, a bioluminescent bacteria, antagonistic to *Armillaria ostoyae*. The related *A. sinapina*, associated with broadleaf trees, will attack birch near the end of their 50-year lifespan.

In 1791 Albrecht Wilhelm Roth noted these strings and named several species *Rhizomorpha*. Armillaria was not put forward until 1857, and thus precedence should be held, at least taxonomically. A recent paper by Stalpers et al, (2021) suggests Armillaria be preserved, as well as opinion on numerous other genera names. This will take several years to sort out, as it moves up the nomenclature ladder.

The parasitic, and edible *Entoloma abortivum* is able to overcome the oxalic acid defense mechanism of *Armillaria* species (Koch & Herr, 2021).

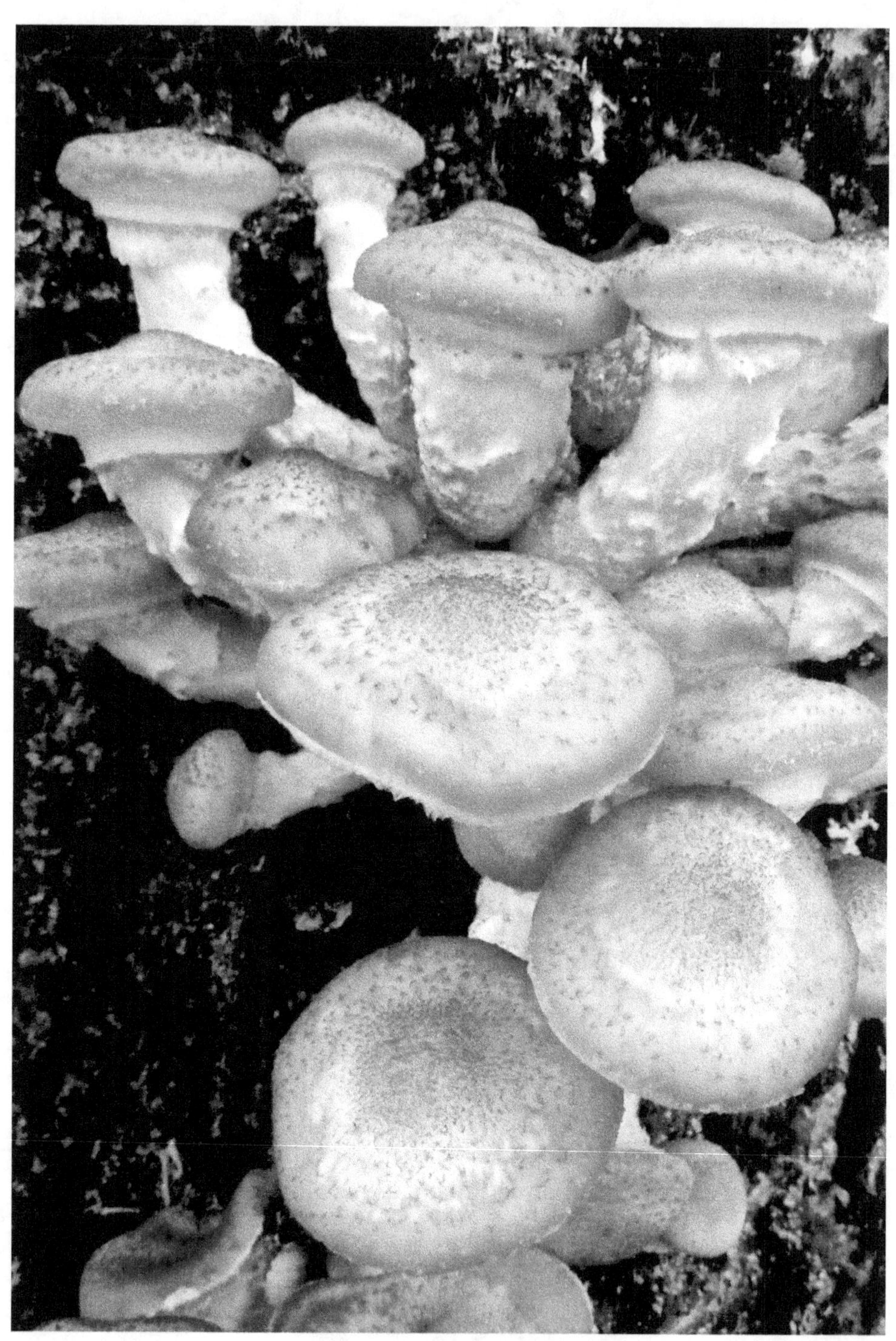

Armillaria mellea

In China, it is known as *Mi Huan Jun*, and in Japan, *Naratake*. Traditional Chinese medicine (TCM) categorizes honey mushroom as sweet, with neutral energy, influencing the liver meridians. It is used to calm the liver, reduce internal wind, and restrain floating yang, according to TCM modalities. It has been used for centuries for treating insomnia, and for calming a hyperactive liver in the book *Cao Ben Shi Yi*.

The mushroom is unique in that the growing mycelium and rhizomorphs glow a blue-green phosphorescence, with maximum intensity at 7:30 pm. Radiation from mushrooms will penetrate cardboard and develop photographic plates.

Why only the mycelium? It appears the complete set of enzymes and substrates for bioluminescence under conditions of free oxygen access. The luciferin precursor, hispidin, and 3-hydroxyhispidin hydroxylase in fruiting bodies is blocked (Purtov et al, 2017).

The emission range in nine species of mycelium varies slightly in intensity from 515-525 nm (Mihail, 2015).

Work by Huang et al, (2017) found the growth of Umbrella Polypore (*Dendropolyporus umbellatus*) sclerotia is related to infection of symbiotic honey mushroom and secondary compounds. In fact, the growth of sclerotia requires the rhizomorphs of honey mushrooms to supply nutrition (Xing et al, 2020).

The fruiting body contains a number of indole compounds including tryptamine, L-tryptophan and serotonin (2.2 mg/100 grams dry weight).

In China, mycelium tablets are easily available for treating a variety of neurological conditions, including headache, insomnia, epilepsy, neurasthenia, after-stroke syndrome, limb numbness and hypertension.

Armillaria tablets given to 43 patients in Shanghai reduced cholesterol, triglycerides and blood pressure levels in the vast majority.

In animal studies, it protected bone marrow cells from the chemotherapy drug cyclophosphamide.

Armillarinin, an aromatic ester, induces apoptosis in human liver and leukemia cell lines, *in vitro*.

Another compound, armillaridin differentiates and activates human macrophages, helping modify inflammatory conditions (Liu et al., 2015).

A xylosyl galactofucan significantly supressed the release of tumor necrosis factor-alpha (TNF-a) and cytokine macrophages, suggesting anti-inflammatory activity (Chang et al, 2018).

Armillaridin inhibits four human esophageal cancer cell lines, via apoptosis. Studies by Chi et al, (2013) suggest it may both inhibit cancer growth but also enhance radiation on human esophageal cancers, in synergistic manner.

Armillardin induces autophagy-associated cell death in human chronic myelogenous leukemia K562 cells, but not in normal monocytes (Chang et al, 2016).

Armillarikin, another compound, induces apoptosis in human leukemia cells, *in vitro* (Chen et al, 2014).

Later work by the same lead author (Chen et al, 2016) found this compound induced apoptosis, *in vitro*, of human hepatocellular (Huh7, HA22T & HepG2) carcinoma cells (HCC).

Melleolides, derived from mycelium, are cytotoxic to HepG2 cells, inducing cell arrest at the G2/M phase (Li et al, 2016).

Melleolides also inhibit 5-Lipogenase, which initiate the biosynthesis of pro-inflammatory leukotrienes from arachidonic acid (König et al, 2019).

Bohnert et al, (2011) compared cytotoxicity of 11 melleolides, against four human cancer cell lines. Armillaridin was the most active against Jurkat T cells; suggesting anti-leukemic activity.

The same team led by Leu et al, (2019) found armillaridin inhibited the growth of above carcinoma cell lines, but not through apoptosis. Instead, armillaridin induced HCC cells through autophagy, suggesting an anti-hepatoma compound.

Ethanol and water extracts show significant reduction of uric acid in a mouse study by Yong et al. (2018). The inhibition of xanthine oxidase suggests potential benefit in the treatment of gout, without the renal toxicity of allopurinol.

Polysaccharides derived with ultrasonic extraction from wild fruiting bodies possess significant anti-oxidant and immune modulating activity (Chen et al, 2020).

Work by Kostic et al. (2017) observed a reduction in *Pseudomonas aeruginosa* biofilm.

Animal studies found honey mushrooms calm heart rates, reduce peripheral and coronary vascular resistance, and increase blood flow and oxygen to the brain.

Mycelium extracts reduce beta-amyloid plaque, in *in vivo* animal studies.

A fermented extract reduced seizure activity in mice. Watanabe et al, (1990) identified a novel N6-substituted adenosine, 1000 times stronger than adenosine in protecting cerebral brain cells.

Mycelium polysaccharides were tested on Alzheimer's disease model mice. The study is intriguing, as movement, and endurance improved. It reduced the apoptosis rate, amyloid beta deposition, oxidative damage and p-Tau aggregations in the AD mouse hippocampus. Central cholinergic system functions improved after a four-week supplementation, as indicated by enhance acetylcholine and choline acetyltransferase concentrations, and reduced acetylcholinesterase levels in blood and hypothalamus (An et al, 2017).

Two separate rodent studies by Lin et al, (2021), and Zhang et al, (2021) suggest potential benefit for treating depression.

The first trial gave water extracts of honey mushroom (*A. mellea*) to rats for 4-5 weeks, and then looked at content of serotonin in frontal cortex. Both acute and chronic anti-depressant effects were noted.

The second mouse study involved protoilludane esters derived from *A. mellea*, given at 1mg/kg, i.p. Marked anti-depressant-like activity was noted, as well as increased levels of hippocampus dopamine and GABA, and decreased levels of glutamate.

Water and alcohol extracts of the mycelium increase both REM (rapid eye movement), and non-REM sleep in animal studies, suggesting possible benefit in the treatment of insomnia (Li et al. 2021).

A fermentation liquor relieves insomnia via alteration of gut microbiota and the serotonergic systems. It enhanced 5-hydroxytryptamine content and the expression $5HT_{1A}$ and $5\text{-}HT_{2A}$ receptor in hippocampus (Yao et al., 2022).

A novel lectin, isolated from *A. luteo-virens*, inhibits proliferation of MBL2, HeLa and L1210 cell lines (Feng et al, 2006).

Gastrodia elata is a perennial, saprophytic orchid that depends upon the hyphae (mycelium) of honey mushroom for nutrients. The orchid was first recorded in early Chinese *Materia Medica* around 100 AD., for insomnia, dizziness, tinnitus and nervous tension. It has been well-studied, and in many cases, both the Tian Ma orchid and honey mushroom exhibit similar neurological benefits.

The endophytic fungus *Epicoccum* associated with this orchid was co-cultured with *Armillaria* species, leading to unique, novel compounds. One constituent showed moderate, *in vitro*, activity against five human cancer cell lines, and weak acetylcholinesterase inhibition (Li et al, 2020).

Work by Ojemann et al, (2006) suggest the orchid, its constituent vanillin, and its symbiotic fungus Armillaria hold great promise for cost-effective and less toxic alternatives to standard epileptic drugs.

The ketone diet was originally devised by Johns Hopkins some 80 years ago, and showed great benefit in many cases of epilepsy. When the first drugs were developed, the research was unfortunately stopped.

HUMAN CLINICAL TRIALS

Tracking down the human clinical trials conducted in China has been a challenge, to say the least. Some lack citations, and others are confusing.

According to a study of 43 patients with hyperlipidemia (high serum cholesterol), armillaria tablets shows a serum cholesterol decline of 48mg% after treatment, with an effective rate of 83%. In those patients with elevated triglycerides, they also declined by 42mg%, and effective rate for lowering triglycerides was 75%.

Other symptoms associated with hypertension also improved, with 86% of patients showing systolic/diastolic pressure reduction, and symptoms such as dizziness, oppression of the chest, nervousness and other symptoms improved. This report was from the Central Hospital of Shanghai, Jingan District, no date or author given.

Armillaria fermentation liquid, prepared as a tablet, was given to 45 patients with dizziness, tinnitus, numbness of limbs and insomnia associated with yin-deficiency or yang excess. Symptomatic curative effect ranged from 60-82% for the various symptoms. (Zhou 1978).

Armillaria fungus tablets (250 mg/tablet) gave a similar result as intramuscular injection (2ml ampule) of Gastrodia tuber for vascular nervous headaches. Fifty-two patients were treated and the effective rates were 81% and 83% respectively. (*Jiangsu Prov Coop Research Group*, 1980).

Another study reported on the use of Gastrodia tuber injection or Armillaria fungus tablets on vertigo. Hypertension, arteriosclerosis, Meniere's syndrome and common vertigo are caused in TCM by liver deficiency and wind. One hundred and sixty-nine patients enrolled and effect rates of 92% for injection, and 79% benefit for the mushroom extract (Jiang et al, 2002; Duan, 2000).

Honey mushroom essence may be helpful in those searching for perpetual or regained youth, and the feeling that life is passing them by too quickly. This can lead to impetuous action and the desire to return to adolescent behavior (Rogers, 2016).

DOSAGE - mycelial tablets are used in China 3-4 grams daily.

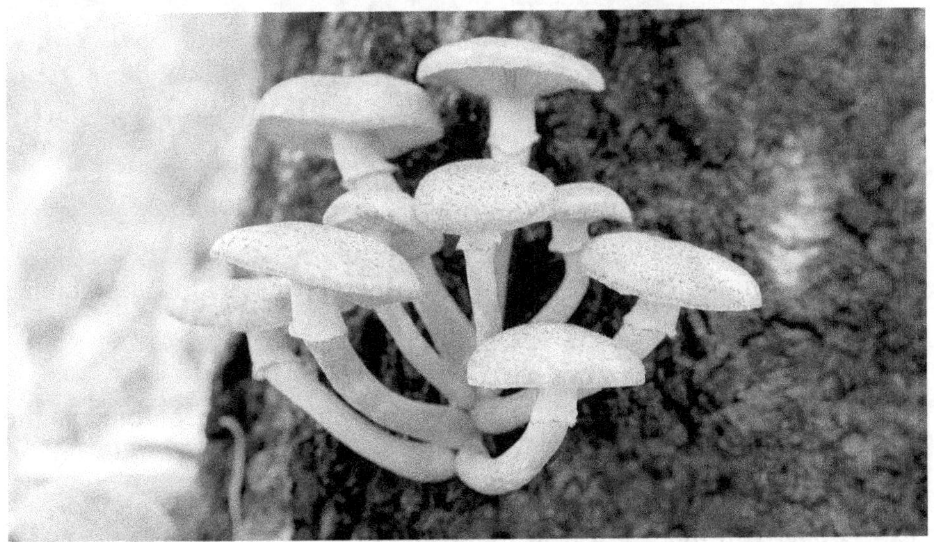

Armillaria mellea

ARTIST'S CONK
(Ganoderma applanatum)

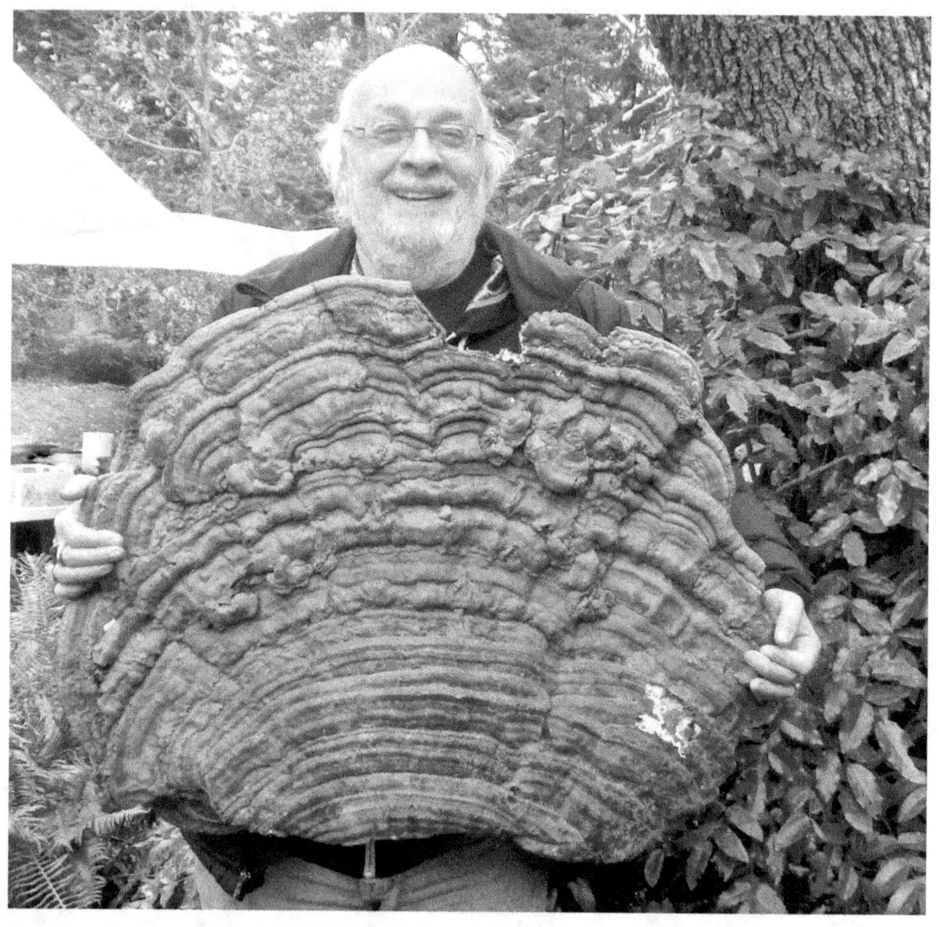

Ganoderma applanatum being held by the author

Living east of the Rockies, in northern Alberta, I have long appreciated this perennial polypore. It is associated with Balsam Poplar, in my region, but with various trees throughout North America.

The fruiting body is bitter and cooling, and has long been noted as the Ancient Ling Zhi, due to its longevity, as opposed to various annual members of the genus.

The largest fruiting body was found on Kulu Island, Alaska in 1951, with a circumference over three metres and weight of over 52 kilograms.

The annual addition of a white ring, like tree rings, helps one surmise it's age. This new growth is rich in polysaccharides and triterpenes. I have long suggested to my students and others, that an annual harvest of this new growth is preferred to removal of the entire fruiting body. Simply carve off the outer portion and return year after year for more medicinal offerings.

In TCM, it was used for excess phlegm, digestive complaints, and relief of inflammation and pain.

The conk contains small (26 ppb) of organic germanium, a rare but important trace mineral.

I have previously written a chapter on this plentiful polypore in both *The Fungal Pharmacy* (2011), and more recently, co-authored *Medicinal Mushrooms of Western North America* (2020) with Duane Sept.

When compared to Reishi (*G. lucidum*), which may itself be a misnomer, the Artist's conk fruiting body has higher levels of phenolics and polysaccharides in ethanol extracts (Raseta et al, 2021).

Significant research has followed in the past five years. Here is some of the more notable contributions, mainly based on in vitro, and in vivo laboratory work.

Water extracts are active against two strains of *Pseudomonas aeruginosa, P. fluorescens, Bacillus subtilis, Staphylococcus epidermidis,* and *Micrococcus luteus* (Hassan et al, 2019).

Both water and methanol extracts of the fruiting body suggest benefit in blood sugar, hyperlipidemia and hepatic liver enzyme markers (Hossain et al, 2021).

Research by Mfopa et al, (2021) on fat-fed, induced obese rats, found hot-water extractions, given orally, increased body weight, but significantly reduce total cholesterol, triglyceride and LDL ; and increased healthy HDL after two months.

Applandermic acid D may be useful in treating obesity and related conditions by inhibiting lipid accumulation in adipocyte and alleviating inflammation (Peng et al, 2021). It appears the compound interacts with formyl peptide receptor 2, associated with inflammation.

Many years ago, my mushroom mentor, Martin Osis, mentioned the benefit of warm foot bath decoctions for gout.

Work by Yong et al, (2018) on hyperuricemia mice, suggests some possible pathways of benefit.

Both ethanol and water extracts were administered orally, and down-regulated the level of CNT2 proteins that elevate uric acid secretions and decline absorption of purine in the gastrointestinal tract.

Renal OAT1 decreased significantly, compared to control drugs allopurinol and benzbromarone; as well as significantly decreased levels of GLUT9. The ethanol extract decreased URAT1 protein, while the water extract was less effective.

Recent work by Yong et al, (2022) identified a methyl ester in the fruiting body, and in work with mice, found down-regulating URAT1, as well as inhibition of xanthine oxidase. Efficacy was similar to drugs mentioned above, without the toxicity and negative effects on liver, kidney, spleen and thymus noted for the pharmaceuticals.

Interstitial fibrosis is present in final stage chronic kidney conditions. A mice study by Susilo et al, (2022) found polysaccharide extracts reduced inflammation, creatinine levels and other markers.

Inflammatory bowel disease (IBD) is associated with disrupted gut microbiota. Polysaccharides, derived from Artist's Conk, promoted and modulated the recovery of induced colitis, repairing intestinal barrier, and reducing inflammation (Li et al, 2022). Reduced levels of *Escherichia, Shigella, Enterococcus* and *Staphylococcus* bacteria were noted.

Triterpenoids, derived from the fruiting body, show potential for treating obesity, due to down-regulation of adipogenesis via various proteins (PPARgamma, CEBPbeta and FAS). Su al., (2021).

Obesity is linked with increased risk of diabetes and cancer. A study with an 80% methanol extract was tested against Caco-2 human colon cancer cell line, in vitro; and Ehrlich tumor in vivo. The apoptotic properties of former were p53 independent, and p53-dependant pathways in solid tumors (Elkhateeb et al, 2018).

Lectins, derived from broth culture (pH 6.5/26⁰C) were cytotoxic and induced apoptosis against Ht-29 human colon adenocarcinoma cell lines (Kumaran et al, 2017).

Cervical cancer is a leading cause of death worldwide and is related to use of oral contraceptives, smoking and oncogenic human papilloma virus (HPV). A sub-critical extraction showed anti-proliferative activity on HeLa cells, but no sign of toxicity on HaCaT human skin cells. The compound 2(5*H*) furanone (IC_{50} of I.99 ug/mL) may be responsible for anti-cancer effect (Kiddane et al, 2022).

Previously, Donatini (2014) found 41 patients with HPV were 88% cleared when given *G. lucidum* and *Trametes versicolor* treatment for two months.

Breast cancer is the number two killer of women at the present time. Work by Hanyu et al, (2020) found polysaccharides induce apoptosis and autophagy through MAPK signaling pathway in MCF-7 human breast cancer cells lines.

A combination of polysaccharides and paclitaxel showed synergistic activity against 4R1 breast cancer cells in vitro. When formed into a thermosensitive gel and combined with paclitaxel injection, mice tumors were significantly reduced, with fewer chemotherapy side effects (Tang et al, 2020).

In mice bearing Dalton's Lymphoma Ascites, doxorubicin (injection) with oral administration of *G. applanatum* methanol extract, significantly reduced drug toxicity. The authors, Laimuansangi et al, (2022) suggest the toxicity reduction could be due to antioxidant properties associated with high phenolic and flavonoid content.

The fruiting body may hold promise for improving and/or restoring brain health.

Triterpenoids show inhibition on nitric oxide release by LPS-induced BV-2 microglial cells (Luo et al, 2020). Work by Jiao et al, (2016) identified similar benefits to microglial cells by the related *Ganoderma curtisii*.

Water and ethanol extracts show binding affinity to receptors, showing potential CNS anti-depressant, anti-anxiety and analgesic effects (Hossen et al, 2021).

Very interesting is the identification of novel cannabinoids (CB1 and CB2) and receptors from this mushroom. Ganoapplanin, sphaeropsidin C and cytosporone C showed best binding affinity to the selected receptors.

Cannabinoid receptors are therapeutic targets for obesity/metabolic, neurological/mental issues and immune modulation.

This follows work by Zhou et al, (2020) identifying novel myco-cannabinoids from five different Ganoderma species, including *G. applanatum*. They showed immune regulation, increased vitality, hormone balance and stimulation of the central nervous system.

As research continues, more secrets from this amazing mushroom are sure to be revealed.

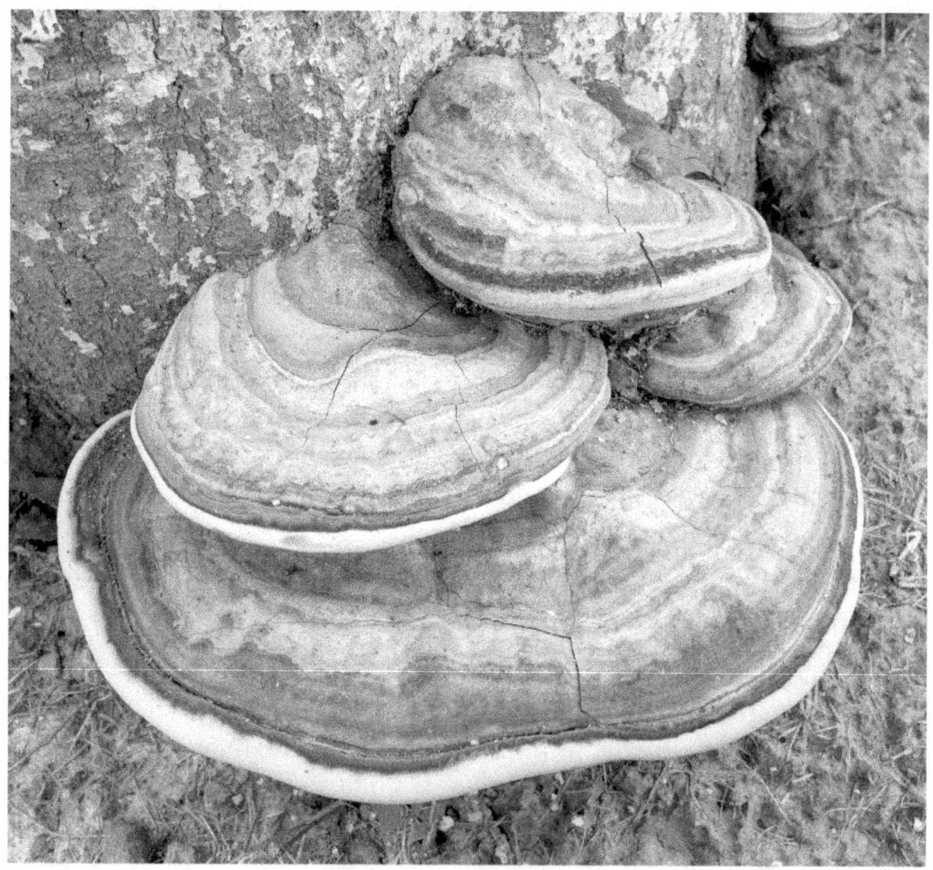

Ganoderma applanatum

BAROMETER EARTHSTAR
(Astraeus hygrometricus)
ODOROUS EARTHSTAR
(A. odoratus)
GIANT HYGROSCOPIC EARTHSTAR
(A. pteridis)

The *Astraeu*s genus contains 15-19 species, with Barometer Earthstar, perhaps the most well-known. The Earthstars of the *Geastrum genus*, on the other hand, number some 350 species.

During the 17th century, a human-like form was drawn of *Geastrum fornicatum* by Seger, who named it *Fungus Anthropomorphos.*

A limerick from an unknown source resulted. Of course.

Said mycologist Linda verbatim
"When it comes to earthstars, I hate 'em"
So asked by her Master
To key a Geaster
She growled out a curse "fornicatum."

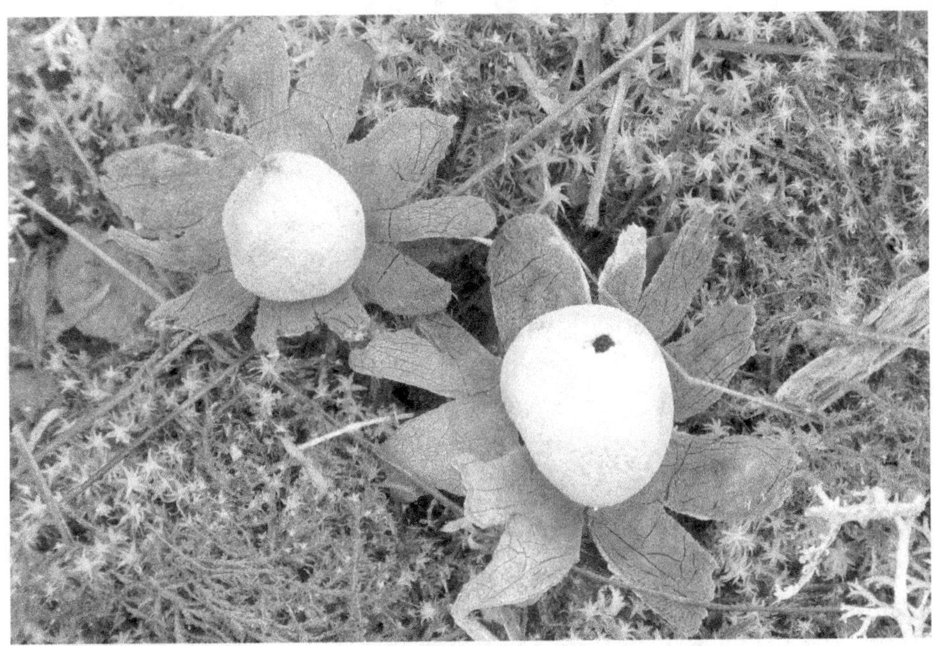

Astraeus hygrometricus

At one time Barometer Earthstar foretold weather, with the radiating segments bending backwards in dry weather, and straightening when dry. The fungi are hydroscopic, opening its rays to rainy weather, to encourage spore release.

When dry, it was traditionally used to staunch bleeding, relieve swelling and reduce internal heat and fever.

The fruiting body contains over 16% protein, and high amounts of potassium (1930 mg/100grams), and D2 (ergosterol).

The fresh mushroom is a delicacy, enjoyed during the monsoon season in south-western India, and elsewhere. In China, the powder was traditionally used for burns, wounds and staunching blood.

Giant Hygroscopic Earthstar is found in western North America, and noted for its quilt-like pattern on rays. Arora notes. "For some inexplicable reason, the fructifications remind me of 'tribbles'—those lovable but relentlessly prolific creatures of 'Star Trek' renown."

Studies suggest numerous health benefits.

A recent study by Khan & Chandra (2019) found inhibition of *E. coli* and *Aspergillus flavus*, and significant anti-oxidant activity.

Polysaccharides, including beta-glucans, and various peptide/protein molecules suggest immune modulation.

Work by Mallick et al, (2010) isolated a polysaccharide (AE2) with a hot alkaline extraction and tested the in vivo potential, on mice.

This heteroglucan (AE2) appears to possess anti-tumor activity. Mallick et al. (2010a) found Daltons lymphoma cells underwent apoptosis (self-programmed death), with a reduction of tumor growth and increased survival rate in the tumor bearing host. Natural Killer cell activity increased, and Th1 cytokine activity increased, the Th2 levels decreased. The authors suggest therapeutic potential for the treatment of cancer or other disease associated with immune suppression.

Macrophages from treated mice showed higher production of nitric oxide and interleukin-1, as well as increased phagocytic potential. AE2 enhanced natural killer cell activation and proliferation of splenocytes, with increased T-helper 1 cells production.

The following year (2011), Mallick et al. investigated the AE2 heteroglucan and suggest macrophage activation might be, in part, via mitogen-activated protein kinases pathway of signal transduction.

Two lanostane-type triterpenes were isolated from the mushroom by Lai et al, (2012). One triterpene significantly inhibited the growth of *Leishmania donovani*, while the other exhibited in vitro toxicity against *Candida albicans*, comparable to standard anti-fungals.

Barometer Earthstar contains an interesting sesquiterpenoid, astrakurkurone. In work by Dasgupta et al, (2019), the compound exhibited cytotoxic activity against hepatocellular carcinoma (HCC) cell lines, at significantly low dose.

Astrakurkurone induced apoptosis, disrupted mitochondrial membrane potential, and induced expression of Bcl-family proteins. This latter includes Bax and the downstream effector caspases 3 and 9. A molecular docking study predicted interactions with the anti-apoptotic proteins Bcl-2 and Bcl-xL, suggesting a potential in cancer therapy.

The triterpenoid astrakurkurol was recently derived from the fresh mushroom. Nandi et al, (2019) examined its potential against the human hepatocellular cancer cell Hep3B. Apoptosis was noted, including DNA fragmentation, chromatin condensation, nuclear shrinkage, membrane blebing, and imbalance of cell cycle distribution. The compound also inhibited migration of Hep3B cells, suggesting inhibition of metastatic potential.

Recent work by Nandi et al, (2022) investigated the apoptotic mechanism of astrakurkol in HepG2 cells, including its anti-migratory and anti-proliferative activity, and increased expression of p53. Cell death was mediated via both extrinsic and intrinsic apoptotic signaling, suggesting a non-toxic substitute of chemotherapy.

Sandflies in many parts of the tropical world carry a protozoa, resulting in *Leishmania donovani* infection. The visceral form, known as Kala-azar is life-threatening, and includes symptoms of fever, anemia, leukopenia and weight loss.

The standard of treatment is sodium stibogluconate, with its attendant significant side-effects and drug resistance.

Astrakurkurone has been investigated for possible benefit by Mallick et al., 2015).

It appears to induce reactive oxygen species, associated with apoptosis.

A frequently disrupted pathway in renal cell carcinoma is inhibited by this compound, suggesting possible anti-cancer possibility (Yadav et al, 2022).

Astrakurkone caused a significant increase in Toll-like receptor 9 expression of L. donovani-infected macrophages, along with proinflammatory response. The compound reduced the parasite burden in vivo by inducing protective cytokines, gamma interferon and interleukin 17. It also is non-toxic toward peripheral blood mononuclear cells of immune compromised patients with visceral leishmaniasis (Mallick et al, 2016).

A 'carbohydrate fraction", named $AH_{f\text{-}Car}$ was evaluated against L. donovani infection both in vitro and in vivo, by Hussain et al, (2021).

The compound induced expression of nitric oxide synthase 2, and pro-inflammatory cytokines such as TNF-1 and IL-12, and down regulation of anti-inflammatory cytokines including TGF-beta and IL-10. Increases of IL-6, IL-1beta, IfN-gamma, and IRF-7 and * were noted in vivo.

It also reduced the parasite burden in the spleen and liver along with proliferation of Ly6C cells in the bone marrow of infected animals. Monocytes increased and the expression of myeloid transcription factor PU.1 suggests the expansion of protective macrophages. The authors suggest the compound is a potent, unique and effect adjuvant.

Ethanol extracts lower blood sugar level in alloxan-induced diabetic mice (Biswas et al, 2013), protect against hepatoxicity due to anti-oxidant activity (Biswas et al, 2011); and inhibit platelet aggregation, prostaglandin synthesis and stimulate nitric oxide synthesis in human blood (Biswas et al, 2011a).

A thorough review by Biswas et al. (2017) contains other studies of interest.

There are two other Astraeus species of medical interest.

Odorous Earthstar is confined to Thailand, Laos and parts of India and Nepal. It is a choice edible, when prepared in curry and fish sauce dishes.

The mushroom possesses blood sugar lowering properties, based on work by Phadannok et al, (2020). Enhanced muscle glucose uptake was determined with in vitro L6 myotubes, looking at glucose transporter types I and 4.

Tuberculosis causes from two to three million deaths worldwide annually, and is often treated with isoniazid and rifampicin, which possess potential hepatoxicity.

Four new lanostane triterpenes, astraodoric acids A-D, were tested against *Mycobacterium tuberculosis* H(37)Ra by Arpha et al, (2012). Both astraodoric acids A and B exhibited moderate activity, as well as cytotoxicity against both KB and NCI-H187 cancer cells. KB is a subline of HeLa, containing human papillomavirus 18, and the latter is a small cell lung carcinoma cell line.

Giant Hygroscopic Earthstar (*A. pteridis*) also contains lanostane triterpenes that exhibit moderate activity against *M. tuberculosis* (Stanikunaite et al, 2008).

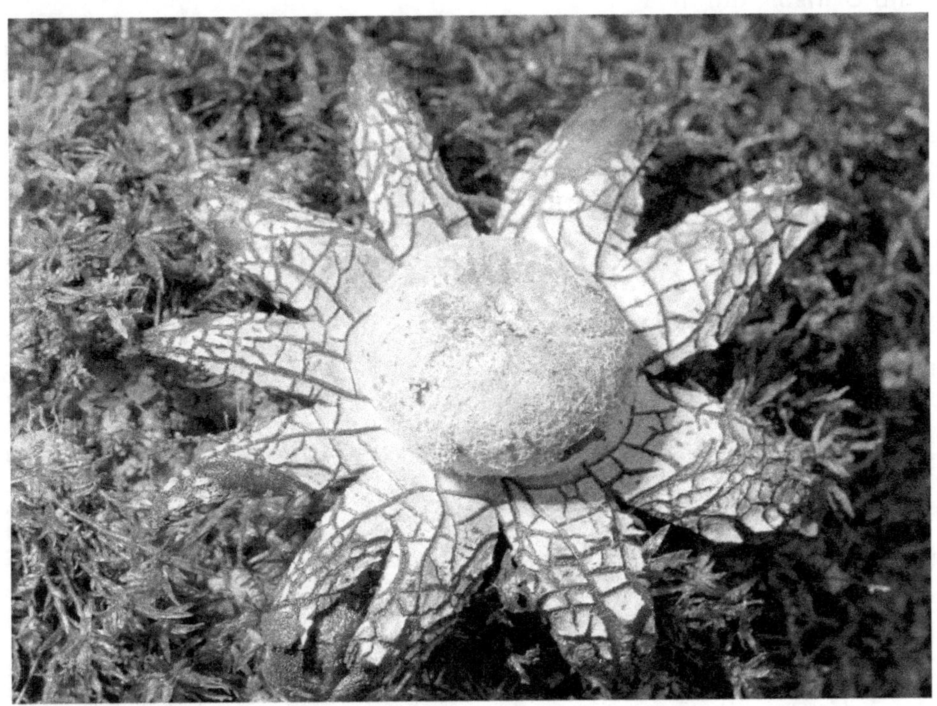

Astraeus hygrometricus

BIG BROWN CAT
IMPERIAL MUSHROOM
(*Catathelasma imperiale*)
SMALLER WHITE CAT
SWOLLEN STALKED CAT
MOCK MATSUTAKE
(*C. ventricosum*)

Catathelasma may derive from the Greek kata meaning "downward", and thelasma for "the act of suckling". It has been suggested that the shape of decurrent gills running down the stem, resembles a teat stretched out during suckling. Or perhaps from katatheo meaning, "I run down."

Imperiale relates to its large, impressive size.

Ventricosum may derive from the shape of stipe, "with a swelling on the side like a belly."

Many years ago I travelled from Alberta, across the Rocky Mountains, into British Columbia.

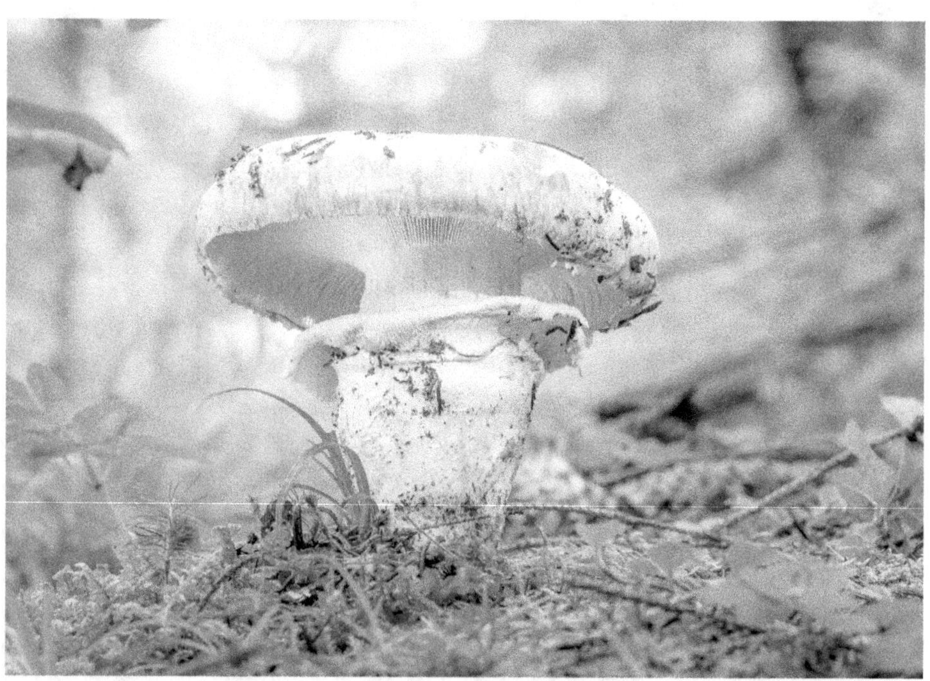

Catathelasma imperiale

I looked forward to hunting the prized western Pine Mushroom (*Tricholoma murrillianum*), as well as White Chanterelle (*Cantharellus subalbidus*) and Lobster (*Hypomyces lactifluorum*) mushrooms, the size of footballs.

I found my first "pines" and remember to this day the distinctive spicy odor.

A few years later, during a wander in woods, east of the Rockies, I found what I believed to be another patch of this prized mushroom.

Alas, I was informed by the brilliant mycologist, Paul Kroeger, it was a Smaller White Cat. I cooked it up, and although quite chewy, was very delicious.

Since that time, I have noted both mushrooms being passed off as pines and sold at Farmer's Markets.

The "true" Matsutake, *Tricholoma matsutake*, is highly prized in Japan, but has experienced lower yields, due to declining health of native pine forests. For years, the North American mushroom was called Tricholoma magnivelare, but that binomial is now reserved for species from Eastern North America.

A third species, Hongo Blanco de Ocote (*T. mesoamericanum*) is recently described from Mexico. (Trudell et al, 2017).

Big Brown Cat can be massive, with firm flesh, with white spores. In Alaska, it is referred to, by Indigenous people, as the potato mushroom.

The other is smaller, with a somewhat longer stipe; both are found under conifers.

Work by Liu et al, (2012) found water extracts of the Imperial mushroom inhibit high levels of alpha-glycosidase, as well as possess significant anti-oxidant activity. The former enzyme breaks down sugars in the small intestine, allowing molecules to pass into the bloodstream and raise blood sugar levels. And hence the interest in its hypoglycemic benefit.

The fruiting body contains catathelasmols, which exhibit inhibition of two isozymes of 11beta-hydroxysteroid dehydrogenases. These compounds help catalyze the interconversion of cortisol and cortisone (Zhang et al, 2009).

The polysaccharides inhibit the growth of sarcoma 180 tumor cells, and promote apoptosis of fibroblast L929 cell lines (Liu et al, 2019). They also promote production of T and B immune cells.

Mock Matsutake is known as Momitake in Japan.

Small White Cat (*C. ventricosum*) mushroom contains polysaccharides that lower blood sugar and lipid levels in streptozotocin-induced diabetic mice. Both anti-oxidant and HDL cholesterol levels were elevated (Liu et al, 2013). A team led by Liu (2016), later identified the glucopyranose-rich heteropolysaccharide responsible for its potential for the prevention and treatment of diabetes.

Early work by Zhan & Yue (2003) identified two glycosphingolipids, cerebrosides B & C, as well as six known ergostane-type sterols and tyrosamine. Cerebrosides compose animal muscle and nerve cell membranes, and play a role in immunity and anti-cancer activity.

Selenium-enriched mycelium has been studied for benefit in diabetes, using induced diabetic mice. Three studies by Liu et al, (2015/2017/2018) examined the benefits of selenium content, including selenium nanoparticles. If selenium content is too high, it damages the triple-helix structure of polysaccharides and diminishes the benefit.

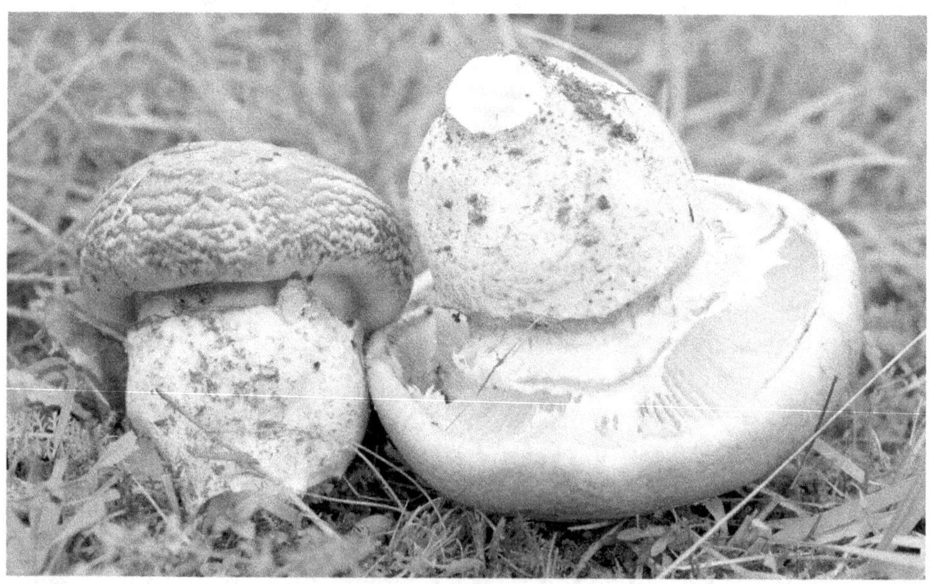

Catathelasma imperiale

CHICKEN OF THE WOODS
(*Laetiporus sulphureus* [Bull.] Murill)

Laetiporus is from the Latin meaning "a wealth of pores, or bright-pored". Sulphureus means, "a bright yellow color". The yellow-orange colored fruiting body can approach red in some specimens.

This yellow-pored mushroom is widely found in eastern United States and Canada on hardwoods. Fruiting bodies on conifers are known as *L. conifericola*.

The pigment color is due largely to laetiporic acid.

There is considerable taxonomic confusion with DNA and other work suggesting at least eight clades. Work by Lindner and Banik (2008) looked at North American species and suggested five major clades, including *L. sulphureus* s. stricto isolates with yellow pores.

Worldwide work by Vasaitis et al, (2009) concluded it is not possible to define *L. sulphureus* s. stricto. Enough taxonomy. Let us move on.

One specimen discovered in England in 2003 measured more than sixteen feet in circumference and estimated to weigh, at that time, nearly 700 pounds.

Older specimens can smell like rotten eggs, but the younger specimens or the newer growths are very pleasant.

The mushroom is generally considered edible. There are a couple of reports in the literature about possible un-toward effects. One case involved a six year-old girl who experienced hallucinations after nibbling on a sulfur shelf. (Appleton 1988).

The Mycological Society of San Francisco toxicology committee reported one ingestion in which an adult experienced a tingling sensation in fingers, a floating sensation, dizziness and disorientation. It was not noted if it was growing on a hardwood, conifer or eucalyptus (*L. gilbertii*). The latter species is considered by a very poor edible, and/or unpleasant dining experience.

Hordenine, tyramine, N-methyl tyramine and two unidentified alkaloids have been reported from western specimens.

The mushroom can be preserved for medicine by drying in thin slices and later decocting a tea, or by preparing a fresh decoction and preserving in minimum 25% alcohol.

Large-scale commercial cultivation is now possible, suggesting the possibility of year round availability. (Pleszczynska M et al, 2013).

A lectin, similar to the mosquito toxin MTX2 (from *Bacillus sphaericus*), and the insecticidal, cyclodepsipeptide, have been isolated from the polypore. I have smoldered a small piece of the dried mushroom as a mosquito repellant in my tent with good success.

Egonol and derivates are used as melanin inhibitors and whitening agents to treat sunburned skin after UV irradiation, and skin pigmentation such as pregnancy mask.

MEDICINAL

CONSTITUENTS - ergosterol peroxide, cerevisterol, sulphureuines B-H, lanostanoid triterpenes including 3-oxosulfurenic acid, laetirobin, melanin, mannitol, trehalose, alpha, gamma and delta tocopherols, oxalic, citric, cinnamic and p-hydroxybenzoic acids, three mycophenolic acid derivatives, seven sulphureuines (B-H), beauvericin (cyclic peptide), laminarin, ergothioneine, GABA (gamma-aminobutyric acid), triterpenoids such as eburicoic acid, sulfurenic acidk acetyl eburicoic acid, acetyl tremaetenolic acid, and 15alpha-hydroxytrametenolic acid, isoprenoid ubiquinone Q9, laetiporic acids (A-C), LSL (lectin), masutakeside 1, masutakin acid A, egonol, demethoxyegonol, egonol glucoside, egonol gentiobioside, sulphureuines B-H, agripilol A, 3beta-hydroxy-11,12-O-isopropyldrimene, sulphurenic acid.

Chicken of the Woods exhibits a number of health benefits.

The antioxidant activity is similar to alpha tocopherol and synthetic preservative BHA. Turkoglu et al, (2007).

The same study found it strongly inhibited gram-positive bacteria and *Candida* species.

Earlier work identified activity against methicillin-resistant *Staphylococcus aureus* (MRSA). (Ershova et al. 2003). In this same submerged cultivation, *Leuconostoc mesenteroides* growth was suppressed. This bacterium is responsible for fermenting sauerkraut and pickles. It is probably not a good idea to try and pickle the mushroom and cabbage in same crockpot.

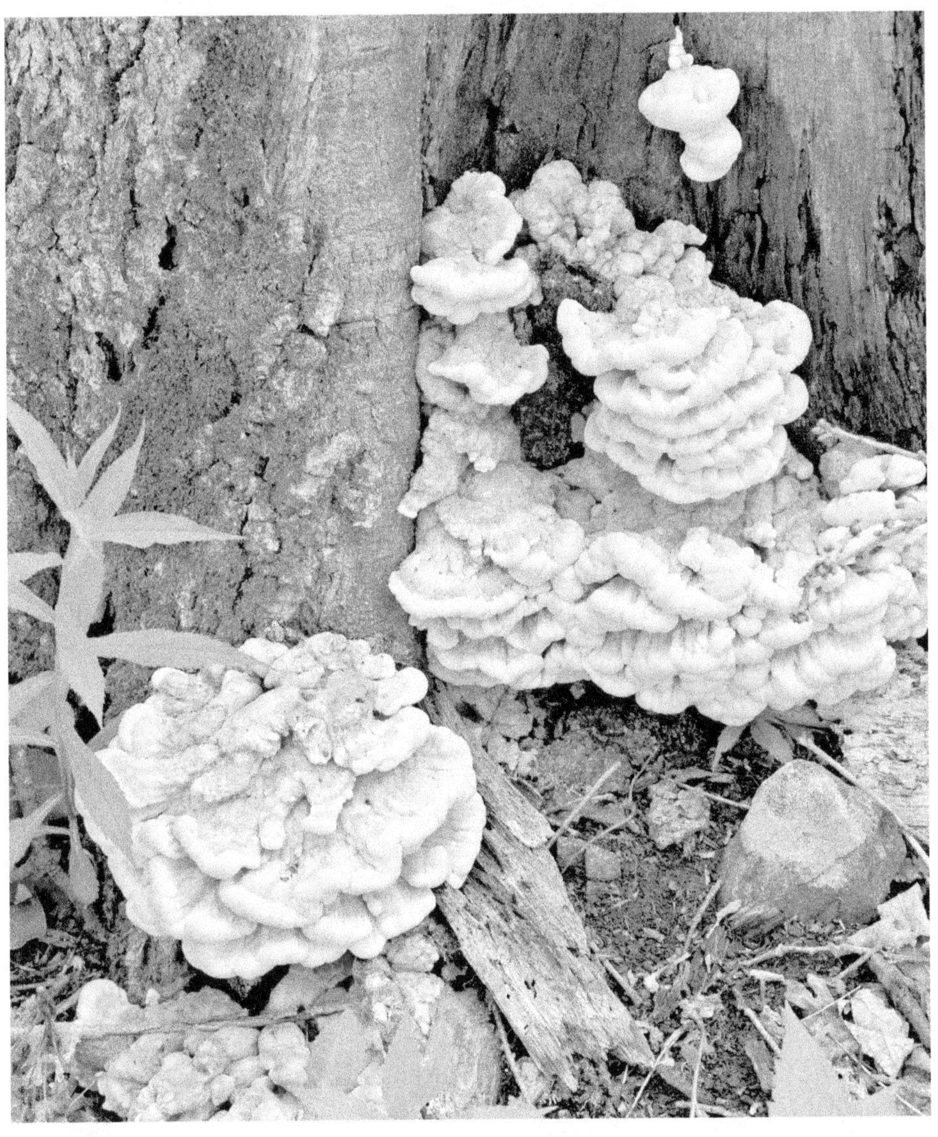

Laetiporus sulphureus

On the other hand, alcohol extracts help preserve foods against *Aspergillus flavus*. (Petrovic et al, 2014).

A screening of 57 wood-damaging fungi found chicken of the woods the most active inhibitor of HIV-1 reverse transcriptase. (Mlinaric et al. 2005).

Eburicoic acid is a potent inducer of apoptosis in HL-60 human myeloid leukemia cell lines. (León F et al. 2004).

Work by Kang et al, (1982) found hot water extracts suppressed the growth of Sarcoma 180 in mice, suggesting anti-carcinogenic activity.

Egonol, demethoxyegonol and egonol glucoside all exhibited cytotoxicity against human stomach cancer KATO III cells. (Yoshikawa et al, 2001).

Egonol gentiobioside promotes the biosynthesis of estrogen by aromatase. Estrogen deficiency is associated with a variety of health concerns including osteoporosis, atherosclerosis and Alzheimer's disease. (Lu et al, 2012).

Exposure to radiation can deplete testosterone-binding globulin, which can affect androgen ligand binding. Lipid polyene preparations from this mushroom have been found to help restore radiation-induced changes. (Popoff & Kapich 2010). This may have application to restoration of hormone health after chemotherapy.

The compound (+/-)-laertirobin was isolated from *Laetiporus sulphureus* growing on the black locust tree. Early studies found it enters into tumor cells, blocks cell division at a late stage of mitosis and invokes apoptosis, or programmed cell death. (Lear MJ 2009).

It has been synthesized and is presently being investigated by Xenobe Research Institute in California for possible treatment on various human cancers.

Mycophenolic acids and sulphureuines have been isolated from the polypore. Moderate cytoxicity has been noted against HL-60 (leukemia), SMMC-7721 (hepatoma), A-549 (lung) and MCF-7 (breast) cancer cell lines. (Fan, 2014; He, 2015).

Eburicoic acid showed moderate activity against five cancer cell lines. HL-60, SMMC-7721, A-549 and MCF-7 mentioned above as well as SW-480 (colorectal) cell lines were inhibited by this compound. (Jiang-Bo He et al, 2015).

Lanostanoid triterpenes induced apoptosis on HL-60 (leukemia) cell lines over ten years ago. (Francisco L et al, 2004).

Work by Ríos et al, (2012) identified lanostanoid triterpenes with potential anti-cancer activity.

Cell wall preparations from the fruiting body effectively induce mutanase, that helps remove *Streptococcus mutans* biofilm from teeth and dentures. The water-soluble glucan produced by the bacterium, inhibits cariogenic pathogens causing dental disease. Mutanase and dextranase, found in chicken of the woods, hydrolyze and remove dental and denture plaque. (Wiater et al, 2008). These two compounds are found Biotene, a dental product used by individuals suffering dry mouth.

Polysaccharides have been shown to inhibit the expression of pro-inflammatory mediators by suppressing NF-$_k$B activity. (Jayasooriya et al, 2011). This suggests anti-inflammatory activity.

Melanin has been isolated from mycelium of chicken of the woods, yielding about 2.49% of fresh weight. Melanin is not only a free radical scavenger, but may play a role in pineal gland health and production of melatonin.

On the other hand, external application may be useful in skin hyperpigmentation disorders, with higher potential than kojic acid and hydroquinone (Pavic et al, 2021).

Chicken of the Woods contains laminarin, a water insoluble polysaccharide more commonly found in seaweed and algae. This linear (1>3)-linked beta glucan

Laminaran inhibited formation of human melanoma SK-MEL-28 and colon cancer DLD-1 cell lines. (Menshova et al, 2014).

Earlier work by Park et al, (2013) found laminarin induced apoptosis in HT-29 colon cancer cells and inhibited the heregulin-stimulated phosphorylation of ErbB2.

ErbB2 is also known as HER2 and is a human epidermal growth factor receptor. An over-expression of this oncogene has been shown to play an important role in development of 15-30 % of aggressive breast cancers. It is also implicated in ovarian, stomach and uterine cancers. HER2 is the target of Herceptin, which increases p27, a protein that halts cell proliferation. One-third of patients respond well to Herceptin cancer treatment.

Type two diabetes is a growing health epidemic. Syndrome X, also known as diabesity is a complex mixture of insulin resistance, high blood sugar, high cholesterol, cardiovascular risk and obesity.

The compound dehydrotrametenolic acid acts as an insulin sensitizer in glucose tolerance tests. (Sato et al, 2002). It induces adipose conversion; activates PPAR gamma, peroxisome proliferator-activated receptor gamma; and reduces hyperglycemia in animal models of non-insulin dependent diabetes. This compound is also found in *Poria cocos*, a polypore widely used in Traditional Chinese Medicine.

Submerged mycelial cultures produce an extracellular polysaccharide (EPS) with insulinotropic properties. The proliferation of animal insulinoma cells increased by 152%; suggesting both cell proliferation and insulin secretion. (Hwang et al, 2008). The same study found EPS protected the cells against strepatzocin-induced apoptosis.

The key enzyme in the metabolism of fat is lipase. In one study an extract of chicken of the woods inhibited pancreatic lipase by 83%, comparable to commercially available lipase inhibitor Orlistat. (Slanc et al, 2004).

Lovastatin is naturally found in Oyster mushroom, and helps block cholesterol synthesis with the side effects of statin drugs.

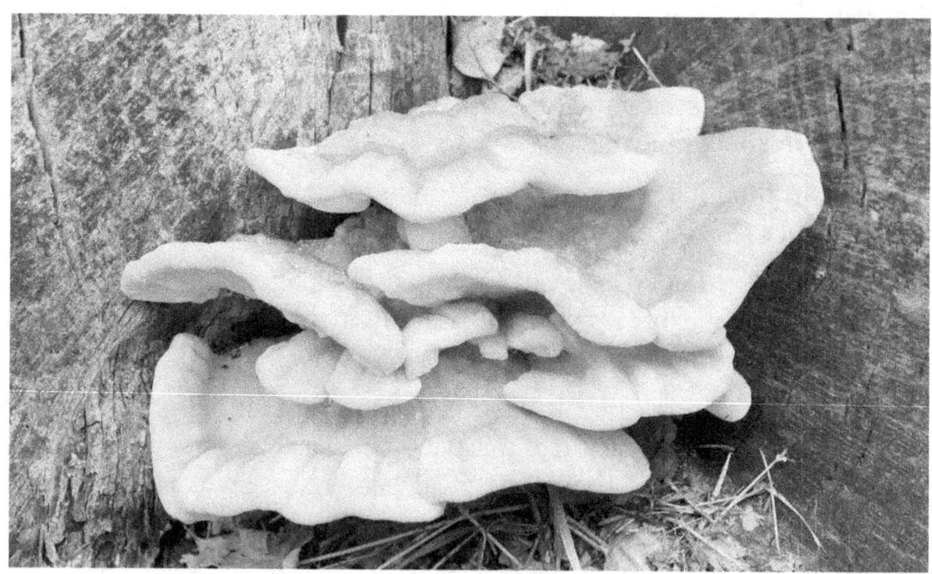

Laetiporus sulphureus

Work by Lee (2006) found mycelial extracts of Oyster and Chicken of the Woods showed the highest inhibition rates of HMG-CoA reductase, the limiting enzyme in biosynthesis of cholesterol, by 37.2% and 29.1% respectively. Chicken of the Woods showed high inhibition activity even though it had a lower level of lovastatin. The authors suggest there may be another compound in the mushroom, with synergistic activity.

Statin drugs (Crestor, Lipitor) decrease blood plasma levels of coenzyme Q10, and can lead to rhabdomyolysis, a rare but serious side-effect. Coenzyme Q10 has been reported to reverse this condition and associated acute renal failure. (Wang et al, 2015).

It is interesting to note that many of the North American studies on the connection between muscle related symptoms, statin use and Q10 show no correlation. One study of fifty patients, treated with statins, and reporting muscle pain, was conducted by Skarlovnik et al, (2014). One group of 25 patients received 100 mg of Q10 daily and the other group of 25, a placebo for thirty days. The supplementation effectively reduced the mild to moderate, statin-induced muscular symptoms. Pain severity scores and Pain Interference scores in placebo group did not change.

Chicken of the Woods contains CoQ9. Research in mice found a reduction of CoQ9 led to brain specific impairment, leading to mitochondrial encelphalomyopathy. (Garcia Corzo, 2013).

The mushroom also exhibits anti-thrombin activity. An unusual study fused chicken of the woods with the edible mushroom *Hypsizygus marmoreus*, resulting in a thrombin time of only 170.5 seconds. (Okamura et al, 2000).

The Conifer Sulphur Shelf (*L. conifericola*) has been less studied. Work by Johnathan et al, 2021 examined in vitro activity against various Gram-positive and Gram-negative bacterium. Ethanol extracts were very effective against *Staphylococcus aureus*, while water extracts were not. Ethanol extracts strongly inhibited *Bacillus cereus* and *Pseudomonas aeruginosa*, while *E. coli* was best inhibited by water extracts.

Some things to think about the next time you sit down to a meal of Chicken of the Woods. Bon Appetit.

CAULIFLOWER MUSHROOM
(*Sparassis crispa*)

Cauliflower mushroom (*S. crispa*) is a choice edible, and medicinal mushroom found in Europe and widely cultivated in Asia. I have had occasion to find and eat the western cauliflower (*S. radiculata*), but no studies have been done on this species, to my knowledge. The eastern species, *S. spathulata*, is more flattened and found in pine forests.

Sparassis is derived from the Greek, "torn apart", an apt description of the loose knit fruiting body, found mainly at the base of old conifers. Work today involves cultivating the mushroom on conifer sawdust.

The fruiting body possesses anti-tumor, anti-carcinogenic, anti-inflammatory, anti-viral, anti-hypertensive, anti-allergenic, anti-diabetic, and anti-coagulant properties, mainly *in vitro*, and *in vivo*, but there are a few human clinical studies.

The anti-microbial activity of sparassol was noted nearly a century ago.

The fruiting body is rich in beta-glucans (up to 43%), of course, but also sparassol, sparoside A, ergosterol peroxide and various benzoate derivatives useful in treating human conditions. Zinc levels are significant, as well as saponins, terpenoids, flavonoids, tannins and cardiac glycosides (Niazi & Ijaz, 2021). Ethanol extracts inhibited *Escherichia coli* bacterium.

A novel compound has been found to inhibit the growth of methicillin-resistant *Staphylococcus aureus* (MRSA), and melanin synthesis (Kawagishi et al, 2007).

Polysaccharides decreased ATP in *S. aureus* cells, and disrupt metabolism of the glycolysis and tricarboxylic acid cycle pathways. This suggests a possible alternative to the widespread overuse and abuse of antibiotics (Lan et al, 2021).

In Japan, it is a choice edible-medicinal mushroom known as *hanabiratake*. In China it is known as *Xiu Qiu Jun*.

When fermented with lactic acid bacteria, the innate immunity increased significantly, albeit in a mice study (Nishioka et al, 2020). The authors suggest that based on this study, that humans could benefit from this fermented product.

Two studies of interest involve anti-diabetic activity (Yamamoto et al, 2010) and (Jeong et al, 2017).

In the first, cauliflower mushroom reduced serum glucose and insulin levels, and increased the body weight of diabetic mice. This study involved both oral and topical application of the mushroom, suggesting possible benefit in diabetic ulceration, a leading cause of leg amputation in un-controlled, human diabetes.

The second, a rat study, noted serum glucose and insulin level reduction, as well as increased nutrition intake, and gain in body weight.

A mice study found the mushroom attenuates the exhaustive exercise-induced reduction of TNF-alpha production (Uchida et al, 2019). Moderate exercise benefits human health, but in excess can create temporary immune depression.

A hot water extract inhibited over 70% of HIV at low concentration of 1mg/ml (Wang et al, 2007).

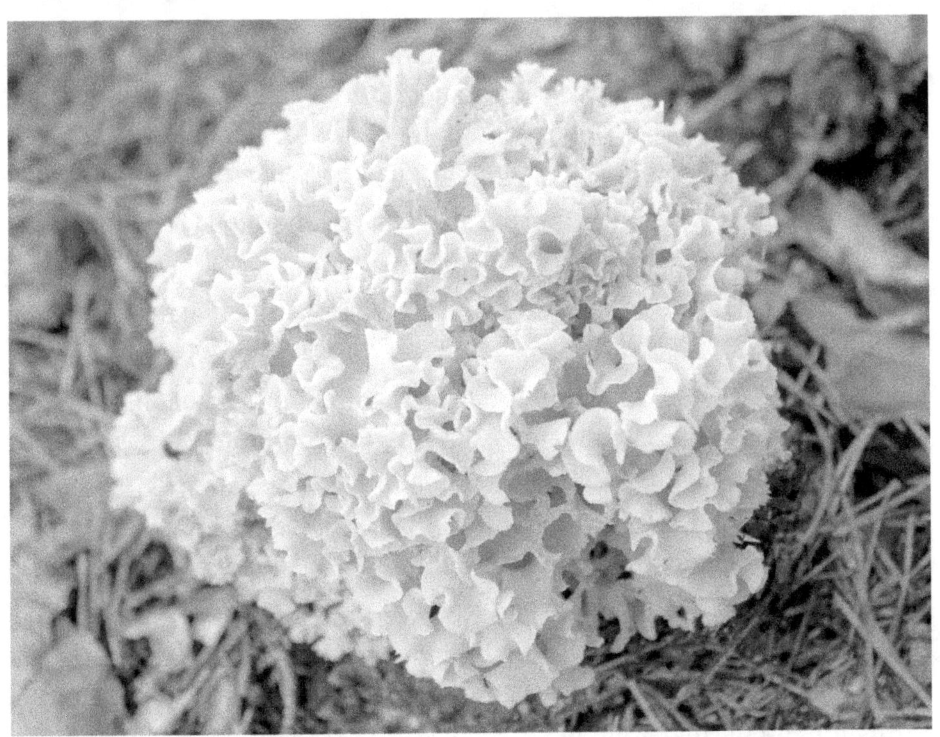

Sparassis crispa

Nineteen studies (Ngoc et al, 2018) were conducted on anti-cancer possibilities. Seven reported anti-tumor activity, five showed inhibition of cancer cell growth, and nine indicated IFN-gamma induction, suggestive of immune regulation.

Four studies found reduction in inflammatory cell survival.

The mushroom may be useful in treating cancer. Work by Nowacka-Jechalke et al, (2021) found polysaccharides non-toxic to normal human colon epithelial CCD841 CoN cells, but destroyed membrane integrity and inhibited proliferation of the human colon cancer cell lines: Caco-2, LS180 and HT-29.

Water extracts (polysaccharides) provided protection of neuron (PC) cells against glutamate-induced toxicity, suggesting possible benefit in neurodegenerative conditions. A recent study by Zhang et al, (2022) identified a purified polysaccharide that protects hippocampal neuronal (HT22) cells by modulating antioxidant enzymes and reducing cell apoptosis.

Another studied looked at the benefit of polysaccharides against L-glutamic acid induced differentiated PC12 cells. A water extract showed promise in this *in vitro* study by Hu et al, (2016), suggesting a promising compound for treating neurodegenerative disease.

Dendritic cell activation and maturation has been noted (Kim, 2010).

Work by Wang et al, (2019) identified 110 components in the fruiting body. They identified sparoside A, and demonstrated its potential to inhibit symptoms associated with allergic rhinitis.

Sparoside A, and hanabiratakelides exhibit potent inhibition on PCSK9 mRNA expression, suggesting an alternative to the statins, for hyperlipidemia treatment (Bang et al, 2017).

Hanabiratakelides A-C possess anti-oxidant, anti-inflammatory and anti-tumor activity against colon cancer cell lines (Yoskikawa et al, 2010).

A rat and human study with cauliflower mushroom was conducted by Kimura et al, (2013). The first part involved oral administration to collagen synthetic activity-reduced rats. Increased turnover of stratum corneum and dermal soluble collagen was observed.

Polysaccharides provide prebiotic benefit to the gut microbiota, promoting beneficial genera, and inhibiting some harmful bacteria (Zhang et al, 2022a).

In a human clinical trial a beta-glucan preparation from cultivated fruiting bodies was given orally to 14 cancer patients, including those with ovarian and uterine cancers. The dose was 300 mg/daily. Results showed a disappearance of all nontarget lesions and normalization of cancer marker level in four cases and partial response in five cases (Ohno et al, 2003). The number of NK (natural killer) cells did not increase, suggesting activation of Th1 and inhibition of Th2 direction. Maybe.

A controlled human study found daily consumption of 320 mg daily of the fruiting body over twenty-eight days significantly reduced trans-epidermal water loss, and improved skin integrity (Kimura et al, 2013).

The authors suggest the mushroom is effective and safe for improving skin conditions. Diabetic patients usually exhibit delayed or slow, impairing wound healing. Oral and topical application may be useful as preventative, and treatment of this serious condition.

DOSAGE - for immune and skin maintenance 300 mg daily shows benefit. For more immediate results in acute cases, from 3-5 grams daily may be warranted.

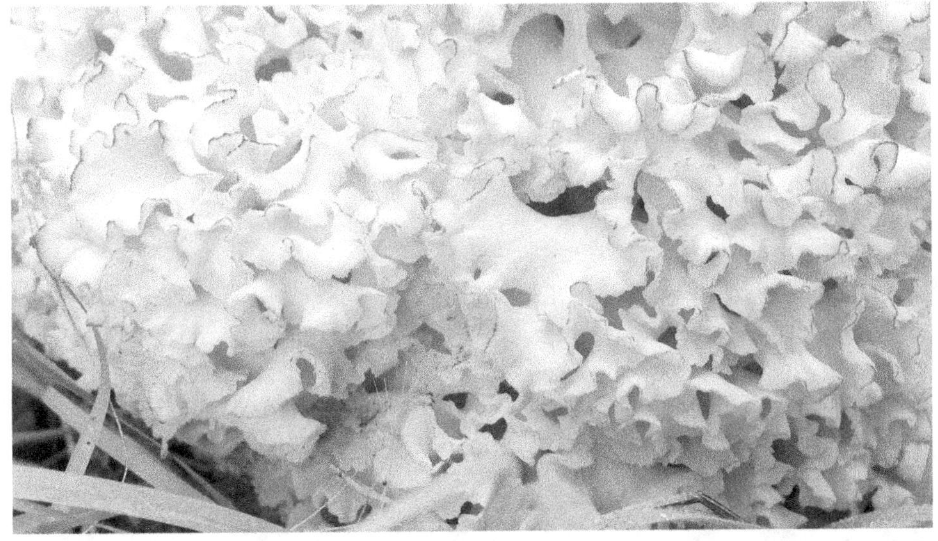

Sparassis crispa

CLOUDED FUNNEL
(*Clitocybe nebularis*)
Club Foot
(*C. clavipes*)
(*Ampulloclitocybe clavipes*)
Trumpet Funnel Cap
(*C. geotropa*)
(*Infundibulicybe geotropa*)
Wood Blewitt
(*C. nuda*)
(*Lepista nuda*)
Alexander's Funnel
(*C. alexandri*)
False Chanterelle
(*C. aurantiaca*)
(*Cantharellus aurantiacus*)
(*Hygrophoropsis aurantiaca*)
Common Funnel
(*C. gibba*)
(*C. infundibuliforms*)
(*Infundibulicybe gibba*)
Funnel Mushroom
(*C. squamulosa*)
(*I. squamulosa*)
Giant Clitocybe
Giant Leucopax
(*C. gigantea*)
(*Leucopaxillus giganteus*)
Orange Funnel Cap
(*C. inversa*)
(*Lepista inversa*)
Large Funnel Cap
(*C. maxima*)
The Sweater
(*Clitocybe rivulosa*)

Clitocybe means "sloping head" and nebularis is derived from the Latin nebula meaning, "mist". At one time there were about 200 species in

North America, but a number have been moved to various genera in the past decade. MacKinnon & Luther (2021) in their excellent *Mushrooms of British Columbia*, note a recent analysis of clitocybes in that province and the US Pacific Northwest. Of the 130 species once assigned to this genus, only about 80 remain.

A few are tasty, some are marginally edible, and a few are deadly poisonous.

Clouded Funnel mushrooms have a sweet, fruit smell to some; turnip-like to others; and a skunk-cabbage or dirty mouse cage odor to some noses. Edible, but not really recommended. Dried, young specimens can add flavor to winter meals.

Clouded Funnel contains nebularine, 9-(beta-D-riboufruanosyl) purine, which inhibits sarcoma 180 cancer cell lines.

It is anti-bacterial, anti-viral and the compound clitocybin shows activity against *Mycobacterium tuberculosis* at water concentration of 1:300,000 *in vitro*.

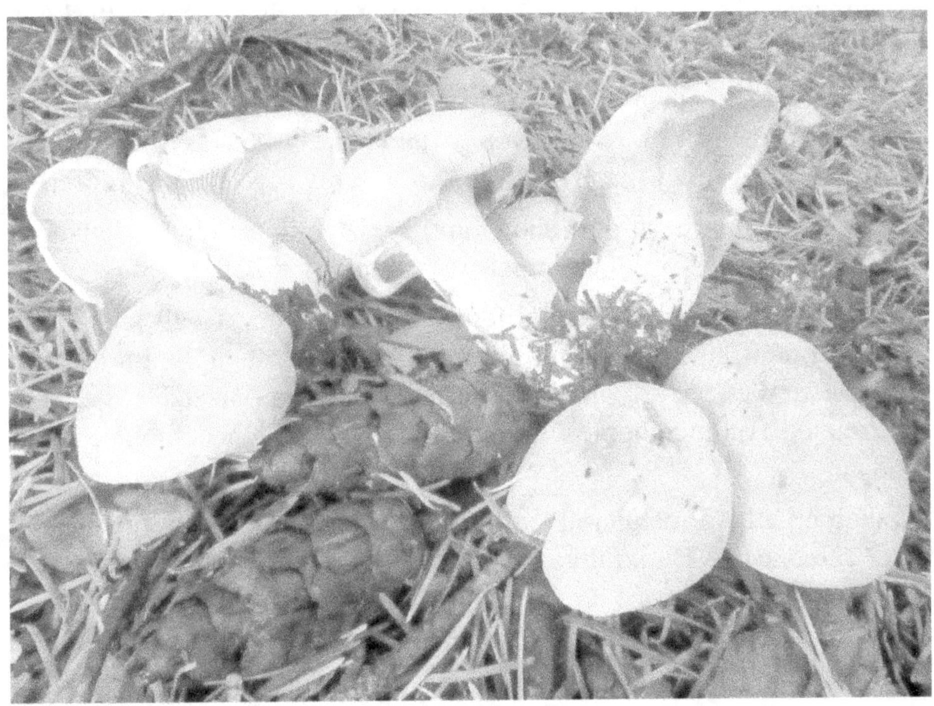

Clitocybe nebularis

The compound was researched shortly after WWII, for tuberculosis, but was abandoned when streptomycin was introduced.

The fruiting body contains aspartic proteases. An example are beta and gamma secretase, two enzymes necessary to release A beta peptides from the Alzheimer's precursor protein. A ricin-B-like lectin brings it to carbohydrate receptors on human leukemic T-cells, suggesting anti-proliferative activity. This lectin is the only one, found so far in medicinal mushrooms, to possess immune modulating properties.

This novel lectin activates, and induces, maturation of human dendritic cells via the toll-like receptor 4 pathway, suggesting strengthened anti-tumor immune response (Sabotic & Kos, 2019).

One compound, cnispin, is highly specific to trypsin, and similar to the serine protease inhibitor in Shiitake (*Lentinus edodes*). (Avanzo et al, 2009).

It contains a compound specific to Lacdi NAc that is common in nematodes and helminths. It is not present in mammals, but is found in human leukemia and tumor cells, targeting glycan cells. It shows activity against Jurkat and Mo-T leukemic T-cell lines.

Nebularine, and phenylacetic acid inhibit various pathogenic fungi, including athlete's foot (*Trichophyton mentagrophytes*), as well as ringworm, nail fungus, and so-called cuddly toy mycosis in children.

A lectin from this mushroom shows anti-proliferation on Jurkat leukemic T cell line, suggestive of apoptosis (Nanut et al, 2022).

Ethanol extracts show antiproliferative activity on HT-29 and MCF-7 cancer cell lines, and inhibit multi-drug resistant Gram-positive bacteria, and effectively inhibit biofilm production (Dizeci et al, 2021). The related Trumpet Funnel Cap also showed similar benefit in the same study.

A submerged, fermentation culture yields sesquiterpenes nebucanes A-G. Nebucane D exhibits antifungal effects against *Rhodotorula glutinis*, and Nebucane G is significantly cytotoxic against MCF-7 (breast), and A431 (small cell lung) cell lines (Schrey et al, 2022).

Club Foot is somewhat edible, but consumed with alcohol it can cause a coprine-like reaction of miserable internal disturbance, similar to Inky Cap.

It contains meroterpenoids, including clavipols and clavilactone H, which shows cytotoxicity against HeLa, SGC-7901, and SHG-44 human cancer cell lines (Sun et al, 2019).

Clavipyrrine, another meroterpenoid, displays anti-glioma activity and induced apoptosis by inhibiting the JAK/STAT2 pathway, and reinforcing SOCS1/3 (Sun et al, 2021).

Clavilactones J-K, and clavipol C exhibit moderate cytotoxicity against the human tumor cell line HGC-27 (Hou et al, 2022). This cell line was obtained from a metastatic lymphatic node, associated with gastric cancer patient.

Trumpet Funnel Cap (*Clitocybe geotropa*) is not overly common, but found along the Rocky Mountains of the Pacific Northwest.

L-amino-acid oxidases from the fruiting body induce apoptosis in Jurkat cells via both intrinsic and extrinsic pathways. The increase in caspase-9, or caspase-8 suggests the former pathway is more predominant (Pislar et al, 2016).

The blue to violet-capped Wood Blewit is one of my favorite edibles, with a nutty flavor and good texture. The fruiting bodies can be found in late summer to early winter, especially on the coast.

When fed to mice as part of high-fat diet for eight weeks, amelioration of diabetic and dyslipidemic states was noted, via various pathways (Chen et al, 2014). A follow-up study by Shih et al, (2014), confirmed the hypoglycemic properties, due to increased muscular glucose uptake, and the reduction in hepatic glyconeogenesis.

Other work suggests water extracts induce dendritic cell maturation, that may be useful as an adjuvant in cancer vaccine immunotherapy (Chen et al, 2013).

Wood Blewitt exhibits anti-oxidant activity, with remarkably low IC50 levels, in a study by Emsen et al. (2020) on human lymphocytes.

C. alexandri is found in Quebec and elsewhere. An ethanol extract of the fruiting body induced cell cycle arrest and apoptosis in lung cancer cell line (NCI-H460). Various compounds were tested, but the whole extract exhibited the strongest decrease in cancer cell numbers. Both caspase-3 and p53 were involved (Vaz et al, 2012).

The False Chanterelle is considered inedible, possibly poisonous. About twenty years ago, I believed I spotted the true Chanterelle in an isolated part of Alberta. But alas, it turned out to be not, and to this day there are no reliable sightings in the province.

It is consumed by Tepehuán of northwest Mexico, after roasting or boiling. It is known as *kia's gio'* meaning, "iguana lard." Doesn't sound that tasty to me!

It may have some application in cosmetics. Clitocybin A, an isoindolinone isolated from mycelium, increased pro-collagen synthesis, and protects from UV irradiation, suggesting benefit in anti-wrinkle products (Lee et al., 2017).

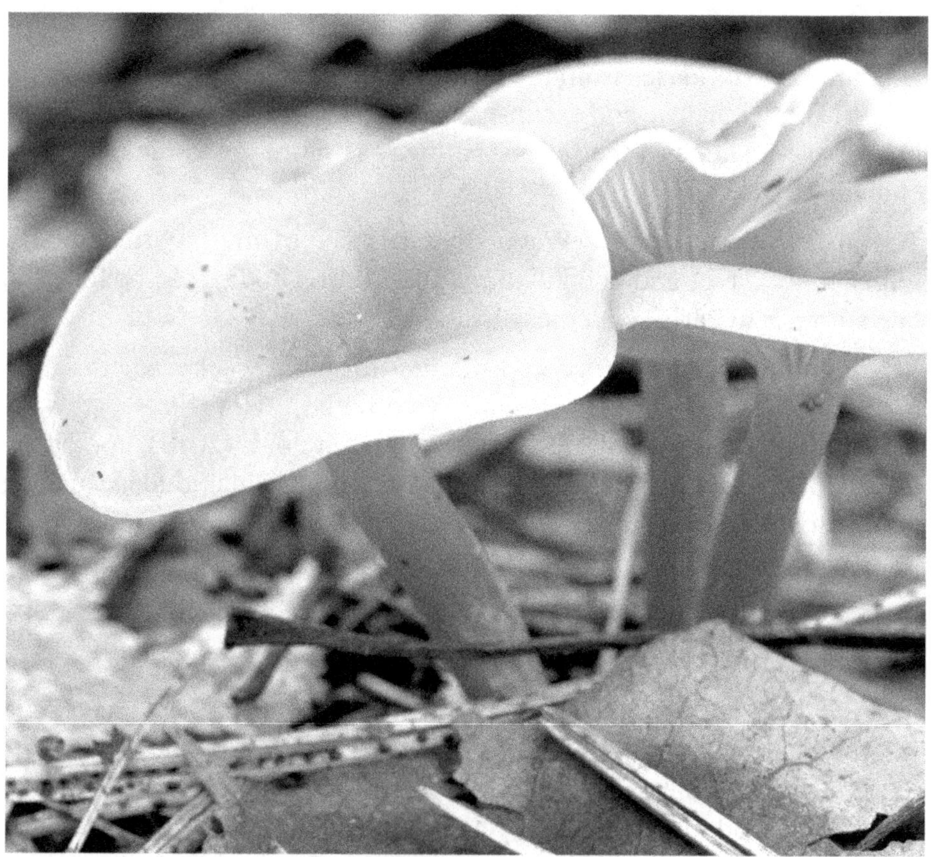

Funnel Cap

The same compound may inhibit vascular smooth muscle cell proliferation. Abnormal growth plays a significant role in atherosclerosis, hypertension and restenosis (Yoo et al, 2012).

The latter condition occurs after angioplasty or insertion of a stent, into a blocked artery. Over time, the inflammation creates another obstruction blocking adequate blood circulation.

The similar compound, Clitocybin B was also investigated by Yoo et al, (2012a). Studies on aortic smooth muscles, derived from rats, suggests it may be an effective anti-proliferative compound involving atherosclerosis and restenosis.

The bright orange-red color is due to pulvinic and variegatic acids, and derivatives. In Boletes, Suillus and other genera the color turns blue upon oxidation.

Variegatic acid inhibits TNF-alpha production, and PKCbeta1 activity in human leukemia cells (Sugaya et al, 2020).

Common Funnel *(C. gibba)* contains a thrombin inhibitor, suggesting possible benefit in preventing blood coagulation (Doljak et al, 2001).

Funnel Mushrooms (*C. squamulosa*) water extract contains novel polysaccharides that promote the growth of RAW264.7 cells and shows potential immune modulation, anti-inflammatory and anti-tumor activity (Guo et al, 2022).

The polysaccharides, when digested and fermented by human microbiota, reduces the proportions of Firmicutes and Bacteriodes, and promotes the growth of beneficial intestinal microbiome. This suggests a functional food prebiotic potential (Guo et al. 2000a).

Clitocine is found in Orange Funnel Cap (*C. inversa*), and *C. gigantea*, now re-named *Leucopaxillus giganteus*. See whole chapter later.

Clitocine is a exocyclic amino nucleoside that exhibits cytotoxicity, and apoptosis, to various human cancer cell lines, including DU145, K-562, MCF-7, and U251 (Fortin et al, 2006). It is also a potent Mcl-1 inhibitor that induces apoptosis in drug-resistant cancer cells both in vitro, and in vivo (Sun et al, 2014).

In a follow up study by Sun et al, (2016), pretreatment with clitocine dramatically enhanced TRAIL lethality in resistant human colon cancer cells. TRAIL (tumor necrosis factor related apoptosis-inducing ligand) is used in cancer treatment due to its relatively low toxicity to normal cells. But cancer cells can quickly develop drug resistance. This study suggests a possible effective adjuvant in cancer therapy. In fact, Friesen et al, (2017) suggest it represents a novel therapeutic modality to treat cancers and genetic diseases caused by nonsense mutation.

A cultivated culture of Large Funnel Cup (*C. maxima*) exopolysaccharides were fed as a daily dose to mice with artificially induced metastatic pulmonary tumors. Not only were sarcoma lesions reduced, but the numbers of total T cells, CD4+ cells, CD8+ cells and macrophages increased, compared to control group (Hu et al, 2015).

The Sweater (*C.rivulosa*) grows on lawns and pastures, and has been mistaken for the edible Fairy Ring (*Marasmius oreades*). It contains muscarine, which can promote liquids from every orifice. Caution is advised.

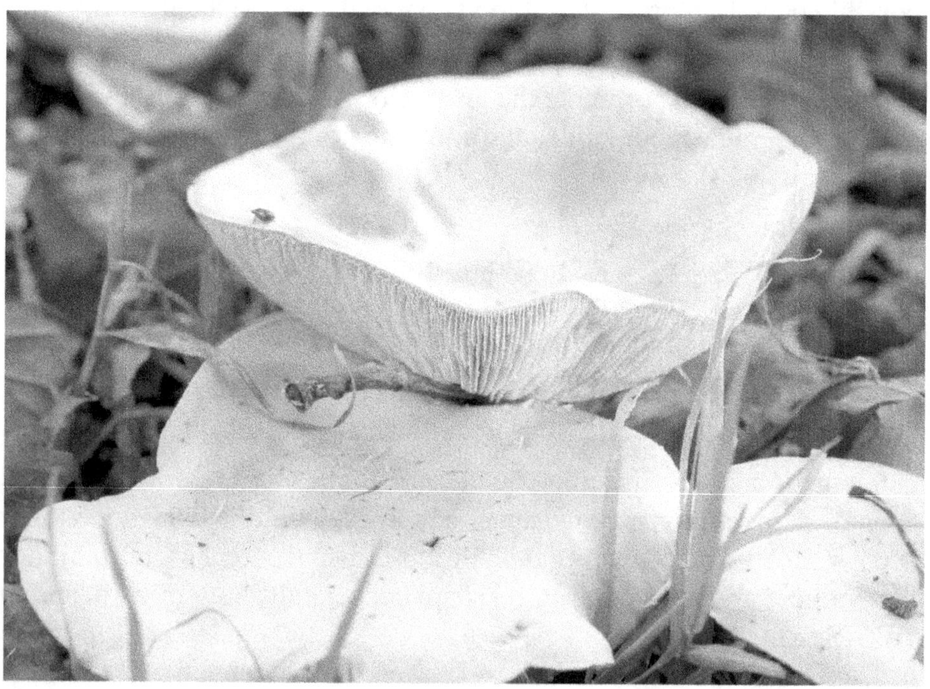

Clitocybe nebularis

COLLYBIA
SPOTTED COLLYBIA
(*Collybia maculata*)
(*Rhodocollybia maculata*)
TUFTED COLLYBIA
(*C. confluens*)
(*Gymnopus confluens*)
(*Marasmiellus confluens*)
OAK LOVING COLLYBIA
JUNE MUSHROOM
(*C. dryophila*)
(*Gymnopus dryophilus*)
ROOTED COLLYBIA
ROOTING SHANK
DEEP ROOT
(*C. radicata*)
(*Hymenopellus radicata*)
(*Oudemansiella radicata*)
SNOWY COLLYBIA
(*C. nivalis*)
(*Gymnopus nivalis*)
(*Marasmius nivalis*)
BROAD GILL
(*C. platyphylla*)
(*Megacollybia platyphylla*)
(*Tricholomopsis platyphylla*)

Collybia derives from the Greek "small coin". They are generally small, inedible and tough, with hollow stipes (often hairy or velvety), and crowded gills (never decurrent), and white (rarely buff) spores.

They usually appear in spring, in tight tufts, generally in forest debris.

Confluens is from Latin, meaning "flowing together", dryophilus from Greek, "oak loving", and maculata from Latin, "spotted."

In writing *The Fungal Pharmacy* (Rogers, 2011), I almost completely ignored the genus.; but attempting to make up for that oversight. The genera is slowly disappearing with new DNA technology.

Spotted Collybia (*C. maculata* or *Rhodocollybia maculata*) is widespread and common in Pacific Northwest. In fact, there are at least five varieties, based on their cap or gill color. Variety *maculata* gills are cream to pale tan color, var. *scorzonerea* has yellow gills, var. *occidentalis* gills range from white to pale orange; var. *nigra* has dark, brown-black caps, var. *fulva* caps are vinaceous red, and var. *immutabilis* is grey-cream in color. They are edible, but not great.

It is difficult to know which variations were used in the following studies.

Lipoxygenase (LOX) is an enzyme that processes arachidonic acid metabolism into leukotriene, which mediate inflammation. Inhibition of LOX thus produces an anti-inflammatory effect, as chronic and persistent inflammation contributes to cancer, diabetes, cardiovascular and neurological disease.

Work by Lee et al, (2014) found extracts of this fruiting body exhibits potent LOX inhibition by 73.3%).

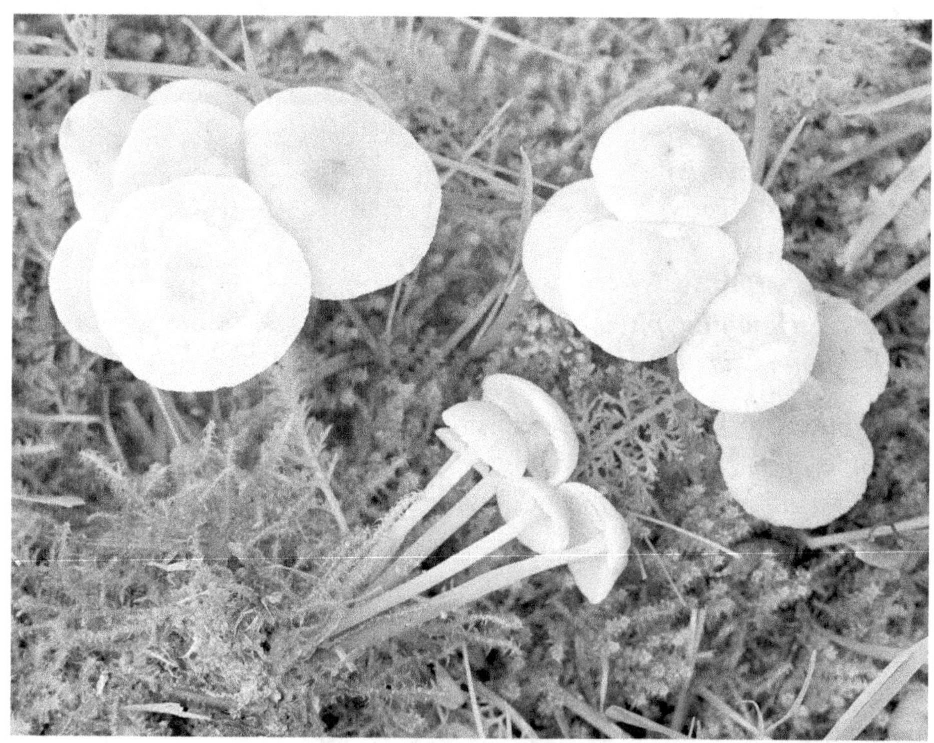

Gymnopus confluens

The mushroom has a high concentration of organic iron (274 mg/kg). (Wang & Hou, 2011).

It contains the sesquiterpene collybolide, a highly selective agonist of kappa-opioid receptors. The compound is very similar to salvinorin A, from *Salvia divinorum*, but differs slightly. Collybolide exhibits ten to fifty fold higher potency in activating the mitogen-activated protein kinase pathway compared with salvinorin A. They both equally inhibit adenylyl cyclase activity, suggesting the mushroom compound behaves as a biased agonist of kappa-opioid receptor. It also exhibits more than a ten-fold higher potency in blocking non-histamine-mediated itch (Gupta et al, 2016).

Three purine derivatives isolated from mycelial cultures exhibit anti-viral, anti-fungal and cytotoxic activity (Leonhardt et al, 1987).

Tufted Collybia (formerly known as *C. confluens*, now *Marasmiellus confluens*) is widely distributed, and like other Collybia and Marasmius species, will often dry up, and revive after rain. Plentiful mycelium is present in the forest duff.

Collybial is an antibiotic sesquiterpenoid derived from the fruiting body. The structure is similar to Koraiol, isolated from *Pinus koraiensis*. Work by Simon et al, (1995) found collybial inhibits the growth of Gram-positive bacteria; and vesiclular stomatitis virus in kidney (BHK-21) cell lines.

The mycelial powder showed anti-diabetic and hypolipidemic effect on streptozotocin-induced diabetic rats. Blood sugar, total cholesterol, triglycerides and LDL cholesterol were all reduced in work by Yang et al, (2006).

A related study on same rat model found reduced plasma glucose levels (259%) compared to controls, as well as lower total cholesterol and triglyceride levels. Artist Conk (*Ganoderma applanatum*) showed similar benefits (22%) in reduction of blood sugar, and hyperlipidemia. (Yang et al, 2007)

Rooted Collybia (*C. radicata*), is also known as *Hymenopellis radicata*, or *Oudemansiella radicata*. It is noted for its distinct "tap root" underground stipe extension.

The mushroom is cultivated, as a functional food, for the market in China.

And polysaccharides have been found to benefit the product quality and unami flavor of shiitake mushrooms post-harvest (Liu et al, 2021a).

Polysaccharides were fed to mice for 14 days, and counts of intestinal flora and immunoglobin A (IgA) improved (Wang et al, 2015).

Water soluble polysaccharides protect from induced liver damage via antioxidant mechanisms (Liu et al, 2017).

Enzyme-extracted polysaccharides alleviate alcohol-induced liver injury, in part by activating alcohol dehydrogenase and aldehyde dehydrogenase, and reducing cytochrome P450 2E1 levels (Wang et al, 2018a).

More recently, Liu et al, (2021) studied the digestibility of polysaccharides and their effect on gut microbiota. Several short-chain fatty acids were formed, including acetic, propionic and n-butryic acids; and increased production of Bacteroides and Parabacteroides.

Polysaccharides from this mushroom possess several functions, including antiviral, anti-aging and hypolipidemic activity (Wang et al, 2018). This research team found a polysaccharide improved proliferation and phagocytosis of macrophages by 2.1 and 3.4 times respectively. It also induced secretion of nitric oxide, inducible nitric oxide synthase and various cytokines, including TNF-alpha (tumor necrosis factor-alpha), and interleukins IL-1B, IL-6 and IL-10, by factor of 2.3 to 3.6. It also inhibited TLR4 (toll-like receptor 4), suggesting potent immune modulation.

Anti-oxidant, anti-inflammatory kidney and lung protection has been noted in work by Gao et al, (1207 and 2018). Mycelium, enriched with selenium, produced polysaccharides that prevent and alleviate kidney and lung damage in mice.

Oak Loving Collybia, or June Mushroom, was formerly known as *C. dryophila*; and now *Gymnopus dryophilus*. Usually found under hardwoods, but under conifers in western North America. It is not edible.

A 1>3, 1>4 beta-D-glucan derived from fruiting body was found to significantly inhibit nitric oxide production, via INOS gene expression. It also significantly increased prostaglandin E2 production in lipopolysaccharide and gamma interferon induced macrophages, compared to control (Pacheco-Sánchez et al, 2007).

Collybia nivalis (*Gymnopus nivalis*) fruiting bodies contain the anti-fungal strobilurins and oudemansin A (Engler et al, 1998). Both have been stabilized and patented for use in organic food production. Strobularins are also found in the tiny Douglas Fir Cone Mushrooms, *Strobilurus tenacellus*, growing on fallen cones.

Broad Gill (*C. platyphylla*) is common, under hardwoods in eastern North America, but also found in the west. It contains type 8 toxins, which upset some individuals.

Lipids, derived from the fruiting body, provoked an increase in erythrocyte membrane fluidity. This suggest possible benefit in the treatment of hypertension and other cardiovascular conditions associated with decreased fluidity of membranes. (Mujic et al, 2011).

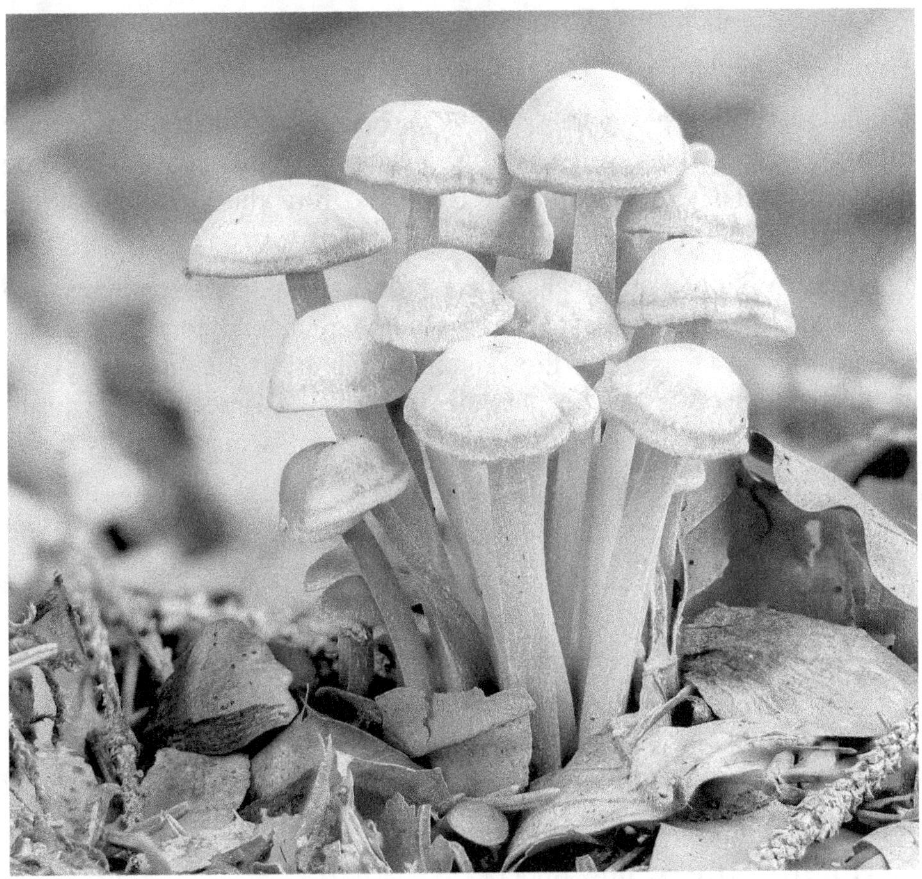

Gymnopus confluens

DIAMOND WILLOW FUNGUS
(*Haploporus odorus*)
CONCEALED POLYPORE
(*Cryptoporus volvatus*)

Two Medicinal Mushrooms with Shared Constituents

C. volvatus constituents- various cryptoporic acids (A, B, D, E, and S), cryptoporol A, 6'-cryptoporic acid E methyl ester, stigmasterol, stigmast-7-en-3beta-ol, stigmast-4-en-3-one, two ergosterols including, (22E,24R)-ergosta-7,22-diene-3beta,5alpha,6beta-triol, and 5alpha, 8alpha, epidocy-22E-ergosta-6,22-dien-3beta-ol; beta-sitosterol, beta-daucosterol, dibutyl phthalate, adenosine, guanosine, uridine, uracil, 1-ribityl-2,3-diketo- 1,2,3, 4-tetrahydro-6,7-dimethyl-quinoxaline, D-arabitol, D-galactitol, D-sorbitol, tetraconsanoic acid.

H. odorus- haploporic acid A, cryptoporic acids.

Diamond Willow polypore (*Haploporus odorus*) is a somewhat rare circumboreal species, often confused with *Trametes suaveolens*, due to their similar anise-like scent. Haplo is from the Greek meaning, "single", and poros, "pores".

Diamond Willow fungus has a great deal of special significance to indigenous people of the northern plains and boreal forest. It grows specifically on Diamond Willow, and the fungus size is directly related to the diameter of its host tree. I gather football-sized specimens in north-eastern British Columbia, on massive willow species, usually Salix caprea.

Across northern Europe and Asia, it is considered near threatened and on the IUCN Red List.

As a teenage Queen Scout, I carved a diamond willow walking stick that I still make use of some 55 years later.

The anise/licorice scent can be easily detected in the boreal forest, or by following one's nose, you are easily led to the cream-white conks.

The Cree call it WIY(H)KIMASIYGAN, or WASASKWETIW, while their northern neighbors, the Chipewyan know it as K'AI TLH'ELHT'ARE (willow tinder).

It is smudged, as part of special ceremonies, and with its special coumarin/anise-like odor, is very pleasing to the mind and body. It is a special gift given to healers conducting sweat lodges, as the fungus is believed to guard and protect against unseen forces. The smoke is used in blessings and as part of cleansing and empowerment events. The smoke is said to help communication with the deceased, or to call in the spirits and expel negative forces.

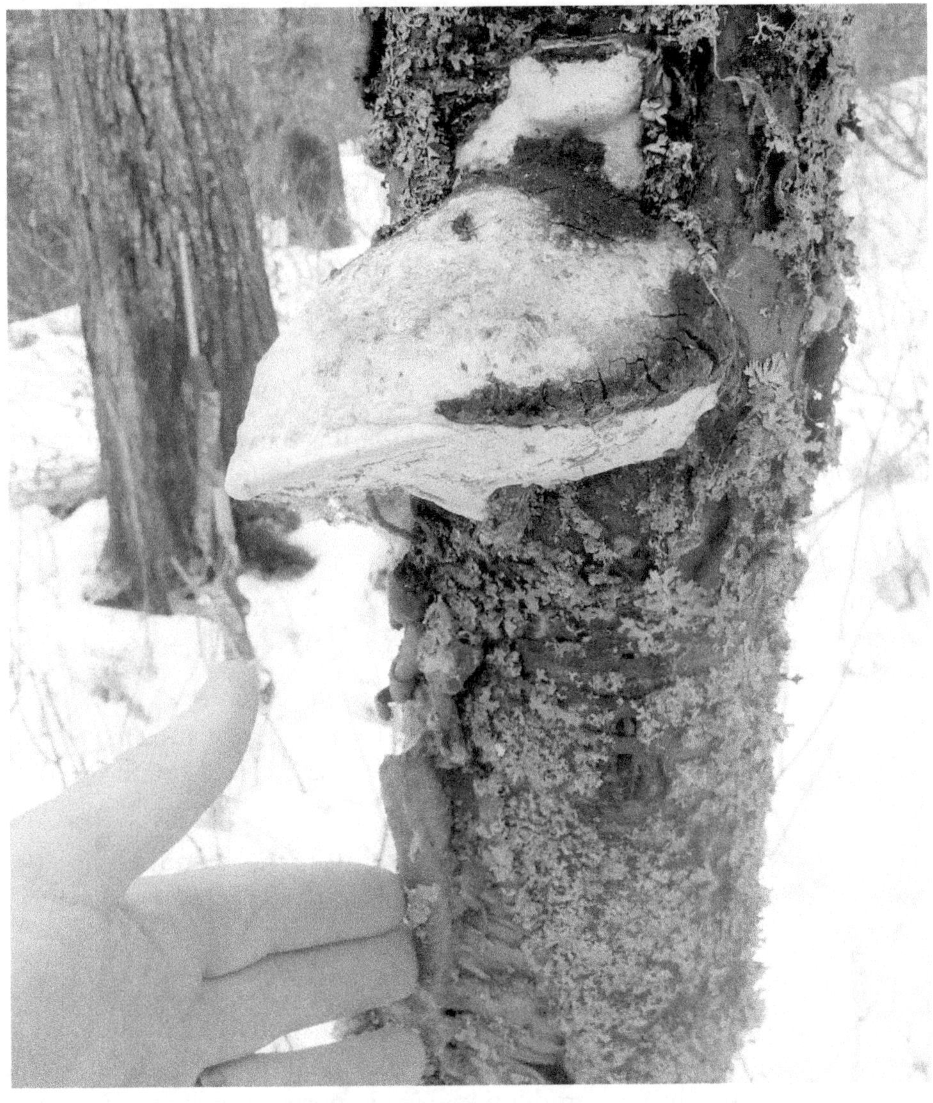

Diamond Willow Fungus

63

It was traditionally used to decorate sacred robes, as a symbol of spiritual power; and found in medicine bundles, along with assorted medicinal plants, for bronchitis and other lung issues.

It is considered to have protective powers and when taken as a steeped infusion will stop diarrhea and dysentery; or it can be combined in decoction with Indian Breadroot (*Psoralea esculenta*) to treat coughs. The smoke is inhaled for treating headaches, including migraine-type, or soaked in water and the resulting juice, squeezed into earaches. Decoctions are taken internally for muscle spasms.

The conk has been used for coughs, diarrhea, various infectious conditions, and to staunch external bleeding. (Blanchette, 1997). He writes, "The exceedingly fragrant anise-like scent of *H. odorus* sporophores appears to be the reason this fungus was selected and revered."

I burned a small piece as a mosquito smudge when camping one summer night. It definitely added a brightened and vivid element to my dream state, similar to the effects of Mugwort (*Artemisia vulgaris*).

The white fungus worn around necks, about the size of tennis balls, has been mistakenly assumed in the past to be puffballs. In fact, this was carved diamond willow fungus, also found attached to robes and blankets.

Mors Kochanski, a close friend and wilderness survival expert, supplied samples of the fungi to Dr. Robert Blanchette, at the University of Minnesota. He compared these samples with museum pieces from the Glenbow in Calgary, to confirm his findings.

I have steam-distilled the fruiting body, resulting in a most pleasant, albeit small yield of essential oil, and a beautiful hydrosol with fragrant scent.

The fruiting body contains a number of drimane sesquiterpenoids, including haploporic acid A, and cryptoporic acids (ethers of isocitric acid). Zmirovich, et al, (2019).

The latter compounds are found in the Pouch Fungus, or Concealed Polypore (*Cryptoporus volvatus*), a leathery annual associated with dying conifers. This suggests a more sustainable option for wildcrafters, and medicinal mushroom production. Cryptoporus means "with hidden pores", and volvatus, "with volva."

The fruiting bodies can be sucked on, and are initially quite fragrant, and then bitter. They alleviate sore throats, and are decocted in traditional Chinese medicine for intestinal bleeding, as well as, tracheitis, asthma and bronchial conditions. A small polypore is given to nursing babies to suck on, helping wean them from breast feeding.

This polypore is unique in that its pores are enclosed by a subtended volva, resulting in the majority of spores accumulating on the inner surface of the sheath. The odor released attracts two sympatric beetles, *Parabolitophagus felix* and *Ischnodactylus loripes*. The fungus provides food and shelter, while the beetles help disperse the spores to other sites. The sporocarp volval chambers become a mating space, with the former beetles using the chamber up to mid-May, and the latter species making use from late May to early June.

Cryptoporic acid E, in vitro, inhibits the development of colon cancer in rat and mice studies. Narisawa et al, (1992).

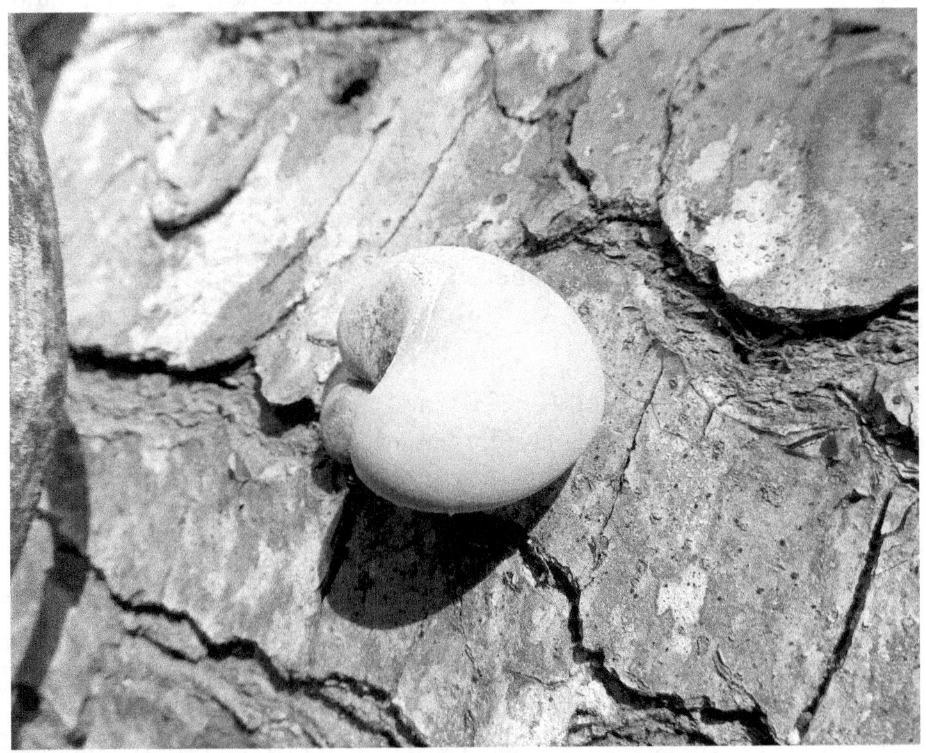

Cryptoporus volvatus

A recent *in vitro* study found Cryptoporic acid E possesses broad-spectrum anti-influenza against H1N1 and H3N2. The compound appears to exerts its inhibition in the middle stages of the virus replication cycle. It inhibits influenza virus RNA polymerase activity and blocks virus RNA replication and transcription in MDCK cells. It impairs the virus by directly targeting virus particles. Gao et al, (2017).

This follows a previous study by same research team (Gao et al, 2014), that found *C. volvatus* extracts significantly decreased viral loads of H1N1 influenza virus in the lungs of mice.

Cryptoporic acid derivatives exhibit cytotoxicity against HCT-116 (human cancer) cell lines (Pham et al, 2021).

Various cryptoporic and isocryptoporic acids exhibit cytotoxicity against five tumor cell lines. One compound ICA-G, exhibits activity comparable to the cancer drug cisplatin. Ling-Yun Zhou et al, (2016).

Holistic veterinarian doctors may be interested to note the compound, 5alpha, 8alpha, epidocy-22E-ergosta-6,22-dien-3beta-ol exhibits activity against the destructive porcine reproductive and respiratory syndrome virus. Wang et al, (2015). This is the most serious economic condition to hit commercial hog operations since swine fever, that reared its destructive head in the late 1980s.

Ergosterol peroxide, extracted from the fruiting body, inhibits porcine delta coronavirus infection, and regulates host immune responses by down-regulating activation of NF-kappaB and p38/MAPK signaling pathways (Duan et al, 2021).

Recent work by Liu et al. (2022) found the same compound inhibits porcine epidemic diarrhea alpha coronavirus. It helps prevent replication and directly inactivates the virus, via ROS production and p53 activation.

Two master's theses, posted on Globalthesis.com, examined the anti-inflammatory and anti-allergenic properties of the fungi.

L. Chen looked at the polysaccharides produced by fermentation culture and found strong reduction of allergic inflammation in a 2009 mouse study.

Five years previously, Z. S. Bao looked at the reduction of allergic-induced asthma in guinea pigs, based on TCM patterns of spleen deficiency.

The compound of most interest to me is uracil. This compound has a wide range of anti-tumor and anti-viral activity, including HIV, herpes viruses, and hepatitis B and C. In fact, the chemotherapy drug 5-FU (5-fluorouracil) is also an uracil derivative. Palasz & Ciez (2015).

Uracil derivates are being investigated for inhibition of acetylcholinesterase and butyrycholinesterase; enzymes associated with senile dementia and Alzheimer's disease. Cavdar et al, (2019).

Uridine is one of five nucleic acids necessary for RNA replication, and promotes new dopamine receptors by acting on D1 and D2 receptor signaling, preventing receptor burn-out, especially in brains with fewer receptors, such as found in Parkinson's disease. A paper by Carlezon et al, (2005), found both uridine and omega-3 fatty acids possess anti-depressant activity. In this in vivo study, the two compounds were synergistic in their anti-depressant like effects.

Recent work by Zhou et al, (2022) found IUNQ is the target of sesquiterpenoids derived from Concealed Polypore. This affects the proliferation of tumor cells by acetylating Lys-144, which blocks Akt binding to downstream PIP3; affecting the proliferation of tumor cells.

An extraction of oil is best accomplished by soaking the mushrooms for one hour, and then decocted for eight hours in ten times the water, weight to volume (Zhao & Liang, 2004). The oil will float to the top and can be skimmed off.

Initial attempts, by myself and colleagues, to produce diamond willow mycelial mass have been disappointing to date. Similar to Agarikon (*Laricifomes officinalis*), an important medicinal mushroom of the Pacific Northwest, cultivation of the mycelium may prove beneficial in the future. Commercial harvesting of this endangered polypore should be strongly discouraged.

Diamond willow mushroom essence helps one discover the true path of the soul, by integrating soul fragments and long hidden parts suppressed by social convention. Fasting rituals and vision quests are enhanced. Rogers (2016).

FAIRY RING MUSHROOM
(*Marasmius oreades*)
HORSE HAIR MUSHROOM
(*M. androsaceus*)

You demi-puppets that by moonshine do the green sour ringlets make, Whereof ewe not bites; and you, whose pastime is to make Midnight Mushrooms.   SHAKESPEARE

CONSTITUENTS - *M. oreades*- marasmone, anhydromarasmone, isomarasmone, dihydromarasmone, various norsesquiterpenes including 0-formlyoreadone, 3alpha-hydroxyoreadone and dehydrooreadone, agrocybin (polyacetylene amide), 4,4-dimethyl-5 alpha-ergosta-8,24(28)-dien-3 beta-ol (an ergosterol precursor) and various drimane sesquiterpenes.

M. androsaceus- marasmic acid; 3,3,5,5-tetramethyl 4-piperidone.

Marasmius is derived from the Greek meaning, "withered", in reference to their ability to revive after a rain. Oreades refers to growing in the mountain, which is not always true. Andrus Voitk suggests androsaceus means, "like a certain algae."

Fairy Ring, or Scotch Bonnet mushrooms are the bane of grassaholics, who worship their pristine Kentucky Bluegrass lawns. Various poisons have been trialed over the years but my considered advice is to gather, dry the caps, and later eat them. That is, if you, or your neighbors do not herbicide the green space.

The rings can be large in size; one encircling Stonehenge believed to be over a thousand years old.

The small amount of hydrocyanic acid, giving a pleasant almond scent, dissipates with cooking. The caps, when cooked fresh in butter have a faint oak smell, and when lightly caramelized are nice addition to salads. The dried and powdered caps add amazing flavour to soups and stews.

The tough stipes are, in my opinion, not worth the trouble of harvesting and drying. About sixty species of mushrooms grow in ring formation, so caution is advised.

Be careful not to pick The Sweater (*Clitocybe dealbata*) which is muscarinic, and will induce unpleasant, yet temporary, symptoms. This white mushroom is funnel-shaped, with fully decurrent gills, sometimes found on the same lawn.

Fairy Ring fruiting bodies are a fair source of protein (12-14%) and fatty acids (7.7-8.4%), mainly linoleic, as well as over 50% carbohydrates, and significant amounts of potassium, sodium, phosphorus, calcium and magnesium. The amino acid score is 1.34, suggesting a good source of quality protein; albeit limiting in tryptophan and leucine. Kayode et al, (2016).

In Germany, the rings are known as Hexen rings, from hexen meaning witches. It was said that on the eve of May Day (Walpurgis Night), the pagan witches would hold their revelry, the rings formed from their dance.

In France, they were known as sorcerers' rings, and said to be sacred to enormous toads with bulging eyes. Today, the choice edible is known as *champignon*.

In Tyrol, the rings were believed caused by a dragon's hot breath, while the Irish believed they were caused by the devil spilling milk, while churning butter. In other parts of Europe, fairy rings were believed formed by spit, sperm or urine of elves.

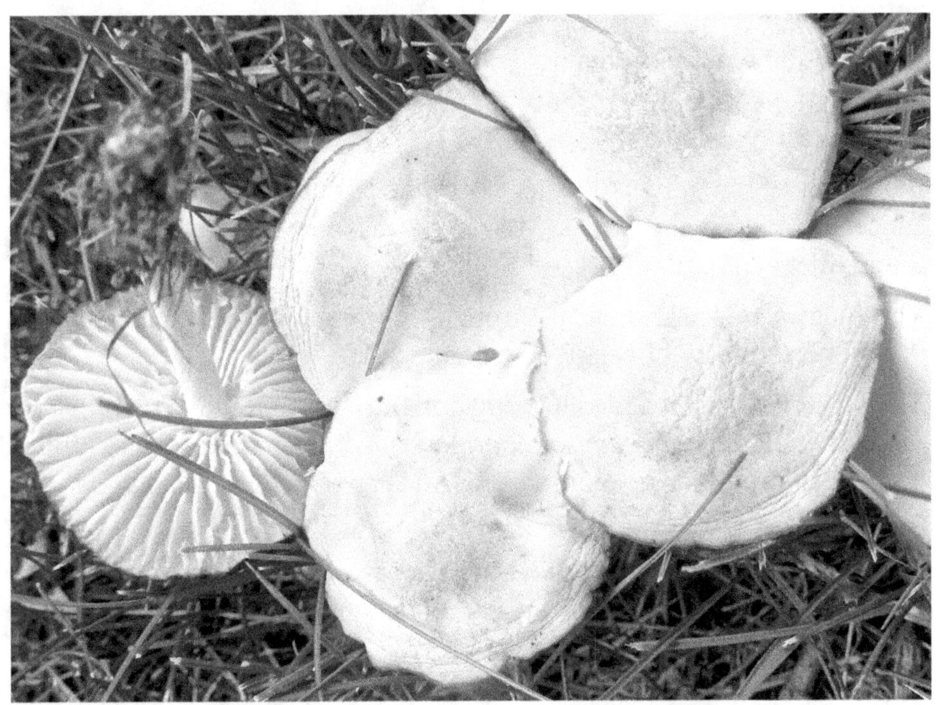

Marasmius oreades

The Blackfoot of Alberta call them *kok-a-tos-i-u,* formerly believing they were formed by dancing bison.

In traditional Chinese medicine (TCM), the dried mushrooms are found in Tendon Easing Powder, used to treat lumbago, leg pain, numbness of limbs, and discomfort in veins and tendons.

Early work by Petrova et al, (2007) found crude extracts inhibit NF-kappaB pathways associated with MCF breast cancer cell lines.

A lectin, agglutinin, may be associated with physiological cell response, such as cytoskeleton re-arrangement, cell detachment and death. Juillot et al, (2016).

Ethanol extracts possess antioxidant activity, with an 8% increase in superoxide dimustase (SOD) anti-oxidant activity.

One interesting study combined the phenolic and polysaccharide extracts of Fairy Ring and King Bolete (*Boletus edulis*) fruiting bodies. Different ratios were trialed, and a 50:50 ratio produced the highest synergistic antioxidant activity. Vieira et al, (2012).

Extracts show activity against triple negative breast cancer cell lines. One fraction, MOC-4, caused significant apoptosis, or cell programmed death. Liao et al, (2017).

Inhibition of three human cancer cell lines; (colon (HT-29), and breast cancers (MCF-7 and MDA-MB-231) was noted in recent work by Shomali et al, (2019).

The fungi act synergistically, through different signalling pathways on 9L glioblastoma cell lines. Ruimi et al, (2010).

The same research team found ethanol extracts inhibited *Enterococcus faecalis* and *Staphylococcus epidermis,* but more importantly, exhibited high biofilm inhibition against MRSA, *S. epidermis* and *Pseudomonas aeruginosa.*

The anti-fungal peptide agrocybin, also present in Agrocybe species, is cytotoxic, and induces apoptosis in human cancer UACC-62 (melanoma), MCF-7 (breast), and TK-10 (kidney) cell lines. It inhibits trypanothione reductase associated with organism responsible for Chagas' disease. Rosa et al, (2006).

Agrocybin, in studies by Ngai et al, (2005), attenuated the activity of HIV-1 reverse transcriptase.

The closely related Horse Hair Mushroom (*M. androsaceus*) is commonly found in woods, on needles, twigs and leaves.

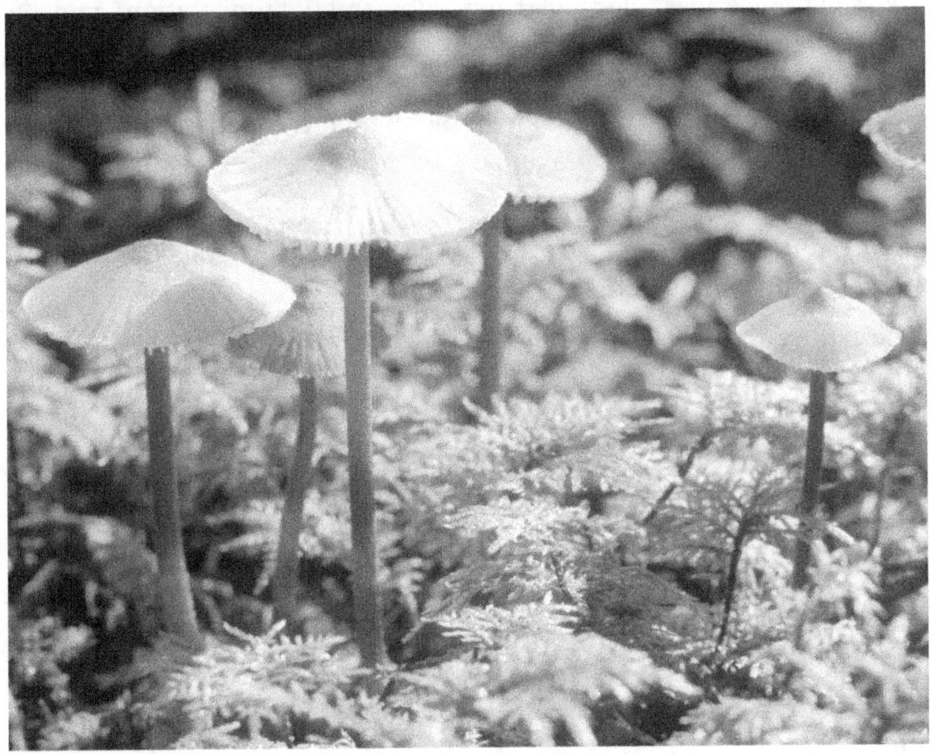

Marasmius androsaceus

Early research by McFarland & Rimmer (1996) found the fungus widely used by birds for nest lining in red spruce/balsam fir forests of Northeastern United States. In fact, 85% of the nests studied contained the horsehair fungus. Whether they are gathered for structure and/or creating a healthy nesting environment is unknown.

In TCM, the mushroom is used for joint pain associated with leprosy and a remedy for injuries from falls, including fractures, contusions and strains. Neuralgia, sciatica, trigeminal neuralgia, as well as some forms of migraine headache respond favorably.

A mouse study by Song et al, (2018) examined the mechanism of oral ethanol extracts on neuropathic pain. The analgesic benefit appears related to the regulation of metabolism by monoamine neurotransmitters and Ca^{2+}/CaMK11-mediated signaling. More research would be helpful.

Exopolysaccharides, derived from submerged fermentation, may be useful for treating depression, based on a rat model study by Song et al, (2017). The oral treatment significantly increased levels of noradrenalin, dopamine, 5-hydroxytryptamine in blood and hypothalamus, similar to the anti-depressant drug fluoxetine (Prozac).

A recent study by Song et al, (2020) found the novel MEPS2 may be involved in catecholamine synthesis and release, and enhances levels of noradrenalin and dopamine.

The extract upregulated protein expression levels of tyrosine hydroxylase in the hypothalamus, suggesting the monoamine neurotransmitter system is involved.

The water extracts of mycelium yield polysaccharides were precipitated with ethanol and show significant anti-oxidant activity. Wang et al, (2006).

Horse Hair contains the anti-hypertensive compound, 3,3,5,5-tetramethyl 4-piperidone, that works via ganglionic blockage. Zhang et al, (2009).

Experiments by Wang et al, (2007) with normal mice found medium to high dosage of polysaccharides increase lymphocyte count, enhance phagocytic function, and immunity regulation.

Marasmic acid is anti-bacterial, anti-fungal and cytotoxic. Abraham (2001).

The eastern NA Pinwheel Marasmius (*M. rotula*) contains peroxygenase that can efficiently produce cyclophosphamide specific drug metabolites (Steinbrecht et al, 2020).

Fairy Ring mushroom essence is taken under the tongue for issues involving birth, fertility, pregnancy, labour and circadian rhythms. Rogers (2016).

FALSE TURKEY TAIL
HAIRY STEREUM
(*Stereum hirsutum*)
GOLDEN CURTAIN CRUST
(*S. ostrea*)

I first discovered my love of mushrooms in the forests of Alberta. Being a novice, I would, more than once, be fooled into thinking I had found Turkey Tail (*Trametes versicolor*), only to be disappointed. Turkey Tail has a fertile surface with visible pores, and white surface.

False Turkey Tail and other *Stereum* species are considered crust or parchment fungi, and not polypores, due to lack of tubes and pores.

Stereum means "tough or rigid", which it generally is not, and hirsutum means "hairy", which it is.

False Turkey Tail under surface is smooth, and dull orange to brown orange. It prefers hardwoods, but I have seen it occasionally on conifers. According to Arora, a bright orange to orange buff spore-bearing surface, suggests Crowded Parchment (*S. complicatum*) or *S. rameale*.

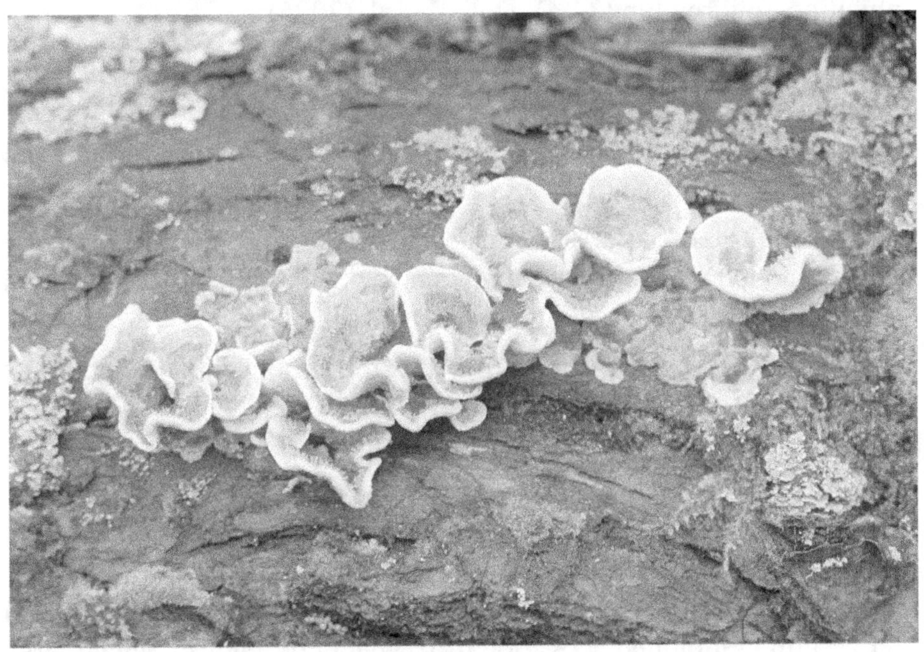

Stereum hirsutum

I have a newly discovered respect for the many medicinal benefits offered by this commonly found forest fungi. That is, I no longer walk by them, but harvest the fruiting bodies.

There are 27 Stereum species, and a thorough review by Tian et al, (2020) examined ten species, looking at the 238 secondary, bioactive metabolites.

False Turkey Tail fruiting body possesses anti-oxidant and cytotoxic activity against HepG2 (hepatic) cancer cells line. Ethanol extracts show potent inhibition of acetylcholinesterase, associated with senile dementia and Alzheimer's disease.

Amentoflavone (also found in the medicinal plant, Saint John's Wort) may be responsible, in part, for the cytotoxic activity (Miskovic et al, 2021).

Ethanol extracts are superior to methanol extracts in anti-oxidant and free radical scavenging activity. Sevindik et al, (2021) suggest the anti-oxidative and anti-inflammatory function, as well as lipid-lowering effects correlate with anti-atherogenic benefit. Not sure I totally agree, but interesting research.

Glycerolipids, extracted from the fruiting body exhibit significant inhibition on thrombin (34%). Doljak et al, (2006).

The extracts show significant activity against *Staphylococcus aureus*, methicillin-resistant *S. aureus*, and *Acinetobacter baumannii*.

An early study by Kleinwächter et al, (2001) isolated the anti-microbial metabolite epicorazine C.

A lanostane triterpenoid, stereinone D, isolated from the fruiting body showed moderate cytotoxic activity against SMMC-7721 (hepatic) and SW480 (colon) cancer cell lines (Yao et al, 2018).

Epidioxysterols 1-4, isolated from the mushroom, show significant activity against *Mycobacterium tuberculosis* (Cateni et al, 2007). Drug-resistant strains of this virulent pathogen are becoming more common, worldwide.

Ten sterhirsutins (heterodimeric sesquiterpenes) isolated from a culture, show cytotoxicity against K562 and HCT116 cancer cell lines. Sterhirsutin K induced autophagy in HeLa (cervical) cells, and sterhirsutin G inhibited activation of IFNbeta promotor in Sendai virus infected cells (Qi et al, 2015).

Cultured mushrooms contain isoprenylated depsides, named sterenins. Work by Wang et al, (2014) found inhibition of alpha-glucosidase, suggesting possible benefit in lowering blood sugar levels.

Hirsutenols E-F, isolated from culture broth, show significant activity against free radicals, suggesting anti-oxidant potential (Yoo et al, 2006).

Myceliated rice contains benzoate derivatives that exhibit activity against methicillin-resistant *Staphylococcus aureus*. One benzoate compound and a sesquiterpene showed cytotoxicity against A549 (small cell lung) and HepG2 (hepatic) cancer cell lines. The authors suggest the use of mycelium as a functional food (Ma et al, 2014).

The mushroom was cultivated on wheat bran, and subsequently developed unique drimane-type sesquiterpenes. The known stereumamides I-K and sterostrein Q showed weak activity against *Mycobacterium tuberculosis* (Pu et al, 2021).

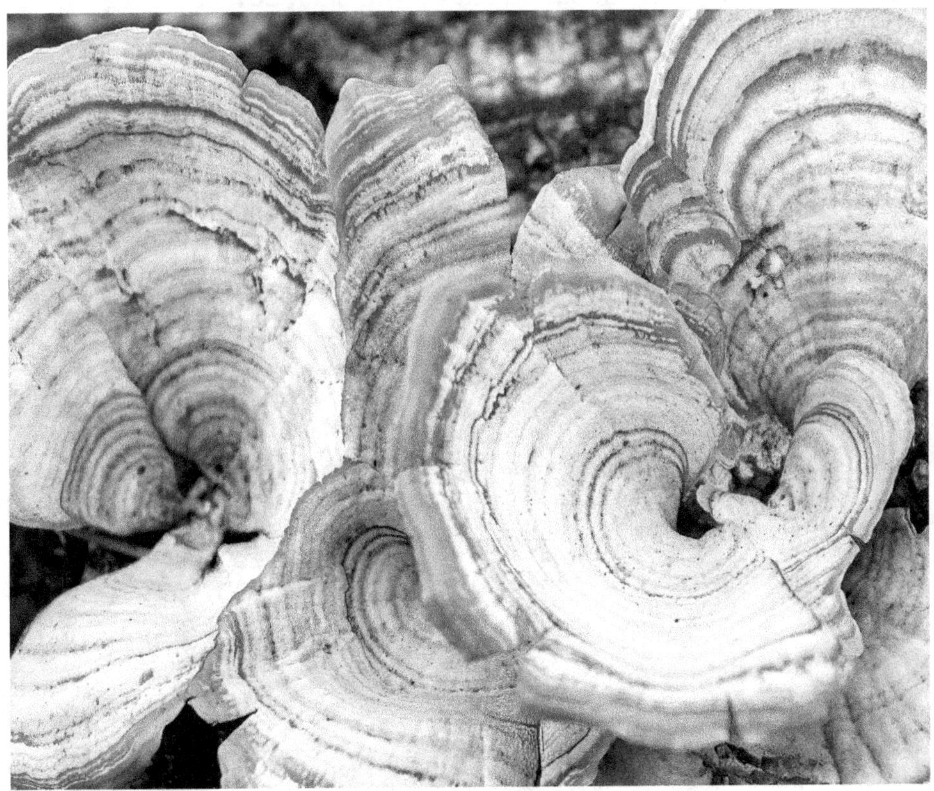

Stereum ostrea

Liquid fermentation of *S. rameale* contains vibralactone and vibralactone B. The latter compound significantly inhibited *E. coli* and *Pseudomonas aeruginosa* (Aqueveque et al, 2015).

Vibralactone and vibralactone B are obtained from *S. hirsutum* and *S. rameale*

Golden Curtain Crust (*S. ostrea*) is often referred to as False Turkey Tail. But is not hairy, tends to be darker red in color and generally found individually, and not in clusters.

It has been less studied, but does contain some interesting chemistry.

The fruiting body contains methoxylaricinolic and laricinolic acids, the latter also found in Agarikon (*Laricifomes officinalis*). Kim et al, (2006).

Thirty-three species of mushrooms collected in Korea, including *S. ostrea*, were examined for anti-oxidant activity, and this species was one of three with exceptional potency (Kim et al, 2012).

Water extracts of liquid culture filtrate shows activity against *Staphylococcus aureus* and Gram-positive bacteria, as well as pathogenic fungi (Imtiaj et al, 2007).

A culture broth yielded three ostalactones A-C, with two displaying potent inhibitory activity against human pancreatic lipase. This suggest possible benefit in anti-obesity products (Kang & Kim, 2016).

The terpenoids, sterostreins, isolated from culture by Isaka et al, (2011) were examined for activity. Sterostrein A exhibited anti-malarial activity (IC50-2.3μg/mL) and cytotoxicity (IC50-5.3-38 μg/mL).

Bleeding Stereum (*S. sanguinolentum*) found on conifers, bleeds red when fresh underside is cut. This species and *S. rugosum* were acetone-extracted and found potent inhibitors of acetylcholineasterase and butyrylcholinesterase, enzymes associated with senile dementia and Alzheimer's disease (Cayan et al, 2019).

The birch-loving *S. subtomentosum* contains botulin and polyporenic acid (Hybelbauerova et al, 2008.)

A jelly fungus, called Golden Ear (*Naemalelia aurantia*, formerly *Tremella aurantia*) is parasitic with Stereum. *Tremella mesenterica*, on hardwoods, is parasitic of Peniophora.

FRIED CHICKEN MUSHROOM
HATAKESHIMEJI
(*Lyophyllum decastes*)
WHITE TUFT
OSHIROISHIMEJI
(*L. connatum*)
HON-SHIMEJI
(*L. shimeji*)

Lylphyllum derives from the Greek, meaning "with loose gills", and decastes from same origin "in numbers of ten." Connatum is from the Latin, "born together."

Many years ago, I was walking up a steep logging road in British Columbia. I turned the corner and in the middle of this gravel-dirt road was a bushel-sized clump of fried chicken. Delicious!

So imagine my surprise just a few autumns ago, while foraging in northern Alberta, when large clumps of white-capped mushrooms appeared everywhere. One of the group Fish G., with Russian ancestry, picked it up, smelled it, and declared it a choice edible.

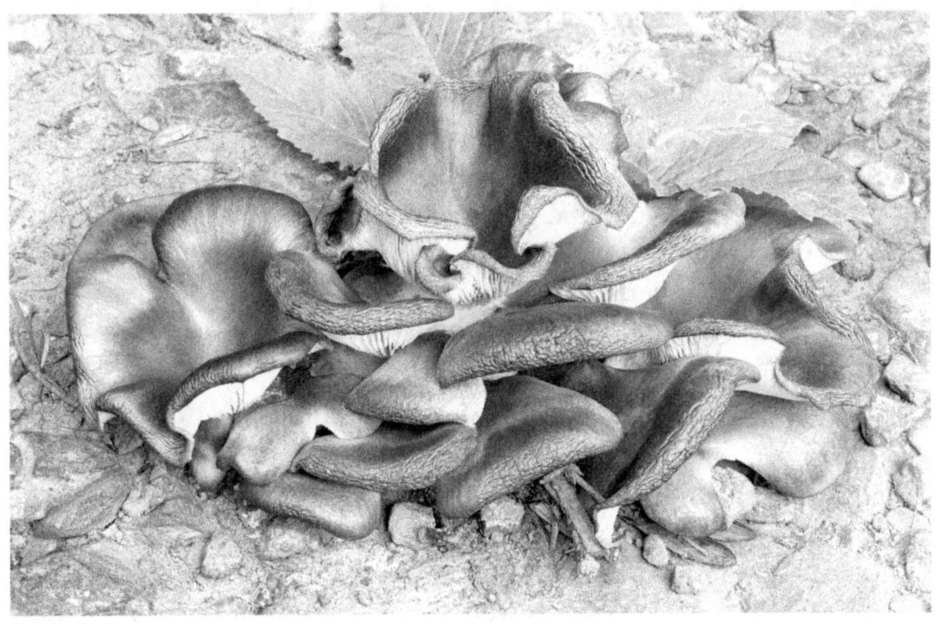

Lyophyllum decastes

We all know the saying about bold and old mushroom hunters, so I was somewhat leery. The Clitocybes, particularly the toxic *C. dilatata*, look similar, and I remember Fried Chicken having a yellow to gray-brown cap. I was leading this foray, so I felt significant pressure to ensure the proper identification.

A quick check identified White Tuft, which is also delicious. Several books and on-line resources suggest it is poisonous. I assure you it is not.

I later found out this species contains beta-hydroxy ergothioneine, a powerful anti-oxidant. All mushrooms contain ergothioneine, which is more stable than L-glutathione, oxidizes less easily, and crosses the blood-brain barrier. Work by Kimura et al, (2005) found the compound protected cultured hepatocytes from injury by carbon tetrachloride.

Fried Chicken is much better researched. The mushroom is difficult to cultivate, due to its mycorrhizal nature, but is highly prized for its umami flavor. Work by Takaki et al, (2014) found applying pulsed electricity to sawdust-based substrate, increasing fruiting body formation by 1.3-2.0 times in total weight. It grows well on aged, cultured waste of previously grown oyster mushrooms, or barley bran mixed with livestock waste.

The $1\rightarrow3$, $1\rightarrow6$ beta-D-glucans increased the number of macrophages and shows marked anti-tumor activity against sarcoma 180 cells. (Ukawa et al, 2000).

Early work by Miura et al, (2002) looked at its anti-diabetic activity in a mice model, designed to exhibit type 2 diabetes and hyperinsulinemia. Water extracts reduced blood glucose after a single administration, and lowered blood glucose and serum insulin after three weeks. The control group showed no change. The researchers concluded the decrease in insulin resistance was due to the increase of GLUT4 protein in the plasma membrane of the muscle.

Serum lipid levels were investigated in a rat study. When the fruit body powder, or hot-water extract were added at a level of 10% in a cholesterol-containing diet, the total serum cholesterol levels were markedly lower than control. On a cholesterol-free diet, the fruit powder at 5% significantly decreased serum total cholesterol. Serum triglycerides and phospholipids were lower. The mushroom significantly increased the activity of cholesterol 7a-hydroxylase, which converts cellular cholesterol to bile acids, and excretion (Ukawa et al, 2002).

Polysaccharides reduced obesity in diet-induced obese mice, by altering gut microbiota and increased secondary bile acids (Wang et al, 2022). Increased levels of *Bacteriodes intestinalis* and *Lactobacillus johnsonii* were noted.

The fruiting body inhibits ACE (angiotensin converting enzyme) and reduces hypertension (Suzuki et al, 2001).

Another mouse study, found oral extracts inhibited atopic dermatitis-like skin lesions. IL-4 production decreased, and both serum IgE and Th2-type immune responses were suppressed. (Ukawa et al, 2007).

Protection from radiation was provided by a hot-distilled water extract in one mouse study. The number of leukocytes, lymphocytes and monocytes was significantly higher in those fed mushroom water extract, than controls. (Nakamura et al, 2007).

Hot water extracts of the fruiting body induced both IFN-gamma and IL-4 production, in a mice study. (Ike et al, 2012).

Recent work by Zhang et al, (2022) found fruiting body polysaccharides protect against induced, acute liver injury by activating the Nrf2 pathway. The proinflammatory factors IL-6 and TNF-alpha were decreased.

The fruiting body contains an unusual amino acid, 6-hydroxytryptophan, that inhibits tyrosinase, an enzyme that controls melanin formation (Ishiara et al, 2019).

Mycelium grown on amaranth flour, showed activity against influenza type A (serotype H1N1) *in vitro*. (Krupodorova et al, 2014).

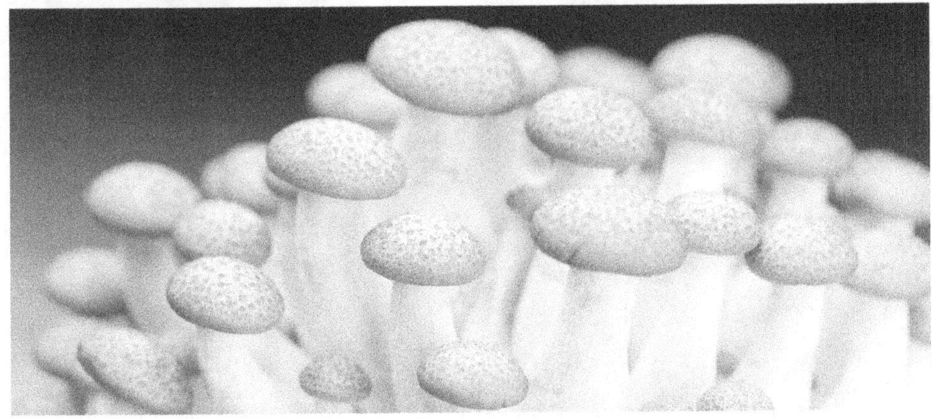

Lyophyllum shimeji

Hon-Shimeji (*Lyophyllum shimeji*) grows naturally in Japan and northern Europe. Patented cultivation practices have led to commercial production. This should not be confused with Buna-shimeji (*Hypsizigus tessulatus/H. marmoreus*), widely cultivated and known on the market as Brown Beech Mushrooms. Bunapi is the White Beech version.

Both are easily available, albeit not always produced organically.

The Elm Oyster (*Hypsizygus ulmarius*- formerly *L. ulmarium*) is often marketed as Hon-Shimeji. I have found this species in the wild, and comparable to oyster mushrooms in flavor, and superior in odor.

Lyophyllum shimeji contains a fibrinolytic enzyme, that may be useful in thrombolytic therapy and helping prevent thrombotic conditions and disease (Moon et al, 2014).

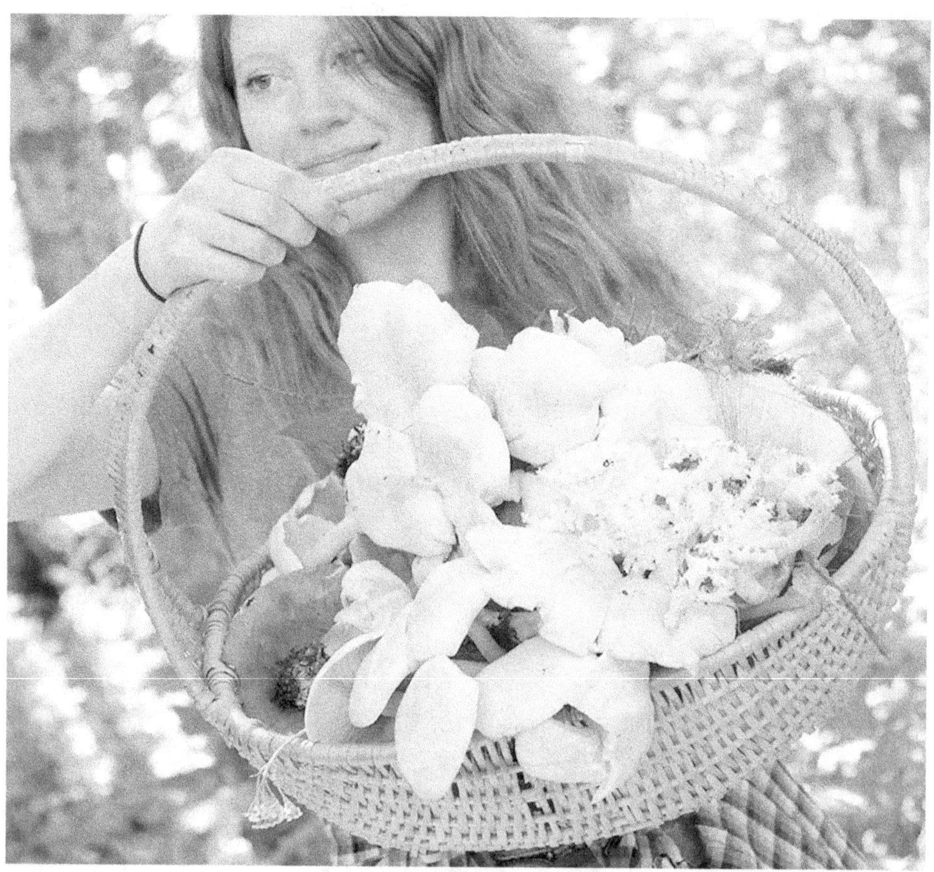

Lyophyllum connatum

GOLDEN CHANTERELLE
(*Cantharellus cibarius* group)

I know, I know. Before you begin typing your letter to the author, give me a moment to explain.

I am well aware that this genus is a taxonomic jungle, and the citation *C. cibarius* is European in origin, with over 30 species identified across the pond, 29 in North America and at least 13, at last count, in India.

In 2010, the chanterelle world-wide market was worth about 1.7 billion US dollars, based on the harvest of up to 200,000 metric tons. Those numbers have likely increased.

And thus, the difficulty with exploring the health benefits and medicinal properties of one of the most popular edible mushrooms on the planet. Bioregional species may or may not contain the compounds in the cited studies.

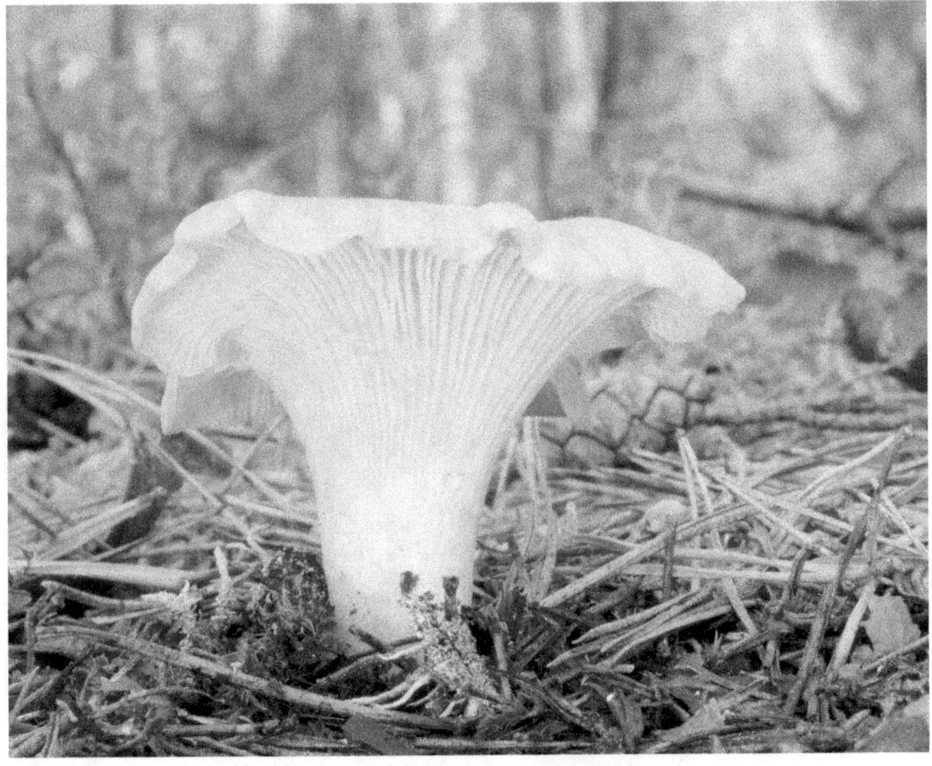

Cantharellus cibarius

The fruiting bodies contain a number of indole compounds, including L-tryptophan, 5-hydroxytryptophan, serotonin, melatonin, 5-methyl tryptophan and tryptamine. Work by Muszynska et al, (2013) found serotonin present in the fruiting body 17.61 mg/100grams dry weight.

They are a rich source of B12 for vegetarians and vegans. Golden Chanterelle, and its cousin Black Trumpet, or Horn of Plenty (*Craterellus cornucopioides*) contain significant levels (1.09-2.65 µg/100g dry weight). Only traces of B12 are present in porcini, parasol or oyster mushrooms (Watanabe et al, 2012).

The fruiting bodies exhibit anti-oxidant, cytotoxic, anti-hypertensive and anti-bacterial properties. Cytotoxicity was noted on human cervix adenocarcinoma (HeLa), breast carcinoma (MDA-MB-453), and human myelogenous leukemia (K562) cell lines. Extracts also show inhibition of ACE (angiotensin coverting 1 enzyme) and various Gram-positive bacteria especially *E. faecalis* (Kozarski et al, 2015).

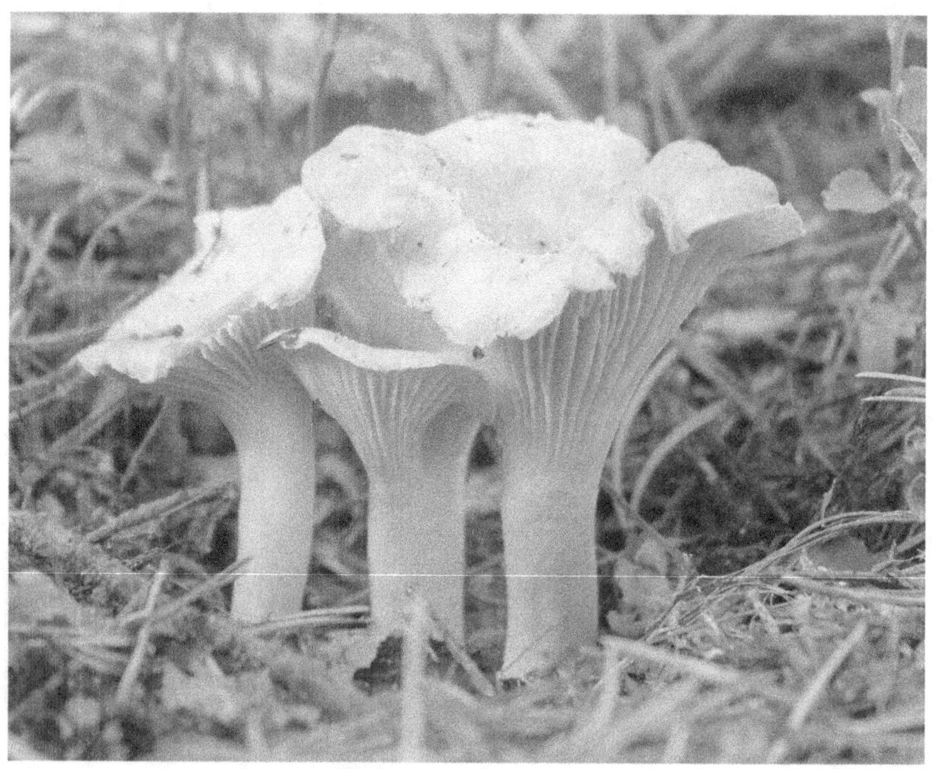

Cantharellus cibarius

Helicobacter pylori bacterium have been implicated in gastric and duodenal ulcers. Work by Kolundzic et al, (2017) found various extracts of the fruiting body active against antibiotic-resistant *H. pylori*. Water extracts were not active against HeLa and N87 cancer cell lines, but showed 68% inhibition of ACE.

The fruiting body contains omega-7 fatty acids, also present in seabuckthorn berry and macadamia nut oil. These fats helps increase HDL, and lower LDL cholesterol levels.

A 2% extract ointment showed significant wound healing, compared to the non-treated control group. Repair of skin epidermal layer, increased collagen production and reduced inflammation were noted (Nasiry et al, 2017).

Work by Lemieszek et al, (2018) found polysaccharide fractions exhibit benefit for neuron viability and neurite outgrowth.

Tumor-associated macrophages, with an M2-like phenotype, are linked with the proliferation, invasion and metastasis of tumors. A novel galactan, isolated from golden chanterelle can convert tumor-promoting M2-like macrophages to tumor-inhibiting M1-like phenotype. This is through the activation of MAPKs and degradation of IkappaB-alpha, through targeting toll-like receptor 2. This natural, and safe polysaccharide could be useful in tumor immunotherapy (Meng et al, 2019).

Small, water soluble, RNA fractions showed strong anti-proliferative activity against human colon adenocarcinoma (HT-29 and LS180) cells lines, while non-toxic to normal human colon epithelial cells. The action was due to p53-dependent cell cycle arrest mediated by p21. Apoptosis was mainly dependent upon the enhancement of p53 expression (Lemieszek et al, 2019).

A heteropolysaccharide was derived by Zhao et al, (2018). It showed significant in vitro antioxidant, and proliferation effect on immune cells, especially B and T cells at various concentrations.

Branched mannan polysaccharides influenced viability and proliferation of human natural killer (NK92) cells, but enhanced activity against human lung (A549) and colon (LS180) cancer cell lines, with affected normal human epithelial cells. Adjuvant benefit is noted, as an increase in fruiting body intake may help promote innate immunity response against cancer via NK cell activity (Lemieszek et al, 2019a).

These branched mannans resulted in perturbation in GO/G and S phases of the cell cycle associated with an increase of DNA fragmentation of colon cancer cells, as well as inhibition of their motility (Lemieszek et al, 2019b).

Qu et al, (2021) found a novel acidic beta-glucan to be a potent natural immune modulator, suggesting golden chanterelle as a valuable functional food. The beta-glucan activated macrophages via the MAPK signaling pathway, and promotion of nitric oxide, TNF-alpha and IL-6.

Angiogenesis is the mechanism by which cancer cells obtain nutrition and grow. Ethanol extracts of the fruiting body show potent lipoxygenase inhibition (nearly double that of ascorbic acid), and anti-angiogenic potential (Marathe et al, 2022).

The polysaccharides show, *in vivo*, potential as a prebiotic, helping change intestinal microbiota, albeit an animal study. (Uthan et al, 2021).

Acidic pH water extracts the highest phenolic content, and strongest anti-oxidant activity (Fogarasi et al, 2021).

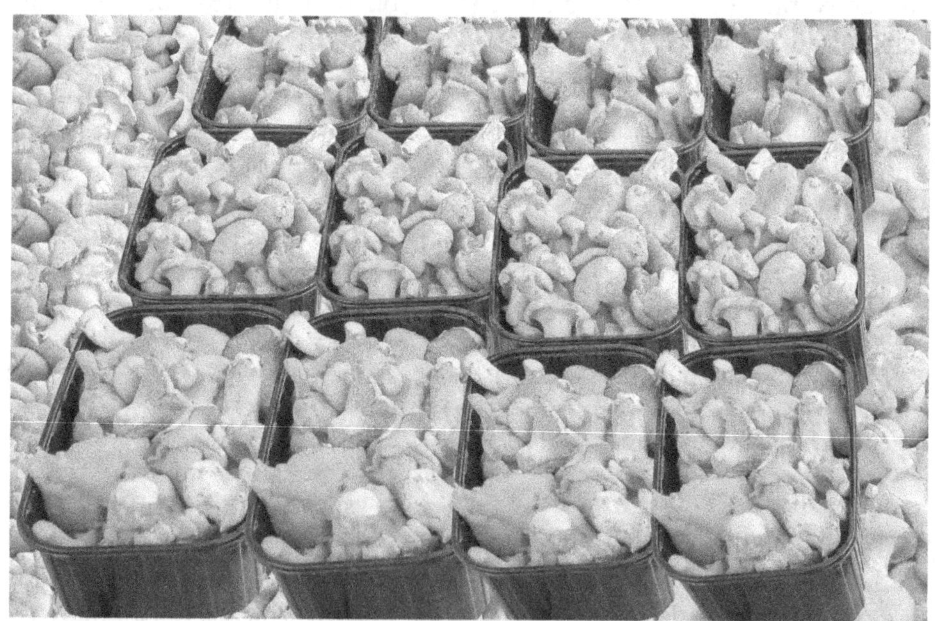

Cantharellus cibarius

HAWK WING
SCALY HEDGEHOG
(*Sarcodon imbricatus*) [L.] P. Karst
(*S. aspratum*) [Berk.) S. Ito
(*S. aspratus*)
SCALY TOOTH
(*S. squamosus*) [Schaeff.] Quel.
BITTER TOOTH
GREEN FOOT TOOTH
(*Hydnellum scabrosum*) [Fr.] E. Laraa., K.H. Larss. & Koljalg
(*S. scabrosus*)

Sarcodon derives from the Greek sarco meaning, "flesh" and odon, "tooth." Hence, a toothed mushroom. Imbricatus is Latin for "covered with tiles or scales."

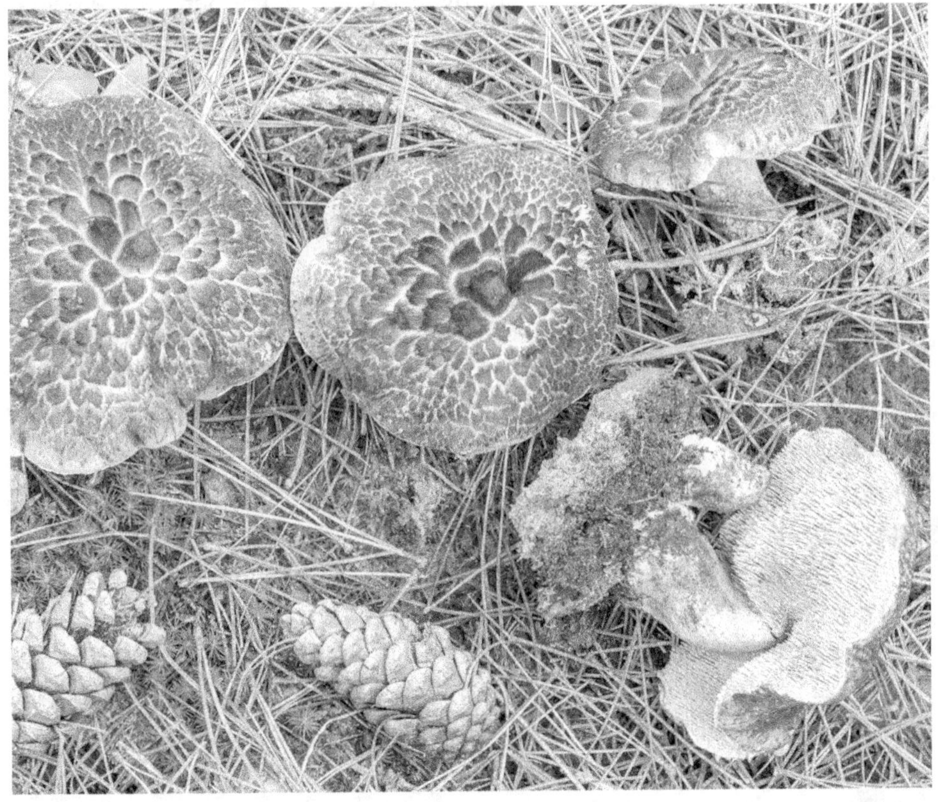

Sarcodon imbricatus

CONSTITUENTS - *S. imbricatus* fruiting body- atromentin, thelephoric acid, dehydrogyrocyanin, 18-26% protein (16 amino acids), 35% total sugars, 26 fatty acids (including a high ratio of unsaturated), polyphenols, sterols, vitamins and minerals. It hyper-accumulates cadmium and mercury, so caution is advised regarding collection sites, such as abandoned mines. *H. scabrosum* fruiting body- scabronines 1-2 and B-F, sarcodonins A, G and M, scabronine H, neosarcodonins A-C. *S. squamosus*- 26% dry weight protein, high in potassium and phosphorus.

Identification is important as similar looking species are very bitter and inedible. The related Scaly Tooth (*S. squamosus*) is commonly associated with pine, whereas fir and spruce hosts are preferred by Hawk Wing. The former does not have an olive-black base on stipe, nor the redder-brown cap of Bitter Tooth. Hawk wing teeth are grey, and produce brown spores.

An article by Johannesson et al. (1999), and more recent DNA work by Larsson et al. (2019) suggests moving several species in this genus to *Hydnellum*, including *H. scabrosum*. When cut open, this species presents a mild watermelon scent to some noses, but a bitter farinaceous odor to others. This species is less common in the Pacific Northwest, and associated with salal, hemlock spruce and Douglas fir.

Individuals dyeing with fungi will note the Hawk Wing produces a gray-beige color, whereas Bitter Hedgehog gives a brilliant blue-green result. In fact, the different color dyes led mycologists to examine if indeed they were different species.

I will admit to mistakenly collecting and cooking various Sarcodons in the past, and unable to get past the extremely bitter taste. I have found fresh parsley added to pan-fried mushrooms helps disguise any mildly unpleasant taste.

An interesting Hawk Wing study looked at acute exercise and chronic fatigue syndrome in mice. Supplementation increased levels of glycogen in liver, and ATP (adenosine triphosphate) in liver and muscle tissue, and decreased lactic acid and blood urea nitrogen (BUN) in both groups. Both superoxide dismustase (SOD) and glutathione peroxidase (GSH-Px) levels improved in the 32-day study. Wang et al, (2018a) suggested the mushroom serves as a novel anti-fatigue supplement.

This may be due in part to the free-radical scavenging rate associated with fatty acid content. In work by Luo et al, (2017), Hawk Wing showed an 81.25% DDPH scavenging ability, with half-maximal inhibition of

0.054 mg/mL. The authors suggest this exceptional anti-oxidant capacity may be related to alpha-hydroxy fatty acids.

Proteus mirabilis is a growing gram-negative bacterial epidemic in long-term care and hospital settings, particularly in immune-compromised patients undergoing catheter treatment. It is increasingly multi-antibiotic resistant as it creates strong biofilms, and in one study (Lubart et al, 2011) is responsible for a 51% mortality rate, associated with chronic urinary tract infections in the geriatric population.

This infection goes largely undetected in senior residences, until the biofilm is well established, and difficult to control.

Extracts of *Sarcodon imbricatus* exhibit a high inhibition (45.4%) on *P. mirabilis* biofilm formation, suggesting adjuvant possibilities (Alves et al, 2014). In the same study, *Leucopaxillus giganteus* extracts inhibited *Escherichia coli* (*E. coli*) microorganisms by 47.8%.

Oral supplementation of polysaccharides significantly increased spleen and thymus indexes in a four-week study of cyclophosphamide-induced immune suppression of Balb/c mice. Work by Wang et al, (2018b) found weight loss alleviated, and NK (natural killer) cytotoxicity and lymphocytes were elevated. The mushroom promoted interleukin-2 (IL-2), IL-6, IL-10, IL-12 and interferon gamma production; and reduced oxidative stress. The authors suggest possible use of the polysaccharides as novel immune modulators, in health foods or medicine.

The same mice study (Wang et al, 2018c) found the mushroom polysaccharides improved blood parameters and found the percentage of B lymphocytes and hematopoietic stem cells significantly elevated in bone marrow.

The fruiting body contains various polyphenols. Work by Shomali et al, (2019) found ethanol extracts possess significant glutathione-S-transferase (GST) enzyme activity. This suggests both alcohol and water-soluble compounds protect the body's major detoxifying agent. Glutathione is so important to human health that fully 7% of daily energy is dedicated to production of this vital anti-oxidant.

A p-terphenyl isolated from the fruiting body showed weak cytotoxicity against colon cancer SW480 and leukemia HL-60 cancer cell lines, in vitro (Zhang et al, 2019).

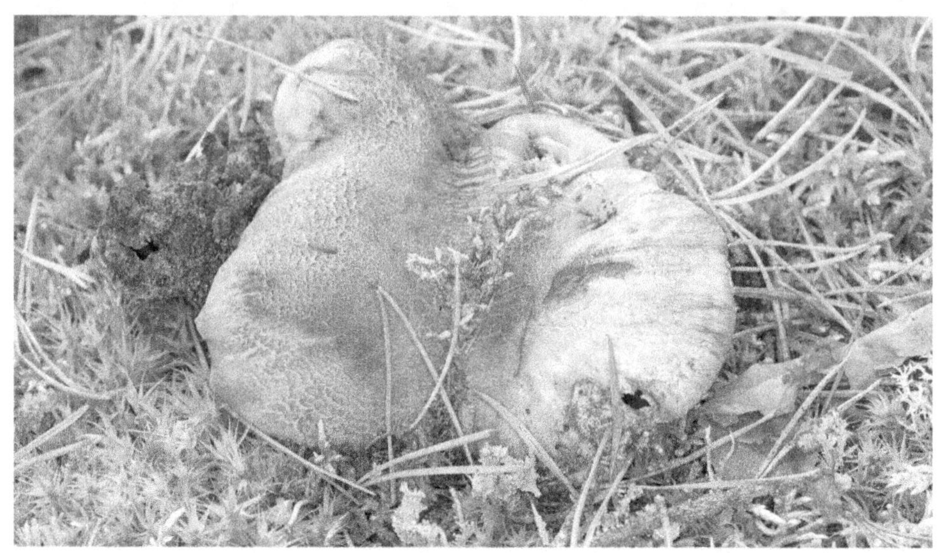

Sarcodon scabrosus

On the other hand, water extracts of the fruiting body, inhibited growth, migration and invasion properties of various breast cancer cells *in vitro*, and reduced tumor growth *in vivo*. (Tan et al, 2020).

Bitter Tooth (*H. scabrosum*) is basically inedible, but contains some very interesting medicinal compounds.

Various cyathane diterpenes, especially sarcodonin G, show significant neurite outgrowth (neurogenesis) promoting activity (Shi et al, 2011).

Much earlier work by Kita et al, (1998) found scabronines B, C and E exhibit stimulating activity of the synthesis in nerve growth factor.

Sarcodonin G, in work by Dong et al, (2009) induced apoptosis (self-programmed death) in HeLa, and five other human cancer cell lines. The mechanism may be possibly via caspase activation.

Sarcodonin A and related derivatives reversed microglia M1 polarization, suggesting a promising candidate against Alzheimer's disease, by targeting neuroinflammation (Cao et al, 2022).

Another compound, neosarcodonin C, showed significant anti-inflammatory activity in an early mouse study (Hirota et al, 2002).

Scaly Tooth (*S. squamosus*) extracts exhibit strong in vitro antioxidant and anti-microbial activity, as well as anti-proliferative and anti-invasive activity, and induce apoptosis (self-programmed death) in HepG2 hepatocellular carcinoma cells (Kaygusuz et al, 2021).

Telomerase activity is an accepted cancer marker and target. Water extracts of *Sarcodon aspratus* exhibit strong positive telomerase inhibition (Xu et al, 2014). Polysaccharides significantly induce apoptosis in HeLa cell lines via mitochondrial dysfunction associated with caspase pathways (Wang, D.D. et al, 2018).

They also enhance immune stimulation, and may be useful as immune modulating functional food (Wang, D.D. 2018a).

Earlier work by Chen et al. (2013) found mycelium polysaccharides active against HeLa cell lines, but with significantly lower cytotoxicity against human liver cell lines than HeLa tumor cells, in comparison with chemotherapy drug 5-FU.

The polysaccharide, in mice, significantly alleviated the toxicity of the drug, suggesting a potential adjuvant (Liu et al, 2020).

Work by Chen et al, (2020) found polysaccharides modulated gut microbiota dysbiosis in mice fed a high-fat diet. This suggests a potential supplement or prebiotic for the prevention or treatment of obesity and related metabolic disorders. A rat study by Zhang et al, (2022) suggests the polysaccharides protect gastric mucosa, and may prevent ulcers and modulate gut microbiota.

The mushroom polysaccharides attenuate oxidative stress, and may have potential for the treatment of pulmonary fibrosis, and related diseases (Dong et al, 2020).

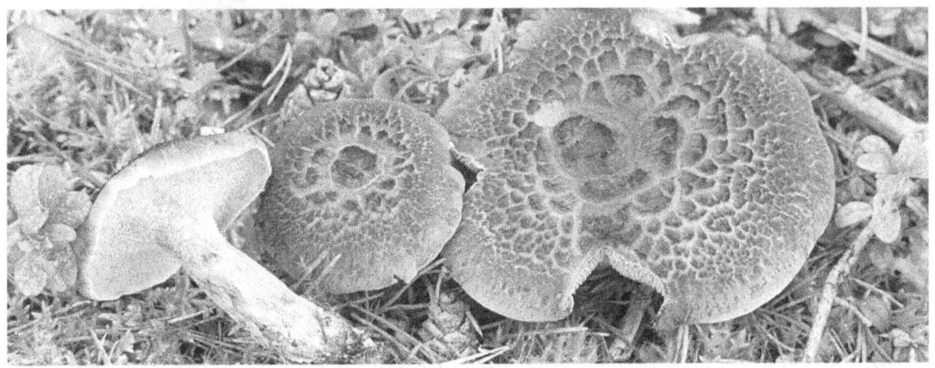

Sarcodon squamosus

A heath beverage, manufactured in Korea contains the dry mushroom as its main ingredient, along with licorice root, and leaves of ginkgo biloba, persimmon and elm.

HELA

HeLa is an "immortal" cancer cell line used extensively in research. It is named in honor of Henrietta Lacks, a 31-year old African-American and mother of five children who died of cervical cancer in 1951. Harvested at Johns Hopkins, the cell line is widely available, and the University never sold it, but has offered it freely to cancer researchers around the world. The cells are noted for active growth associated with the enzyme telomerase during cell division.

Telomeres stop the ends of chromosomes from fraying or sticking during cell division, like the plastic tip at the end of shoelaces. The cell's DNA repair system includes a single strand overlap that "looks like" damaged DNA.

It makes sure that DNA is copied accurately, and telomerase helps reverse the loss of DNA from each round of replication.

Longer telomeres are associated with anti-ageing and are encouraged by healthy lifestyles, including intermittent fasting, and dietary intake of legumes, nuts, seaweed, omega-3 fatty acids, vitamin D, fruit, dairy and coffee. On the other hand, alcohol, red and processed meat shortens them. A longitudinal 10 year follow up study of 1014 elderly patients, looked at telomere lengths and physical activity, and found higher leisure time physical activity in women, but not men, was associated with more rapid telomere attrition (Jantunen et al, 2020).

The discovery of telomerase led to awarding the 2009 Nobel Prize in Physiology/Medicine to three scientists, Elizabeth Blackburn, Carol Greider, and Jack Szostalc.

Telomerase is widely expressed in 85% of human cancers, which are immortal because the telomere mechanism is damaged. Human cells are not, and are subject to apoptosis (self-programmed death).

Too much telomerase increases the number of cancer cells, and too little also increases cancer by depleting healthy regenerative potential, and shortening of telomeres. It is a fine balance.

HEMLOCK VARNISH CONK
(*Ganoderma tsugae*)

Hemlock Varnish Conk may be the most common wild Ganoderma in North America. It is particularly well-established in the east and southeastern United States, and possibly, but rarely, in the Pacific Northwest. The polypore is found in north-eastern China, and known as Song Shan Shu Zhi, meaning "pine or fir tree fungus."

Work by Jiang et al, (2021) suggests this species diverged from of *G. sinense* and *G. lingzhi* about 21 million years ago.

I am frequently asked if this polypore is equal in medicinal benefit to the so-called *G. lucidum*. This binomial is mentioned in thousands of studies and may actually refer to one of the species mentioned above.

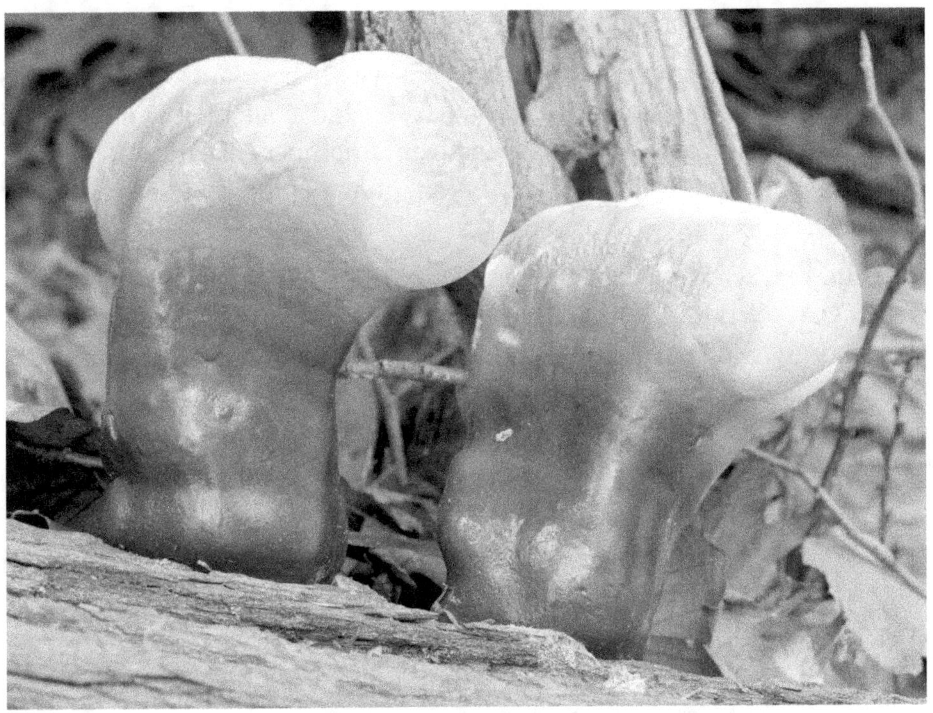

Ganoderma tsugae

It is now well known that *G. lucidum* sensu stricto has limited native distribution in Europe and some parts of China. Loyd et al, (2018) took 20 products off the store shelves, and 17 grow your own kits, all labeled

G. lucidum. When tested, 93% of products, and almost half of kits, were identified as *G. lingzhi*, native to Asia. None of the products contained *G. lucidum*, and it was detected in only one kit. Other species, including *G. applanatum, G. austral, G. gibbosum, G. sessile* and *G. sinensis* were also present.

According to Yao et al, (2020), "The European mushroom name, *Ganoderma lucidum*, has been misapplied to this species for over 100 years, until recently re-identified as *G. sichuanense*. Soon after this, a new species name, *G. lingzhi*, was also proposed for the fungus." The taxonomic discussion is heated but unresolved.

A global meta-analysis by Fryssouli et al, (2020) of ITS rDNA sequences created five main lineages (Clades A to E). The 92 Ganoderma-associated names correspond to at least 80 taxa. *G. lucidum*, for example, was insufficiently and/or incorrectly identified in 78% of entries.

Returning to the question the answer is yes. There are of course less studies, but the polysaccharides and triterpene content is similar. And the research suggests potential benefit in a number of cancer cell lines, including endometrial, prostate, colon, lung, epidermoid, breast, and ovarian.

Ethanol extracts suppress the proliferation of endometrial cancer cells HEC-1-A, KLE and AN3 CA. Work by Tsai et al, (2021) found extracts induced G1/S phase arrest and mitochondria-mediated apoptosis (self-programmed death) and suppressed the Akt signaling pathway. This suggests an adjuvant therapy for treating this difficult, serious drug resistant disease.

Hot water extracts of the fruiting body inhibited proliferation of C6, Hep 3B and HL-60 cancer cells lines. Work by Chien et al, (2015) noted both mature and baby fruiting bodies show activity, through necrosis, apoptosis or differentiation.

An extract of the fruiting body inhibited the growth of HER-2-overexpressing cancer cells, both in vitro and in vivo; and enhanced inhibitory effect of anti-tumor drugs such as taxol and cisplatin (Kuo et al., 2013).

Ethanol extracts significant reduce cell viability and G2/M arrest in K562 human chronic myeloid leukemia cells (Hseu et al, 2019).

Epidemiological studies suggest increased particulate matter in the air is related to increased myocardial infarctions. These particles come into close proximity to capillary endothelial cells. When pre-supplemented with DMSO extract of this mushroom, increased glutathione levels were noted, as well as a decrease in transmigration of particulates into the bloodstream (Tseng et al, 2016).

Triterpenoids prevent stress-induced myocardial injury and provide cardioprotective activity, in a mouse study by Kuok et al, (2013).

Although not proven in human DB, PC randomized trials, this finding suggests prophylactic potential for individuals working or living in poor air quality environments.

Triterpenoid extracts significantly suppress histamine secreted from activated EL4 cells, and Th2 cytokines IL-4 and IL-5, but showed no effect on Th1 cytokines IL-2 and interferon-gamma. This suggests triterpenoids, which are more alcohol soluble, may alleviate allergic-related asthma (Chen et al, 2015).

A D-galactose-induced aging rat study involving oral DMSO mushroom extract for 25 weeks, monitored oxidative stress and memory deficits. Significant improvement in locomotion, spatial memory and learning was noted, and reduced loss of dendritic branching in brain neurons of the hippocampus and cerebral cortex. Brain-derived neurotrophic factor (BDNF) increased and reduced advanced glycosylation end products (Kuo et al, 2022).

Compounds in the fruiting bodies inhibit xanthine oxidase, suggestive of benefit in gout, by preventing the build up of uric acid (Lin et al, 2016).

Lipogenesis, or the activation of lipid biosynthesis is linked with prostate cancer. Ethanol extracts of the fruiting body significantly inhibit the expression of SREBP-1 a regulator controlling lipogenesis. The extract also down-regulated the expression of androgen receptor and prostate-specific antigen suggesting benefit in treating prostate malignancy (Huang et al, 2018).

An in vitro and in vivo study involving ethanol extracts on metastatic prostate cancer cells by Huang et al, (2019) found blockage of signaling pathways associated with cell growth, survival and apoptosis.

KING BOLETE
PORCINI
CEPE
PENNY BUN
(*Boletus edulis*)
QUEEN BOLETE
(*B. aereus*)

King Bolete is considered by many mycophiles the best-tasting mushroom. The Romans prized *boleti* and cooked them in special vessels called *boletaria*.

The taste and aroma of previously dried fruiting bodies is superior, in my opinion. The buttery, roasted, smoky elements are richer and deeper. The drying increases the roasted volatile elements, and reduces the grass-like, earthy notes, according to work by Zhang et al, (2018). Adulteration with *Suillus* species is often detected in products from Asia.

However, the fresh mushroom, sliced thinly and drizzled with salt and olive oil is an amazing gustatory treat! However, this should be limited to a few snacks as ribotoxin-like proteins show toxicity to both normal and tumoral human cells (Landi et al, 2021). The toxicity is abolished after cooking at 90 degrees Celsius.

Lumberjacks working in Bohemia believed eating the prized edible mushroom helped prevent cancer. They were likely correct!

Various *in vitro* studies have found compounds cytotoxic to a variety of human cancer cell lines.

Byerrum et al. (1957) identified tumor inhibition over six decades ago.

RNA fraction BE3 inhibited HT-29 human colon cancer cells, by inducing apoptosis (self-programmed death (Lemieszek et al, 2016 and 2017).

The same team (Lemieszek et al, 2017a) found this fraction contains no toxic natural killer 92 (NK92) cells, but significantly stimulated their proliferation and cytotoxicity against myelogenous leukemia cells.

Ethanol extracts of the stipe show the most potent activity against MCF-7 human breast cancer cell lines (Novakovic et al, 2017).

More recent work by Meng et al, (2021) found a cold-water polysaccharide caused mitochondrial membrane potential collapse, and induced apoptosis of breast cancer cell lines MDA-MB-231 and Ca761.

Mice studies suggest water-soluble polysaccharides possess potential immune modulation and prevention/treatment of kidney cancer (Wang et al, 2014).

Fungal lectins have gained some attention for their anti-tumor, anti-proliferative and immune modulating properties (Rogers, 2020).

A protein, derived from dried mushroom induced apoptosis and arrest of A549 (non-small cell lung) cancer lines, in vitro, and significantly suppressed growth of A549 solid tumors in vivo (Zhang et al, 2021).

A novel BEL beta-trefoil lectin was derived from porcini fruiting body by Bovi et al. (2013). It possesses potent anti-proliferative effect on various human cancer cell lines.

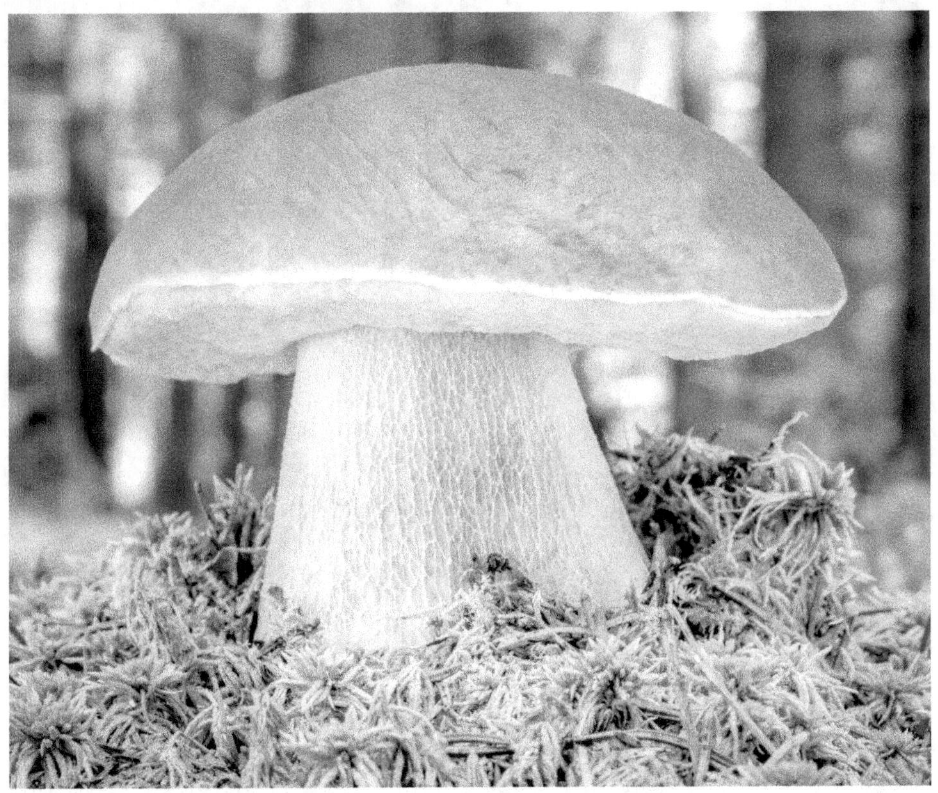

Boletus edulis

RUNX2 is over-expressed in several cancer cells, and in melanoma it promotes cell migration, invasion and angiogenesis. Mortality rates from melanoma are high.

A study by Valenti et al, (2020) found BEL beta-trefoil spreads in tissue and reduced the formation of metastases in melanoma xeno-transplanted zebrafish. The authors suggest the lectin could be an effective molecule for treating melanoma.

Antioxidant capacity is usually measured with FRAP, TEAC and DPPH scavenging ability. Work by Witkowska et al. (2011) found *Boletus edulis* and *B. chrysenteron* measured the highest scores of polyphenol content and anti-oxidant activity of mushrooms tested.

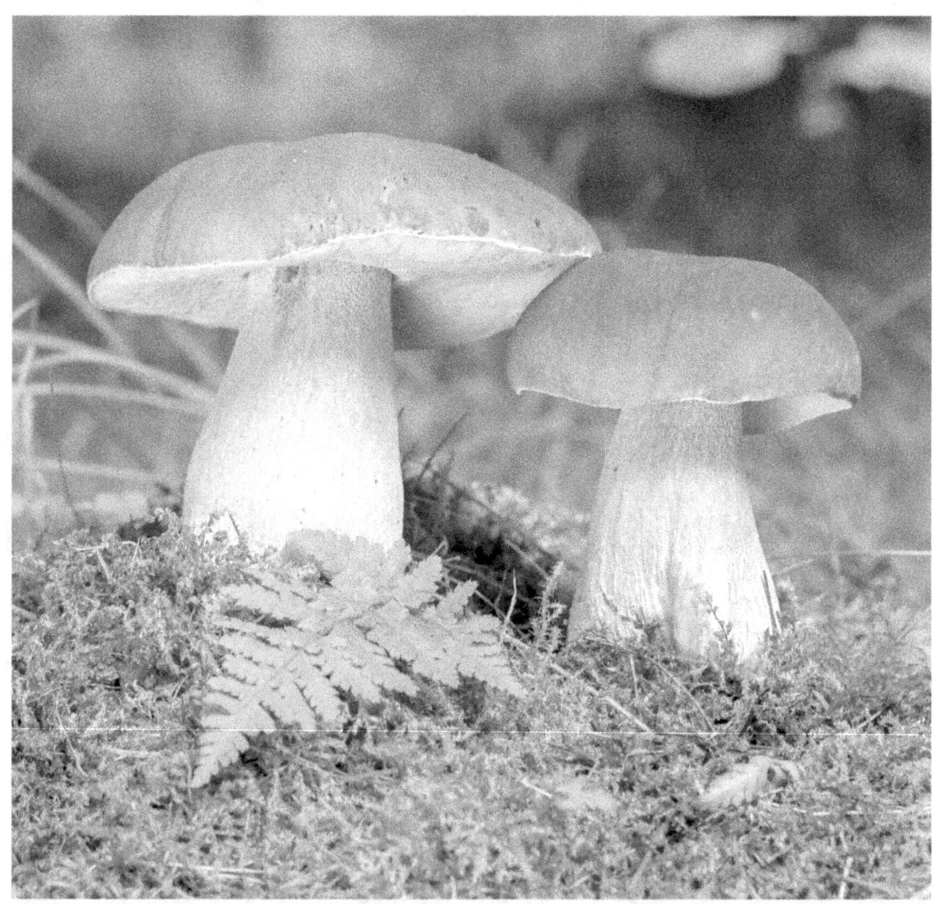

Boletus edulis

Methanol and ethanol extracts were obtained from cold and hot water dried fruiting bodies, in work by Vamanu & Nita (2013). Ethanol extracts produced the highest anti-oxidant capacity, likely due to high content of rosmarinic acid (7-56 mg/100 grams).

Rosmarinic acid is a potent compound showing possible benefit in diabetes, hepatitis B, Parkinson's disease, hypertension, various cancers and inflammatory disease. Over 1900 studies have been reported to date.

When tested against five species of bacteria and fungi, methanol and acetone extracts showed strong inhibition against all microbes (Kosanic et al, 2012).

A recent study by Rosa et al, (2020) found strong activity against *E. coli* and *Staphylococcus aureus*, especially from water extracts, and moderate inhibition of *Klebsiella pneumoniae* microbes.

Porcini contains a number of neurotransmitter compounds that influence human brain health. Work by Muszynska et al, (2011) identified 5-hydroxytrypophan, serotonin, L-tryptophan, melatonin, and tryptamine in the fruiting body.

Alcohol extracts of the fruiting body exhibit inhibition of alpha-glucosidase, suggestive of benefit in diabetes (Younis et al, 2019). By preventing the breakdown of sugars, and their transport from the small intestine to the bloodstream, diabetics require less insulin, or reduce insulin response.

Polysaccharides reduce inflammatory response in mouse models of asthma, in part due to an increase in Treg cells and IL-4 response (Wu et al, 2016). Caution is advised, however, as a study by Helbling et al. (2002), found a digestion-resistant allergen in fruiting body, may cause an IgE mediated food allergy in some individuals.

Multi-drug resistant pathogens are a growing concern worldwide, causing skin and soft tissue infections. Work by Garcia et al, (2022) found water and methanol extracts of King Bolete and Scarletina Bolete (*Neoboletus luridiformis*) exhibit anti-microbial and anti-biofilm activity. This group of bacteria named ESKAPE, includes *Enterococcus faecium, Staphylococcus aureus, Klebsiella pneumoniae, Acinetobacter baumannii, Pseudomonas aeruginosa,* and *Enterobacte*r species.

I love pickled porcini and was pleased to see that this mushroom inhibits nitrite production during the fermentation cycle. The enzyme responsible, nitrite reductase, also eliminates nitrite from the blood after ingestion of sodium nitrite (Zhang et al, 2015).

The Queen Bolete is a choice, delicious edible mushroom.

A polysaccharide derived from a water extract induces apoptosis in sarcoma 180 tumor cells and shows significant synergistic anti-tumor effect when combined with chemotherapy drug, cyclophosphamide (Zheng et al, 2021).

The fruiting body shows effectiveness in ameliorating alcohol-induced liver injury, albeit in a mice model (Zhang et al, 2020).

The eastern *B. speciosus* contains a water-soluble polysaccharide that inhibits L929 cells in vitro, and S180 tumor cells, in vivo. The polysaccharide, named BSF-X, promotes the proliferation of T cells, B cells and macrophages by promoting the cells into S phase from GO/ G1 phase. They also enhance the phagocytes and cytokine secretion of macrophages (Zhu et al, 2019).

The Red and Yellow Bolete (*Baorangia bicolor*) is a choice edible, but should not be confused with Curry Bolete, which turns blue instantly upon touch. The former mushroom contains a novel protein that shows cytotoxicity against non-small lung cancer cell lines (Zhang et al, 2021a).

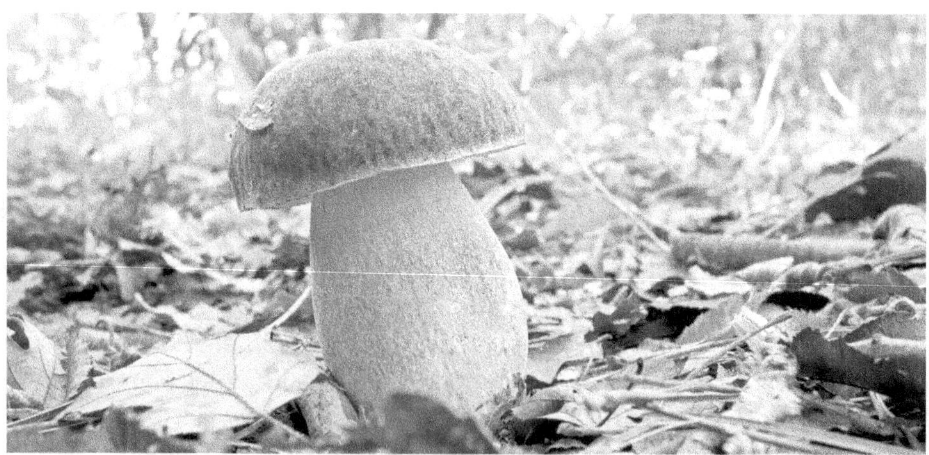

Boletus aereus

LESSER-KNOWN MEDICINAL POLYPORES OF THE PACIFIC NORTHWEST

When *The Fungal Pharmacy* was published (Rogers, 2011), many lesser-known medicinal mushrooms, due to space considerations, had to take a back seat.

With each new discovery of health benefits from fungi, I get quite excited, and love to share the new information and knowledge.

Here are some of the more interesting studies of the past few years, keeping in mind that interesting compounds found in a PNW polypore, does not automatically mean they are safe to ingest, nor recommended for personal experimentation as "natural" medicine. Fully one-third of new molecule-based medicines approved by the FDA are derivatives of natural products. Newman et al, (2016).

The Concealed or Veiled polypore (*Cryptoporus volvatus*) is widespread on dying conifers. Ma et al, (2013) found water extracts show potential to treat porcine reproductive and respiratory syndrome, a serious and contagious viral infection affecting swine. This illness costs the pork industry around $664 million annually.

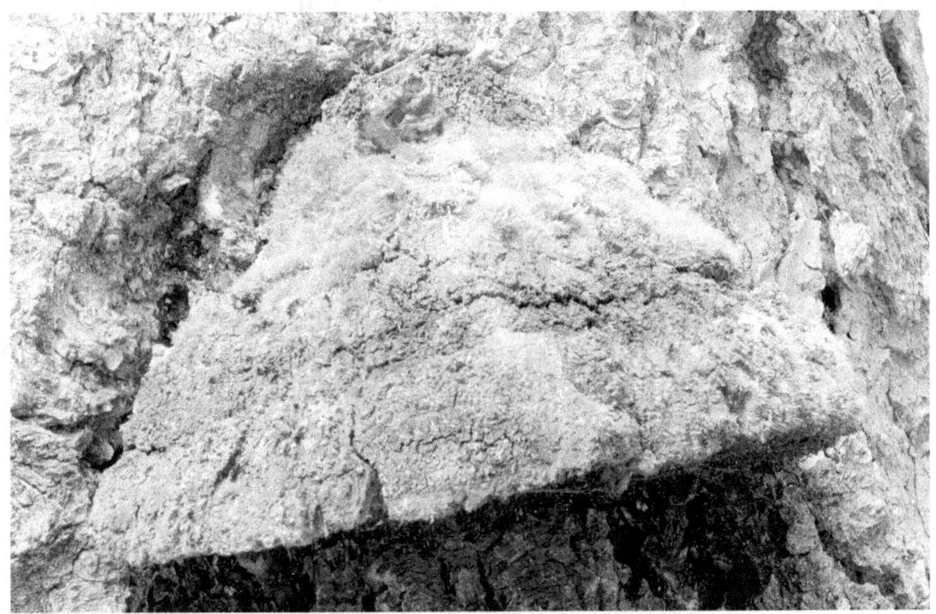

Echinodontium tinctorium

The following year Gao et al, (2014) found inhibition of influenza virus replication; including protection against H1N1/09 in mice with significant reductions of viral load, and decreased lesions in lungs. Recent work by Gao et al, (2017) identified cryptoporus acid E, which exhibits broad-spectrum activity against the above virus, as well as H3N2 and H1N1 strains. The compound directly targets virus particles.

Coriolopsis gallica is commonly found on poplar and willow throughout western North America. Work by Fakoya & Oloketuyl (2012) found extracts from the fruiting body show inhibition of *Pseudomonas aeruginosa* and *Proteus vulgaris* bacterium.

Wastewater from hospitals, pharmaceutical companies, as well as animal and human discharge releases antibiotics into environment. A study by Ayed et al, found this fungi helps biotransform levofloxacin.

The Mossy Maze Polypore (*Cerrena unicolor*) is often covered in algae, giving a green color to its surface. Recent work by Mizerska-Dudka et al, (2015) found extracts exhibit immune modulation, anti-viral activity and cytotoxicity to cervical carcinoma cell lines.

Extracellular laccase from this polypore was found to significantly induce apoptosis in chronic lymphocytic leukemia cells. Matuszewska et al, (2016). Matuszewska et al, (2018) identified secondary metabolites that show strong inhibition of MDA-MB-231 breast carcinoma cells at concentration that did not affect normal human fibroblast cells. And in (2019), the same group identified anti-tumor activity against human colon (HT-29) cancer cells.

An isolated compound may act as a fibrin glue drug carrier enhancer, improving the wound healing process; and reduced proliferation of the HT-29 cell lines mentioned above (Stefaniuk et al, 2021).

The pale, pink-brown spore surface of *Aporpium caryae*, helps identify this polypore found on dead balsam poplar, from Yukon to California. Levy et al, (2003) identified aporpinones, which show weak to moderate anti-bacterial activity against *Bacillus subtilis*, *Staphylococcus aureus* and *Escherichia coli*.

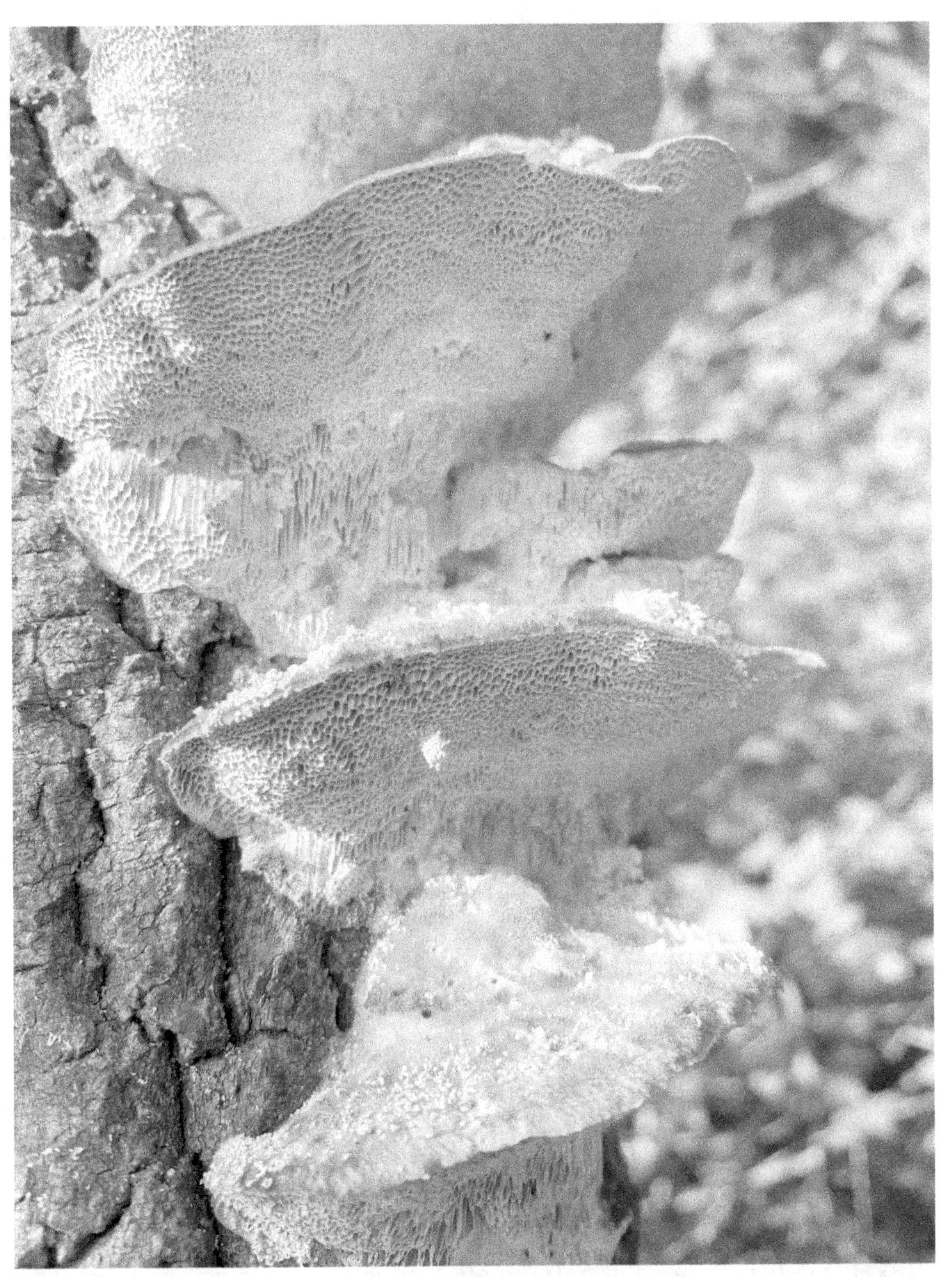

Porodaedalea pini

Antrodiella semisupina causes white rot on hardwoods, but also grows on the fruiting bodies of *Fomes*, *Fomitopsis* and *Trichaptum* species. A most unusual experiment by Deng et al, (2008) used this polypore to cross-couple sinomenine, an alkaloid used to treat rheumatoid arthritis with guaiacol. The resultant metabolites showed more potent inhibition of IL-6 production (reduction of inflammation) than sinomenine, in human synovial sarcoma cells (SW982).

Biotransformation by this fungus created 5-methoxycurvularin and curvularin. The former shows moderate cytotoxicity against CaSki (human cervical) and Hep-G2 (liver) cancer cell lines; the latter is selectively active against MDA-MB-231 breast cancer cells. Deng Z et al, (2015).

Analogs of anti-fungal indoles from this polypore show activity against sudden-death syndrome in soybean crops. Bertinetti et al, (2011).

Auriporia aurea causes brown cubical rot on conifers. The mycelia shows anti-viral activity against both influenza type A, and herpes simplex type two, in cell culture. Turkey Tail (*Trametes versicolor*) also showed a very high therapeutic index against both viruses. Krupodorova et al, (2014).

A more recent study by Krupodorova et al, (2016) involved cultivating both mushrooms on amaranth substrate. When tested against Guerin's carcinoma, in rats, significant size reduction was noted, from administrating oral doses, of both fruiting bodies and mycelium water extracts.

The Asian polypore species *Antrodia cinnamomea* (*A. camphorata*) is widely studied and marketed for its wide-ranging therapeutic value. (Rogers, 2020).

Antrodia species from the PNW are less studied, but do contain interesting compounds.

Antrolactones A and B, as well as polyporenic acid, extracted from *Antrodia heteromorpha* exhibit inhibition on receptor activator of NFkB (nuclear factor-kappaB) ligand-induced osteoclastogenesis. This suggests possible benefit in osteoporosis prevention and/or treatment. Kwon et al, (2016).

Antrodia malicola, found on Arbutus and other hardwoods; as well as *Antrodia xantha*, more common on conifers, contain various polysaccharides studied by Chen et al, (2005). The latter polypore showed greater anti-angiogenesis activity than the more well-known, and researched A. cinnamomea. Angiogenesis is the process by which cancer cells grow blood vessels to feed themselves. Reducing this pathway is one of several strategies employed in holistic oncology.

The Thin-Walled Maze Polypore (*Daedaleopsis confragosa*) is commonly found on birch and willow. When young, they will often stain red-purple when squeezed. Hot water extracts exhibit the highest anti-oxidant activity, but the highest level of phenols is found in a 70% ethanol extract. Overall, the polypore exhibits weak anti-fungal activity. Knezevic et al, (2017).

A methanol extract shows anti-bacterial activity against *Helicobacter pylori*, with the demethylincisterol A3 exhibiting the most potent inhibition. This compound is widely found in the Fungi kingdom (Na et al, 2022).

However, work by Teplyakova et al, (2012) found anti-viral activity against H5N1 and H3N2 in mycelial water extracts.

Hossen et al, (2021) found significant analgesic effect from methanol extracts, as well as cytotoxic action.

Datronia mollis, found on hardwoods, exhibited anti-viral activity against the two influenza strains, in the same study.

Dichomitus squalens is found on living and dead conifers. It contains a unique immune-modulating protein, identified as FIP-dsq2. Work by Li and Xin (2017) found the compound inhibits proliferation of human lung adenocarcinoma A549 cells, by inducing apoptosis (cell-programmed death) and interruption of cancer cell migration (metastasis).

Fomitiporia punctata (synonym *Phellinus punctatus*) causes white rot in hardwoods. Ethanol extracts show activity against large lung cancer cell line (NCI-H460), and exhibit anti-oxidant activity. Water extracts bind to human fibrogen, suggesting the use in wound healing. Yuan et al, (2011).

A polysaccharide, identified by Liu et al, (2017), inhibits HIV protease and integrase, in addition to significant anti-oxidant potential.

When co-cultured with chaga (*Inonotus obliquus*), metabolites showed increased inhibition of HeLa 229 cervical adenocarcinoma. Zheng et al, (2011).

Rosy Conk (*Rhodofomes roseus/Fomitopsis rosea*) is usually found on dead conifers such as spruce and Douglas fir; occasionally on poplar. It contains a variety of lanostane triterpenes and sterol derivatives that possess activity against Staphylococcus aureus bacterium. Popova et al, (2009).

The similar-looking *Fomitopsis cajanderi* (*Rhodofomes cajanderi*) has been studied by Sitkof et al, (2017). Both hot water and, particularly ethanol extracts of the fruiting body exhibit cytotoxicity against Jurkat cells, a line of T lymphocytic leukemia cells.

Work by Hossen et al, (2021) found methanol extracts possess analgesic benefit, binding to COX-1 and COX-2.

Gloeophyllum odoratum is found on spruce, as well as timber, and cut lumber. It has a distinct anise odor. Various triterpenes have been found to selectively inhibit thrombin, but not trypsin. Cateni et al, (2010).

Recent work found fruiting body extracts inhibit the cytopathic effect of the H3N2 influenza virus at non-cytotoxic concentrations. Trametenolic acid B was highly active against the Hong Kong/68 strain, as well as the 2009 pandemic H1N1 flu strain. The compound binds to cell-free viruses and neutralizes their infectivity. (Grienke et al, 2019). Work in the same year by Tel-Cayan (2019) identified the major compound as fumaric acid. Results found moderate inhibition of acetylcholinesterase, but significant inhibition of BChE (butyrylcholinesterase) activity, suggestive of benefit in Alzheimer's disease and related senile dementia concerns.

Milk White Toothed Polypore (*Irpex lacteus*) is widespread on dead hardwood. It has a number of interesting triterpenoids, and seco-tremulane sesquiterpenoids that show significant inhibition against nitric oxide production in macrophage cells (Tang et al, 2018); cytotoxicity against four human cancer cell lines (Tang et al, 2018a); and water soluble polysaccharides that inhibit human hepatocellular carcinoma, and HeLa tumor cells. Zhang et al, (2012). Anti-nephritis (kidney protecting) activity was also found, based on murine mesangial cells (HBZT-1) *in vitro*.

A water-soluble compound ILN3A, exhibits anti-inflammatory activity against glomerulonephritis. Wang et al, (2016).

Care in handling and inhalation of spores must be observed, as a fruiting body was isolated from a lung abscess in a nine year-old girl with acute lymphoblastic leukemia. Buzina et al, (2005).

Irpex lacteus is endophytic to *Cordyceps hawkesii*, a mushroom with high homology to *C. militaris*. Work by Liu et al, (2022) found the endophytic fungi can produce cordycepin. The yield is low compared to *C. militaris* but may provide another choice for enhanced cordycepin in future.

Pine Conk (*Porodaedalea pini*- synonym *Phellinus pini*) is found on living conifers, especially pine species. The fruiting bodies have been studied for anti-dementia and anti-inflammatory activity. Acetyl cholinesterase and butyryl cholinesterase inhibition with methanol and hot water extracts were found comparable to galantamine, the standard drug used in early stage Alzheimer's disease. Im et al, (2016).

Pine Conk shows considerable activity against herpes simplex virus 1. Dogan et al, (2018). Hispidulin has been identified as a major anti-oxidant compound in the mushroom. Kaur et al, (2019).

The oxidative stress reduction may be useful in protective from heart disease and cardiovascular issues (Ryang et al, 2021).

Aromatic cadinene sesquiterpenoids, derived from the fruiting bodies, inhibited the SARS-CoV-2 spike-ACE2. Li et al. (2021).

Rats fed a high fat and cholesterol diet, along with extracts of the fruiting body, showed significantly reduced total cholesterol, LDL and triglycerides compared to rats fed high fat/cholesterol diet. Im et al, (2018).

The fruiting body contains a water-soluble polysaccharide that inhibits alpha-glucosidase, suggesting potent in vitro blood sugar regulation (Yang et al, 2021).

Variants of water-soluble Beta-1,3-glucans from this polypore inhibit both herpes simplex and coxsackie virus B_3. Lee et al, (2010).

When in clinical practice, I treated several cases of myocarditis associated with the later virus, very successfully with *Astragalus membranaceus*, an important TCM herb.

Turkey Tail (*Trametes versicolor*) is well-studied as an important medicinal mushroom. Several Trametes species, including Hairy Turkey Tail (*T. hirsuta*), growing on alder, birch and some cherry trees; and *T. gibbosa*, more common on balsam poplar; possess medicinal properties. Work by Knezevic et al, (2018) found all three species were cytotoxic against human cervix, lung and colon cancer cell lines; with mycelium showing stronger effect than fruiting bodies. Turkey Tail showed the strongest inhibition of acetylcholinesterase, a measure of benefit for prevention of senile dementia and Alzheimer's disease, more so than the other two species.

Hairy Turkey Tail is a source of podophyllotoxin, which exhibits potent anti-oxidant, anti-cancer and radiation protective properties. Chand et al, (2006).

Lumpy Bracket (*Trametes gibbosa*) exhibit higher anti-oxidant activity than Turkey Tail in recent work by Pop et al, (2018).

The University of Northern British Columbia (UNBC) is supporting graduate student research on regional medicinal mushrooms.

A recent paper by Smith et al, (2017) looked at the cytotoxic and immune modulating activity of twelve regional mushrooms. *Trichaptum abietinum*, commonly found on living and dead conifers, and easily identified with its deep purple ridge, showed strong anti-inflammatory activity.

The fresh polypore 85% ethanol extract inhibited lipopolysaccharide-induced tumor necrosis factor (TNF)-alpha production. Hot water extracts were found immune stimulating; and both fractions exhibited anti-proliferative activity against cancer cells. Barad et al, (2016).

Sumreen Javed (2019) a student at UNBC wrote his master thesis on wild mushrooms of British Columbia. He identified significant anti-inflammatory, and micro-circulation activity in Indian Paint Fungus (*Echinodontium tinctorium*), a distinct brick red polypore traditionally used for dyes and paints.

Work by Smith (2017a) at UNBC found fruiting body extracts inhibit cervical, breast, ovarian, liver, lung and colon cancer cell lines, in vitro.

Very recent work by Deo et al, (2019) looked at the anti-proliferative, immunostimulatory and anti-inflammatory activity of 17 mushroom species collected in Haida Gwaii. Anti-proliferative activity, for example, was found in the poisonous Sulfur Tuft (*Hypholoma fasiculare*), the delicious Hedgehog (*Hydnum repandum*) and *Amanita augusta*, formerly *A. franchetti*, but misapplied, and renamed in 2013.

Zeb et al, (2021) identified an immune-stimulating polysaccharide containing 10% glucuronic acid, and a novel polysaccharide (Zeb et al, 2022) showing anti-proliferative activity against multiple cancer cell lines.

My good friend, and remarkable herbalist Darcy Williamson from Idaho, gifted me an ale she produced with this mushroom. It was very tasty!

Apricot Jelly (*Guepinia helvelloides*) exhibited strong immune-stimulating activity.

Hedgehog or Sweet Tooth Mushroom (*H. repandum*) ethanol extract shows anti-proliferative effects against the MCF-7 and HT-29 human cancer cell lines. It also displays anti-microbial and anti-biofilm activity against MRSA, *Staphylococcus epidermidis*, *E. coli*, and *Pseudomonas aeruginosa*.

Synergistic interactions were observed when antibiotics such as kanamycin and ampicillin were used together (Dizeci et al, 2021).

Dryad's Saddle (*Polyporus squamosus/Cerioporus squamosus*) is an edible found on hardwoods, containing nearly 19% protein, and treholose as main free sugar.

This unique sugar may be useful in Huntington's and Parkinson's disease. Rogers (2019).

Work by Mocan et al, (2018) found the fruiting bodies possess anti-biofilm potential, reducing the formation of *Pseudomonas aeruginosa* pili.

A lectin inhibits protein synthesis and induces apoptosis in HeLa (cervical) cancer cell lines. Manna et al, (2017).

Work by Doskocil et al, (2016) found cytotoxicity against both Caco-2 and HT-29 colon cancer cell lines, suggesting possible benefit for immunological gut disorders.

The Pacific Northwest is rich in fungal resources that have only begun to be explored.

Future studies are sure to identify more exciting compounds, and move additional members of the Fifth Kingdom to their rightful place in the Fungal Pharmacy.

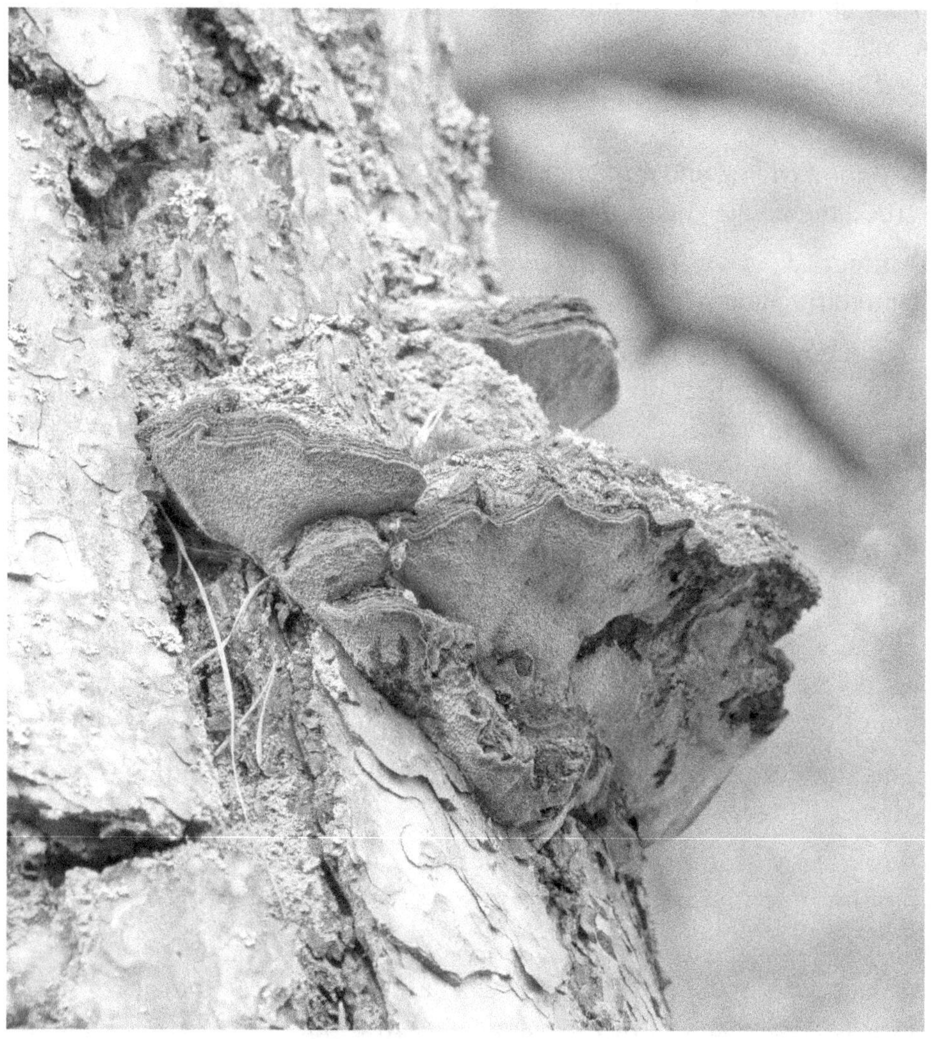

Porodaedalea pini

LEUCOPAXILLUS
GIANT LEUCOPAXILLUS
(*Leucopaxillus giganteus*)
BITTER BROWN LEUCOPAXILLUS
BITTER FALSE FUNNEL CAP
(*L. gentianeus*)
LARGE WHITE LEUCOPAXILLLUS
(*L. albissimus*)

Leuco is derived from the Greek meaning "white", and paxillus is a "small peg or pole." Giganteus is obvious, and albissimus is from the Latin, meaning "superbly white."

Giant Leucopax is great, choice edible when young and tender. They often are found growing in large circles. The odor varies from turnip-like to slightly bitter almond.

Large White Leucopax is inedible, and Bitter Brown, according to David Arora, smells like creepy crawlers and tastes like a mildewed army tent.

Giant Leucopax has been used traditionally for resolving fever states in children, and helping bring to the surface measles, chicken pox and similar afflictions.

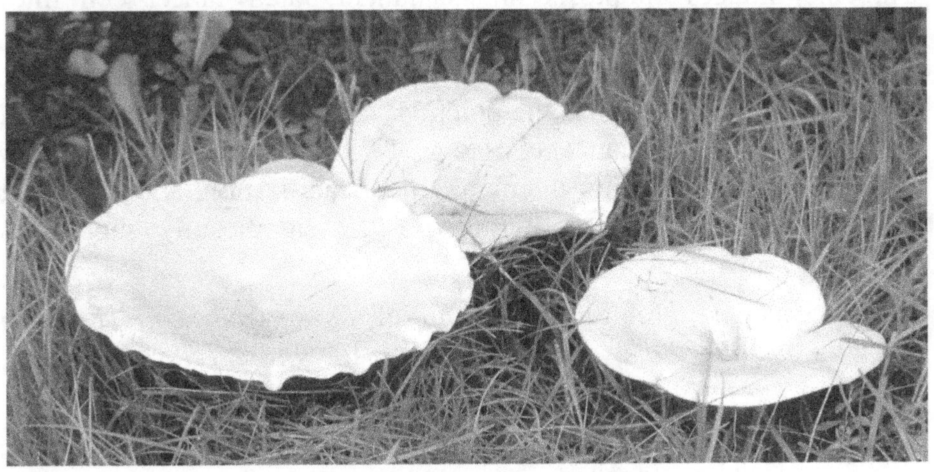

Leucopaxillus giganteus

The dried fruiting body, decocted with ginger root, helps shorten the duration of colds and influenza.

Liu et al, (2012) looked at the mineral content of ten, dried wild mushrooms and found this one highest in organic chromium (6.3 mg/kg) and iron (510 mg/kg).

It has multiple benefits including immune, anti-tumor and anti-bacterial activity.

The compound clitocine shows cytotoxicity in multi-drug resistant cell lines. It helps increase the sensitivity and intracellular accumulation of the chemotherapy drug doxorubicin in R-HepG2 (hepatic carcinoma) cells. The authors suggest clitocine could reverse P-gp associated MDR via down-regulation of NF-kappa B, and inhibited the express of NF-kappaB p65 in human uterine (MES-SA) carcinoma (Sun et al, 2012).

Nonsense mutations occur in critical tumor suppressor genes in many of our most common cancers. Clitocine can induce production of p53 protein harbouring p53 nonsense-mutated alleles; representing a novel therapy to treat cancers and genetic diseases. In the cells, clitocine restores production of full-length and functional p53. It also progresses cells into apoptosis and in work by Friesen et al, (2017) impeded growth of nonsense-containing human ovarian cancer tumors in xenograft tumor models.

Clitocine induces apoptosis in six human colon cancer cell lines accompanied by suppression of Mcl-1. It also significantly enhances the ABT-737 mediated lethality by inducing apoptosis. Work by Sun et al, (2014) determined Mcl-1 is the potential target by which clitocine can sensitize human colon cancer cells to ABT-737 induced apoptosis. It also activates Bak by inducing membrane permeabilization, and in animal models clitocine combined with ABT-737 significantly suppresses xenograft growth.

Giant Leucopax inhibits the growth of *Escherichia coli* (*E. coli*) and *Proteus mirabilis*, and bactericidal for *Pasteurella multocida*, *Streptococcus pyogenes* and *S. agalactiae* (Alves et al, 2012a).

The same team (Alves et al, 2014) looked at synergistic benefit with various commercial antibiotics, and found Giant Leucopax extracts combined for additive benefit in extended spectrum beta-lactamase-producing *E. coli*. This suggests that mushroom extracts could reduce doses of standard antibiotics and reduce micro-organism's drug resistance.

Bacterial biofilms present serious problems, especially when dealing with multi-drug resistance. Medical devices are colonized, leading to local and systemic infections, including catheter-related blood stream, and endocarditis.

Work by Alves et al, (2014) found extracts of this mushroom inhibited *E. coli* biofilm by 47.8%.

A cold water-soluble polysaccharide fraction inhibited, in vivo, the proliferation of H22 solid tumors on mice. Work by Niu et al, (2021) determined the polysaccharide induced apoptosis via S phase arrest and mitochondria-mediated pathway. It also effectively protected immune organs.

Seven identified compounds showed significant inhibition against Axl and immune checkpoints (PD-L1, PD-L2) in the human A549 alveolar epithelial cell line (Malya et al, 2020). Axl and its proteins are expressed on many cancer cells and its pathway promotes proliferation, survival, migration, invasion, angiogenesis and immune evasion.

Large White Leuxopaxillus is common under conifers, with a mealy, farinaceous odor.

The mushroom was studied by Pfister (1988), who first identified and isolated 2-Aminoquinoline (2-AQ).

This fungal compound was later identified by Alves et al, (2012) as possessing the highest antimicrobial activity, against Gram-negative bacteria. Plectasin peptide, derived from the mushroom *Pseudoplactania nigrella* was identified with the highest activity against Gram-positive bacteria. Shiitake showed activity against both Gram-positive and Gram-negative bacteria.

This compound shows modest activity against nine *Burkholderia* species, including *B. cepacia*, and multi-drug resistant strains (Schwan et al, 2010).

Burkholderia species are both beneficial and harmful. The *B. cepacia* complex, for example is an opportunistic pathogen causing severe infections in cystic fibrosis and immunocompromised patients. On the other hand, various species have a competitive advantage in acidic soil. The association of *B. terrae* and *Lyophyllum* species of fungi involves the bacteria using the hyphae for transport and dispersal but also using the fungal exudates as nutrients. *Burkholderia* species are among the main consumers of carbon released from arbuscular mycorrhizal fungi (Eberl & Vandamme, 2016).

The study by Schwan et al, (2010) found 2-AQ showed a weak response against *Acinetobacter baumannii*, an opportunistic Gram-negative bacterial pathogen. It is increasingly drug-resistant and associated with hospital acquired infections. It acquired the moniker "Iraqbacter" due to the high levesl of multi-drug resistant bacteremia (bloodstream infections). Howard et al, (2012).

Bitter Brown Leucopaxillis (*L. gentianeus*) mushroom contains two cucurbitane triterpenes, as well as leucopaxillones A-B.

Clericuzio et al. (2004) discovered cucurbitacin B active against MCF-7, HepG2, A549 and CAK-1 cancer cells, in vitro. Both hepatoblastoma and breast adenocarcinoma cells were particularly susceptible.

Leucopaxillone A, although somewhat less active, specifically showed activity against MCF-7 breast cancer cell lines. This compound is also found in Giant Leucopax as well.

The mycelium contains the triterpene 18-deoxyleucopaxillone A, not found in the fruiting body. Various isolated triterpenes were compared for activity against the NCl-H460 human tumor cell line, and compared to topotecan, the well-known topoisomerase I inhibitor (Clericuzio et al., 2006).

The mushroom is incredibly biiter and inedible.

Three-Color Leucopaxillus (*L. tricolor*) has a brown cap, pale yellow gills and white stipe. It has a strong phenolic or coal tar smell, according to Michael Kuo.

Work by Geng et al, (2015) isolated a angiotensin 1-converting enzyme (ACE) inhibitory protein, from the fruiting body. Both the isolated protein and water extract of fruiting body exhibits clear anti-hypertensive effect on rat models.

A novel acidic alpha-galactosidase has been identified. This enzyme degrades non-digestible and flatulence-causing oligosaccharides, and may be useful for various food applications, involving stachyose, raffinose, melibiose, locust bean and guar gum (Geng et al, 2018).

MILK CAPS

DELICIOUS MILK CAP
SAFFRON MILK CAP
(*Lactarius deliciosus group*)
RED HOT MILK CAP
(*L. rufus*)
BLEEDING MILK CAP
(*L. rubrilacteus*)
CANDY CAP
CURRY MILK CAP
(*L. rubidus*)
SPICY MILK CAP
(*L. camphoratus*)
PEPPERY MILK CAP
(*L. piperatus*)
(*Lactifluus piperatus*)
FLEECY MILK CAP
(*L. vellereus*)
FLEECY-LIKE MILK CAP
(*L. subvellereus*)
FENUGREEK MILK CAP
BURNT SUGAR MILK CAP
(*L. helvus*)
(*L. aquifluus*)
FALSE SAFFRON MILK CAP
ORANGE MILK CAP
(*L. deterrimus*)
WEEPING MILK CAP
TAWNY MILK CAP
APRICOT MILK CAP
(*L. volemus*)
INDIGO MILK CAP
(*L. indigo*)

I am often asked my favorite, edible mushroom. And it largely depends upon what culinary dish I would like to prepare.

Delicious Milk Cap fits into this category, due to its crisp, nutty texture and flavor.

Lactarius derives from the Latin "lactate", and hence milk, based on the latex or sap. This quickly helps one differentiate from similar-looking Russula species.

I have a favorite spot less than a kilometre from my home, that produces lots of Western Saffron Milk Caps every fall.

The entire section *Deliciosi* is taxonomically complex. Many of the studies on medicinal and health benefits of this species were conducted worldwide.

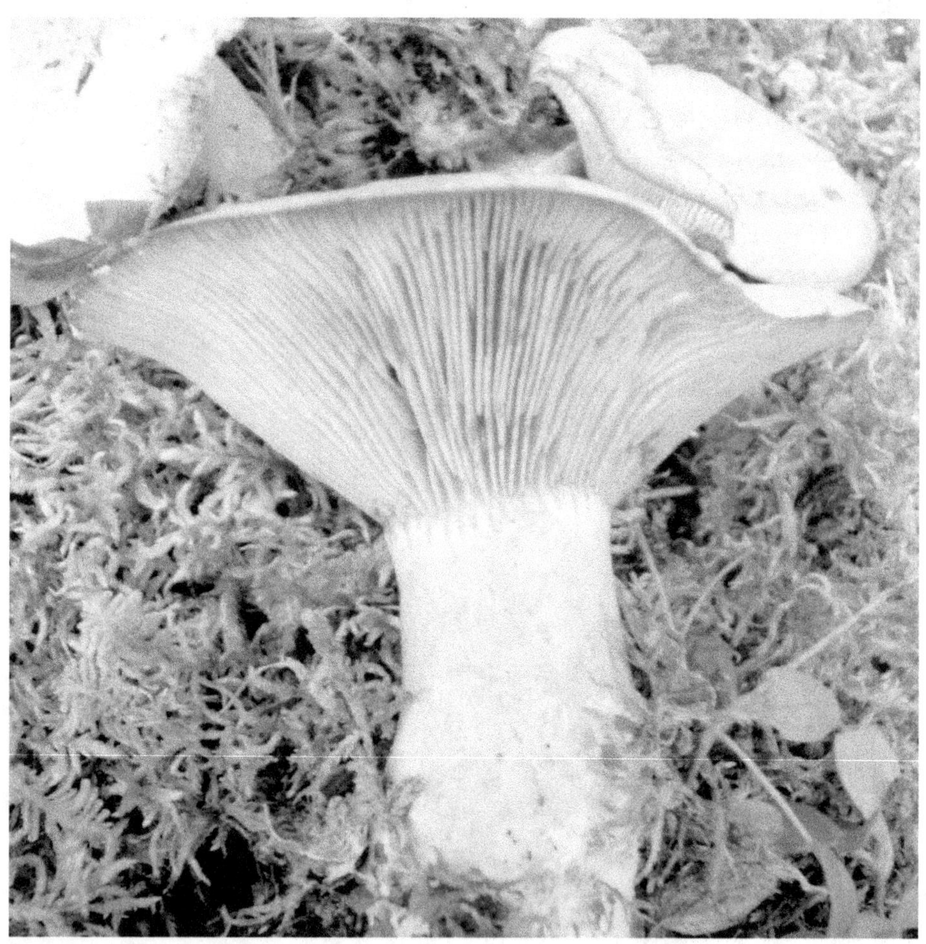

Lactarius rubrilacteus

Work in New Zealand suggests pine (*Pinus radiata*) plantations, mycorrhized with Delicious Milk Cap, may yield up to 300 kilograms per hectare of fruiting bodies by the third year (Guerin-Laguette et al, 2014). The concept of gourmet mushroom orchards, associated with tree planting, after timber harvest, should be encouraged worldwide.

As the fruiting body of Delicious Milk Cap matures, the content of protein, monounsaturated and polyunsaturated fatty acids increase, while carbohydrates, saturated fatty acids and anti-microbial contents decrease (Barros et al, 2007).

The fruiting body exhibits anti-microbial activity, as well as cytotoxicity against human epithelial (HeLa), human lung (A549), and human colon (LS174) carcinoma cell lines (Kosanic et al, 2016).

When supplemented to animals subjected to oxidative stress of carbon tetrachloride, the mushroom ameliorated, and protected from liver and kidney lesions (Dogan et al, 2022).

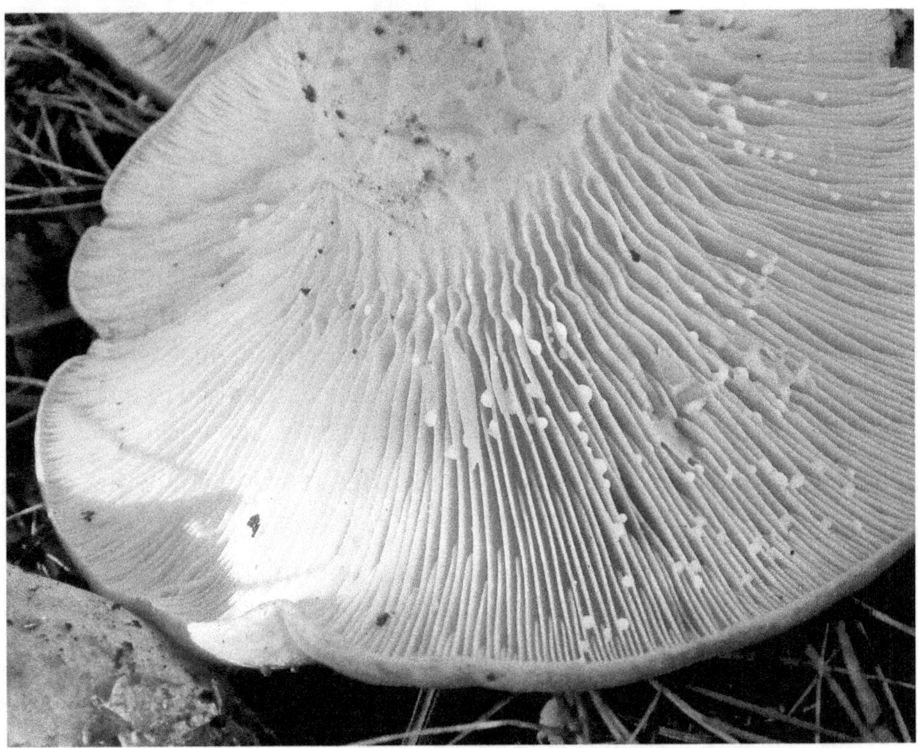

Lactarius rubrilacteus

Work by Nowakowski et al, (2021) looked at four species and found ethanol extracts of *Lactarius deliciosus* and Shaggy Mane (*Coprinus comatus*) with the greatest anti-glioma (brain and spinal cord cancer) potential. These included U87MG, and LN-19 glioblastoma. Inhibition of cancer cell proliferation and induction of apoptosis was associated with arrest of cells in subG1 or G2/M phase and inhibition of metalloproteinases.

Polysaccharides from the fruiting body help proliferate macrophages, with cytokines of TNFalpha, IL-1beta and IL-6 increasing 4.83, 17.8 and 11 times the control, respectively (Cheng et al, 2019).

A novel polysaccharide was found to promote proliferation of B cells, and macrophages (Hou et al, 2019).

A partially, purified lectin shows in vivo immune-modulation, and phagocytic activity towards macrophages and neutrophils (Esseddik et al, 2020).

Derivatives of sesquiterpenoid alcohols were found to inhibit herpes simplex virus type 1 and PHA-induced T lymphocyte proliferation (Krawczyk et al, 2006).

Ethanol extracts of the fruiting body show inhibition on alpha-amylase and alpha-glucosidase, suggestive of anti-hyperglycemic benefit (Xu et al, 2019).

Peppery Milk Cap (*L. piperatus*) is considered edible in parts of the world, after repeated boiling and changes of water. It is also dried and powdered as a seasoning. It is occasionally found in eastern North America under deciduous trees. The white latex is applied to viral warts, in a manner similar to the sap of dandelion stems.

The taste is acrid, hot and peppery, and tasted raw will affect the tongue for an hour or so. Not recommended.

Extracts exhibit strong anti-oxidant, anti-microbial, anti-cancer and neuroprotective effects, the latter due to its ability to inhibit acetylcholinesterase (Kosanic et al, 2020).

Fleecy Milk Cap (*L. vellereus*) fruiting body is edible, and contains catechin, ferulic acid, p-coumaric acid and cinnamic acid. In work by Dogan et al, (2013), the mushroom extracts exhibited anti-oxidative activity, and inhibition of *Klebsiella pneumoniae*.

The similar looking Fleecy-Like Milk Cap (*L. subvellereus*) contains unusual lactarane sesquiterpenoids, that exhibit cytotoxicity against human lung (A549), colon (SK-MEL-2) and melanoma (HCT-15) cancer cell lines (Kim et al, 2010).

Red Hot Milk Cap (*L. rufus*) fruiting body contains 1>3, 1>6 beta-D-glucans, stearic acid, 3beta-hydroxy-ergosta-5,7,22-triene, sotolon, lactarorufin A, rufuslactone and D-allitol.

The water-soluble beta glucans potently inhibit inflammation and pain. (Ruthes et al, 2013).

Rufuslactone exhibits anti-fungal activity, while sotolon decreased production of *Pseudomonas aeruginosa* biofilm, in vivo (Aldawsari et al, 2021). In another study, by Abbas et al, (2021), the biofilm of *Serratia marcesens*, a hospital-acquired infection, was strongly inhibited by sotolon. This bacterium is highly infectious and multidrug resistant.

It should be noted that sotolon is the aromatic molecule that gives Candy Cap (*L. rubidus*), its maple syrup-like flavor. Found in western North America, the caps have a more pronounced odor and taste when dried. The eastern *L. fragilis* mushroom cap odor is more maple syrup-like when fresh.

The related *L. helvus*, found often in spruce bogs, contains up to 1.4% sotolon, but the mushroom is considered mildly toxic, or considered inedible. Burnt Sugar Milk Cap (*L. aquifluus*) may be North American equivalent, a synonym, or distinct species.

Weeping or Tawny Milk Cap (*L. volemus*) is a choice edible found in the eastern United States. The latex is white, but stains a persistent brown on hands. In West Virginia, it is known as a Bradley or Leatherback. The taste is mild, but it has a strong fishy odor.

Polysaccharide extracts exhibit immune modulation, and stimulate macrophage-mediated immune response. They inhibit proliferation of human breast (MCF-1) and H1299 cancer cell lines (Zhong et al, 2021).

A single report of acute pancreatitis in a couple, after eating this mushroom is cited in the literature (Karahan et al, 2016). I am skeptical, but it is reported they had been collecting and eating this species for several years.

False Saffron Milk Cap (*L. deterrimus*) is a bright orange-capped, edible, but bitter mushroom found in Europe. The species name derives from "deterior", meaning the worst or poorest; compared to the more desired Delicious Milk Cap.

Work by Mihailovic et al, (2015) found the extract reduced blood sugar levels in diabetic-induced rats. The most interesting find was a positive effect on pancreatic islet, decreasing AGE formation, and increasing the expression of chemokine CXCL12 protein, that mediates restoration of beta-cells.

Stomach cancer is the 4th most common cancer diagnosed worldwide. A phenolic fraction was found by Król et al, (2021) to inhibit gastric cancer cell proliferation, via an effect on stromal cells. Synergistic and potential activity with cisplatin/5-fluorouracil is noted.

Indigo Milk Cap (*L. indigo*) is a choice edible, and easily identified by its blue fruiting body and latex. It is popular in Mexican farmer's markets.

The blue color is due to azulene derivatives, and also found in German Chamomile, Wormwood, and Yarrow. Various benefits include anti-inflammatory benefit for peptic ulcers, anti-neoplastic with leukemia, anti-diabetic, anti-retroviral with HIV-1, anti-microbial including anti-microbial photodynamic therapy and anti-fungal activity (Bakun et al, 2021)

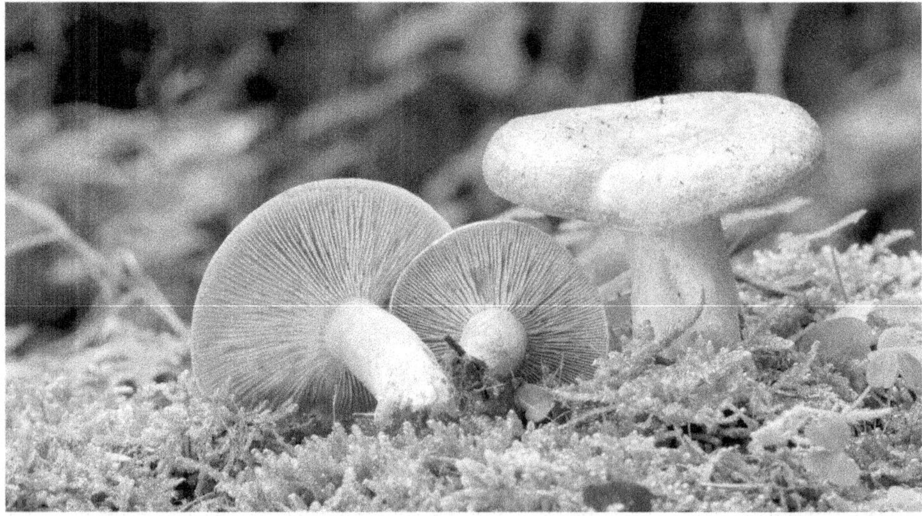

Lactarius deterrimus

MILKY WHITE MUSHROOM
(*Calocybe indica*)

Calocybe derives from the Greek *Kalos*, meaning, "pretty" and *Cubos*, for "head".

My first introduction to Milky White was courtesy of Tradd Cotter (Mushroom Mountain), a close friend and exceptional mycologist.

I was visiting in May and as a far northerner, was complaining about the heat and humidity; which this mushroom originally identified in India, loves. In that country, it is the third most important commercial species, known as Kuduk or White Summer Mushroom, after buttons and oysters.

In fact, it grows best in temperatures between 25 and 35 degrees Celsius, and enjoys humidity of 60-70%.

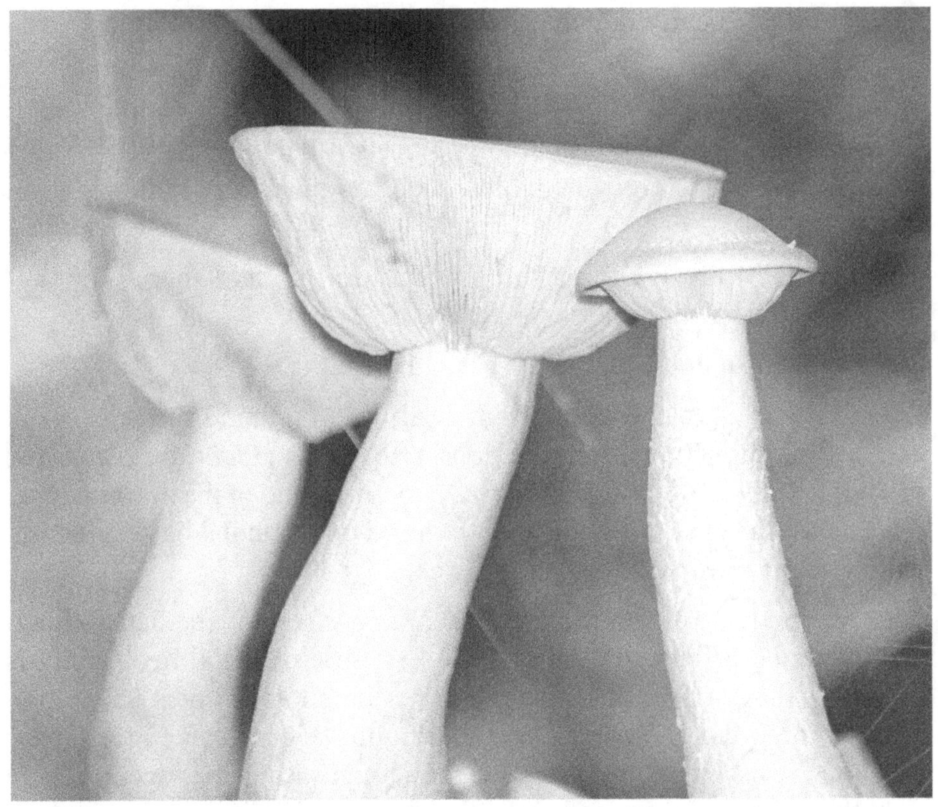

Calocybe indica

Milky White is a choice edible, firm like a King Oyster, with a faint radish scent, and a mild, oily coconut flavor. It is a good source of protein (12.48%)

Commercial cultivation is easy, as it grows well on various substrates, including wheat straw, but does best on rice straw and 30% corn powder. Loamy soil, sand and spent oyster or paddy mushroom substrate can be used as casing material (3 centimeters). Amin et al, (2010a & b). Primordia appear within 18-20 days, and fruiting bodies in 45 days. A yield of 70-85 kilos can be expected per 100 kilograms of substrate.

I have long proposed organic, trace mineral supplementation from edible and medicinal mushrooms, including the important micro-mineral selenium.

When cultivated with wheat straw optimally enriched with 5μ/ml of sodium selenite, the fruiting bodies accumulated organic selenium, and in extracts nearly doubled the anti-oxidant capacity (Rathore et al, 2018).

When exposed to UVB radiation (or the sun), the fruiting bodies increased vitamin D2 considerably, but also the content of 17 amino acids, beta-glucan, and flavonoids such as quercetin (Rathore et al, 2020).

This makes Milky White mushrooms an ideal protein source for sub-tropical and tropical locations.

Add to this its numerous potential health benefits.

An in vitro/in vivo study by Singh et al, (2017), found the mushroom actively inhibits alpha-amylase, superior to Oyster (*Pleurotus ostreatus*) or Paddy Straw (*Volvariella volvacea*), in vitro. And in the accompanied mice study, the extract significantly reduced postprandial blood glucose, similar to acarbose.

Another interest of mine is the synergistic effect of medicinal fungi and plants with standard antibiotics. Very little financial investment is presently allocated for pharmaceutical research into the next generation of these important medicines, considering the widespread concern over antibiotic resistant strains of bacteria. This catastrophe has occurred due to both human over-use and abuse, and the unconscionable addition to livestock feed. In fact, 80% of antibiotics end up on our dinner plates.

Methanol extracts of Milky White mushrooms act synergistically with ciprofloxacin, increasing their efficiency, significantly (Datta et al, 2020).

Fluoroquinolones, including ciprofloxacin, are associated with potentially irreversible, and serious adverse reactions including tendon rupture, peripheral neuropathy, pyelonephritis, arthralgia and exacerbation of muscle weakness in patients with myasthenia gravis. This class of antibiotics is rightly reserved for urinary tract infections in patients that do not respond to less harmful medications. This study suggests investigating a possible adjuvant therapy.

Ethanol extracts show efficacy, in vitro, on two pancreatic cancer cell lines, PANC-1 and MIAPaCa2 cells. Anti-proliferation, inhibition and apoptosis were induced, and p53 protein levels increased (Ghosh & Sanyal, 2020). Considering the low survival rate (1%), with the present protocols, for this cancer; and the relative safety of the edible fruiting body, a human clinical trial is warranted.

One of the water-soluble polysaccharides in Milky White shows immune enhancement and cytotoxicity against the HeLa cancer cell line (Mandal et al, 2011).

Recent work by Nataraj et al, (2022) found the polysaccharides prolong activated partial thromboplastin time, thrombin time, but not prothrombin time. The same study found anti-proliferative activity against the HeLa, PC3, HT29, HepG2 and Jurkat cancer cell lines, in vitro.

Ethanol extracts show effective zone inhibition, in vitro, against Gram-positive and negative bacteria (Shaskikant et al, 2022).

A protein fraction exhibits anti-proliferative activity against several tumor cell lines through induction of self-programmed death (apoptosis). And shows stimulatory effect on splenocytes, thymocytes and bone marrow cells; stimulates macrophages to produce nitric oxide, and enhances natural killer cell cytotoxicity (Maiti et al, 2008).

Work by Mishra et al, (2014) suggests the caps have higher antioxidant properties than the stipe.

In many ways, this is the perfect hot, humid climate mushroom, to grow and consume.

MUSHROOMS AND BEES

In my mid-twenties, I became fascinated with bees. For several years I had four hives, and one year collected nearly 600 pounds of honey.

I was self-taught, but learned that a bee smoker was important, and found that several polypores served the purpose, especially dry Amadou (*Fomes fomenatarius*) and various puffballs.

I never fully understood why, but was told the cool smoke makes them eat honey, in response to a colony-damaging fire. I would experiment, and found that adding pine needles, and hop strobiles to the smoker resulted in even calmer reactions. Smoking wild or commercial bees, to calm them, while removing their food source, is a worldwide practice.

A paper by Harris & Woodring (2002) helps explain the phenomenon, at least in part. When guard honey bees smell smoke they release the pheromone isopentyl acetate. Bees injured during a hive exam, or removing full frames of honey, also release this excitatory volatile.

More recent work by Gage et al, (2018) suggests bees, when provoked, release a venom droplet, which is reduced under smoke conditions.

I attempted to over-winter my hives in northern Canada, resulting in varroa mite infection and massive colony deaths. It was very distressing.

Various factors, including industrial agriculture and the use of herbicides, pesticides and fungicides, has led to bee colony collapse worldwide, during the last decade. Feeding pure sugar water may be a health issue, and so is feeding antibiotics to honeybees, disrupting their microbiota (Raymann et al, 2017).

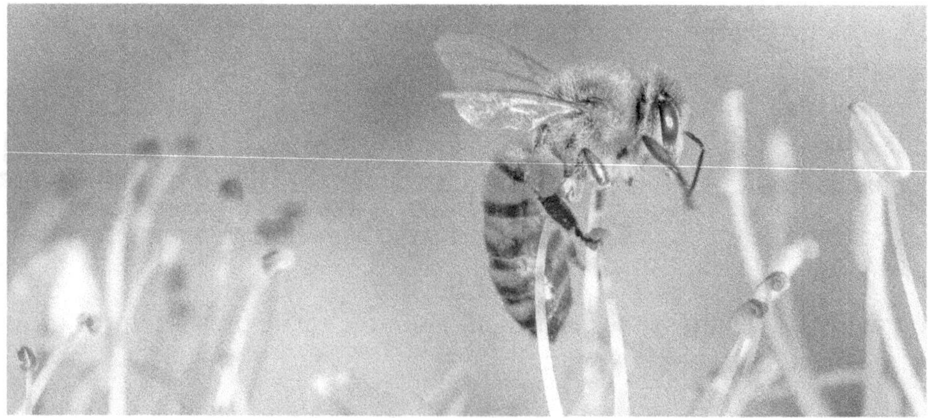

Like humans, the disruption of gut health, negatively impacts survival rates in bees.

Paul Stamets observed bees visiting mushroom mycelium for many years before speculating they were gathering medicine, and not simply sugars. Wild and honey bees will visit Wine Caps (*Stropharia rugoso-annulata*) and cut open the mycelium mats to suck out the sugars (cytoplasm).

His inquisitive mind led to testing mycelium from various polypores, with known anti-viral properties. Extracts from Amadou (*Fomes fomentarius*), and *Ganoderma resinaceum*, reduced levels of honey bee deformed wing virus and Lake Sinai virus significantly. When tested in field trials, the Ganoderma mushroom extract exhibited a 79-fold reduction in the former, and a 45,000-fold reduction in the latter virus (Stamets et al, 2018). An article on this exciting find is found in *Fungi* magazine 2018 11(4): 48.

A Bee Mushroomed Feeder™ is now available as a delivery system for beekeepers wishing to use this holistic approach to apiary.

This innovative work has led to research on other mushrooms for possible benefit to bee colonies. The contribution of bees to human health cannot be underestimated. A number of agricultural crops, including almonds, depend upon bee pollination for optimal crop harvests. Worldwide, the Varroa mite is the single greatest threat to apiculture, threatening $238 billion in bee-related crops on an annual basis.

A team of Washington State University entomologists bred a strain of *Metarhizium* (*M. brunneum*) fungi that can survive, germinate and grow in bee hive temperatures of 35 degrees Celsius. The new strain JH1078 can kill *Varroa destructor* mites, that weaken a bee's immune system and contribute to Colony Collapse Disorder.

Paul Stamets did some initial work, but he gives much credit to Jennifer Han and the team, in developing this specific culture strain (Han et al, 2021). Two years of work, and screening over 27,000 mites helped develop the new, temperature-resistant strain. Approval from the EPA is the next step, towards its use in apiculture.

The parasitic, fungi *Nosema ceranae* has a detrimental effect on honey bee colonies. Recent work by Glavinic et al, 2021) compared fumagillin treatment with a hot water extract of *Agaricus blazei*. A protective effect was detected from the mushroom extract, without any side effects, but also an immune stimulating benefit in preventive applications.

Fumagilin-B is a widely used "antibiotic" veterinary product to prevent the spread of nosema.

This follows the work by Stevanovic et al, (2018) feeding this mushroom extract to honey bees. Initially 640 bees were given the sugar syrup and proven safe. Then a three-year field experiment was conducted on 28 colonies with a single dose of extract (100 mg/kg/day) added to syrup. They were treated once in autumn and twice in spring and significantly strengthened colony strength, as well as improvement in brood rearing, and adult population growth.

Nosema and varroa mites make hives more susceptible to viruses.

Glavinic et al, (2021a) turned their attention to the common button mushroom (*Agaricus bisporus*). Water extracts were tested on honey bees and in cage experiments a concentration of 200 µg/g, with *Nosema* infection was observed. Survival rate of *Nosema*-infected bees was significantly greater in those fed *A. bisporus*-enriched syrup, compared to those fed pure sucrose syrup. The benefit was greatest when applied after the third day of infection.

Commercial button mushroom production is still significant in North America, although being challenged for market share by other functional and medicinal mushrooms (Bunyard, 2021).

The waste product could easily create a value-added opportunity.

Only in the past decade has the human microbiome received due attention, and its relationship to health. While much of the focus has been on healthy and unhealthy populations of bacterium; research into the human mycobiome is still in its relative infancy. It is well-known in the biomedical community that anti-fungals pose a much greater risk to human health, and survival, than anti-biotics.

Work at the University of Canberra, Australia is looking at probiotics for preventing and treating fungal chalkbrood (*Ascosphaera apis*). A healthy honeybee will have between 10^5 to 10^6 gut bacteria.

Dr. Svjetlana Vojvodic Kruse from Rowan University in New Jersey has identified a particular strain of gut bacteria in bees that influences learning, memory and gene expression in the brain. Like humans, the health of the microbiome influences brain health.

A combination of Irish seaweed, thymol and lemongrass oil appears to prevent, and treat nosema, varroa mites and viral infections in treated hives. The product known as *HiveAlive* has been shown effective in numerous trials.

A product derived from hops, HopGuard III, is a liquid miticide.

Lemongrass (*Cymbopogon nardus*) essential oil exhibits activity against mite Varroa destructor, as well as low toxicity against bees (Gimenez-Martinez et al, 2022).

The widespread belief of fungi as pathogens is slowly disappearing as more studies examine symbiotic relationships in nature.

In fact, honey bees fed fungal spores increased longevity, and perhaps consumption may help them compensate for poor-quality plant pollen diets (Parish et al, 2020).

A Brazilian stingless bee, *Scaptotrigona depilis*, requires the fungus *Zygosaccharomyces*, to provide ergosterol for ecydsteroid production that helps modify pupal growth. Another fungus, a *Candida* species, produces volatile, organic compounds that stimulate *Zygosaccharomyces* development. And a third fungus, *Monascus ruber* inhibits *Zygosaccharomyces* growth by producing lovastatin, which blocks steroid synthesis (Paludo et al, 2019).

The latter fungi play a role in the production of Red Yeast Rice, a natural supplement with proven efficacy in reducing total cholesterol levels in numerous human trials. It contains monacolin K, which reduces LDL levels from 15% to 25% within six to eight weeks (Cicero et al, 2021).

Daily consumption of 3 to 10 milligrams of monacolin K is safe, well tolerated, and only mild myalgias in the frailest patients, who cannot tolerate even moderate amounts of statin drugs (Cicero et al, 2019).

Red Yeast Rice also contains GABA (gamma-aminobutyric acid), a neurotransmitter related to calmness, perhaps explaining part of its role in reducing blood pressure, as well as mild dyslipidemia (Minamizuka et al, 2021).

Bee Well and Prosper!

NAMEKO

Nameko (*Pholiota nameko* (T. Itô) S. Ito & S. Imai) is a small, brown gelatinous mushroom that is one of Japan's most popular, cultivated varieties. The name means "viscid mushroom."

The mushroom is rapidly gaining popularity in North America, where it is sometimes known as "butterscotch mushroom." It is organically grown on various soft and hardwoods and more widely available on this continent the past few years. Organic sawdust spawn is available from a few suppliers. Conifer sawdust fruiting is possible with the addition of 15% bran. McCoy (2016).

An excellent short video on growing Nameko outdoors with Tradd Cotter (2014) is found on YouTube. His book is a personal favorite on organic cultivation of mushrooms. They are extremely easy to propagate, indoors or out, depending upon the climate in your area.

For greater, in-depth detail on cultivation, research Chang & Hayes (1978). At one time, it was believed lightning and thunder improved fruiting yields. Research shows that pulsing high voltage to logs increases the fruiting yield by 50%. Takaki et al, (2009).

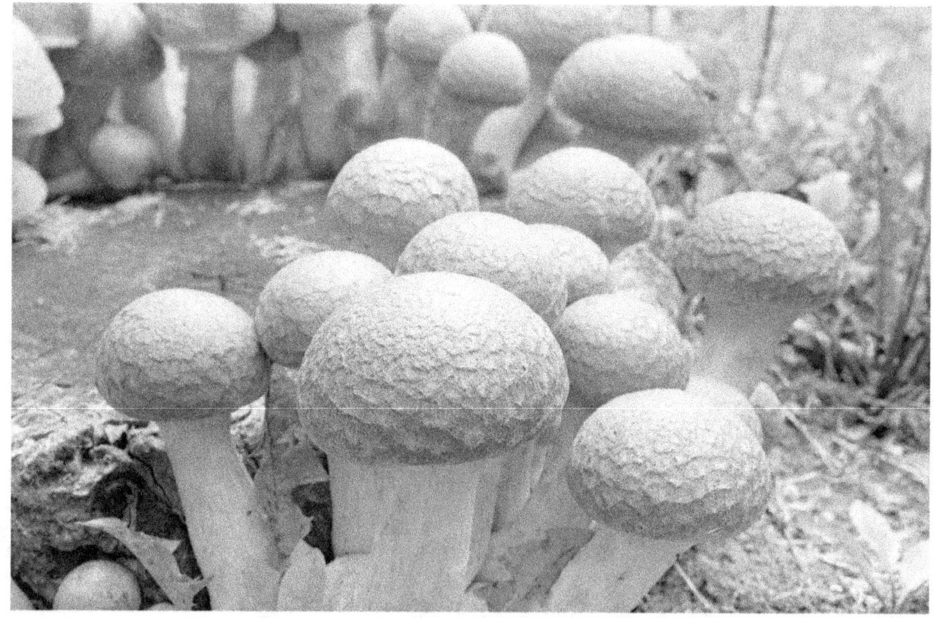

Pholiota nameko

The mushrooms contain nearly 21% protein, and are popular in Japan when added to miso soup, steamed in a pipkin, cooked with grated daikon radish, or stir-fried vegetable dishes.

In China, the Mandarin name is Pinyin: huá gu; or Pinyin: huá zi mó.

Not only is the fresh mushroom delicious, but also rich in medicinal benefits.

I caution readers to purchase only organic certified fresh and dried mushrooms, and even then to be careful with product from some countries. The fresh are far more delicious than the re-constituted dry, fruiting bodies.

Eleven years ago, when finishing my book (Rogers 2011), there was not a lot to share about the health benefits of this delicious fruiting body. In the 1990s, most of the information was related to hypersensitivity and pneumonia, from the spores, associated with cultivation. Inage et al, (1996).

Li et al, (2012) studied the polysaccharide content, and the cytokine response in blood serum of healthy volunteers. The results found significant anti-inflammatory activity on both innate and adaptive immune function, as well as hematopoietic stem cells. The latter reside in the bone marrow and give rise to different blood cell types in the range of 10^{11}- 10^{12} new cells daily.

Both *in vitro*, and *in vivo* anti-oxidant effects of intracellular polysaccharides were confirmed by Zhang et al, (2015).

An area of increasing interest is modification of the substrate, to change or enhance myco-availability of trace nutrients and minerals. In work by Zheng et al, (2015), the transformation of zinc by mycelium polysaccharides, led to a product that is a natural antioxidant that slows, *in vivo*, the progression of ageing. Enrichment of medicinal, edible mushrooms with selenium, chromium, iron and other important trace minerals is coming.

The zinc-rich mycelium polysaccharides may also be effective in lowering cholesterol and protecting against high-fat diet-induced hyperlipidemia and non-alcoholic fatty liver. Zheng et al, (2014). The latter condition is rapidly rising in North America, due in part to the consumption of high fructose corn syrup and trans-fatty acids.

Work by Diyabalanage et al, (2009) tested lipid soluble extracts of nameko, shiitake and oyster mushroom fruiting bodies for peroxidation. Nameko was the most active, with inhibition of 81%. Inhibition of COX-1 and -2 enzymes, suggesting anti-inflammatory activity, was noted.

Early laboratory work by Li et al, (2010) on hyperlipidemic Wistar rats, at different rates, given orally, found amelioration of pathological changes in coronary arteries and significant suppression of hyperlipidemia. The polysaccharide supplementation also lowered body weight and visceral weights of heat, liver and kidney, but not lungs.

Advanced glycation end products induce oxidative stress and inflammation, and are major risk factors in cancer and diabetes. Lin et al, (2021) found polysaccharides mitigate skin cell damage, suggesting benefit in skin care products.

The polysaccharides also promote L929 fibroblast proliferation and migration, suggesting benefit in wound healing (Sung et al, 2020).

They may also protect against UVA-induced skin aging (Lin et al, 2022).

The (1>3) beta-D-glucans possess a gel-like viscosity that inhibits inflammation and pain in a mice study (Abreu et al, 2019).

The fruiting bodies contain various water-soluble proteins. Work by Qian et al, (2016) found an anti-oxidant protein that exhibits anti-tumor activity against breast cancer (MCF7) cell lines, by inducing apoptosis.

Novel anti-tumor proteins were identified by Zhang et al, (2014) and found to induce apoptosis (self-programmed death), *in vitro*, against human breast cancer (MCF7) and cervical cancer (HeLa) cell lines. Activation of caspase-9 and caspase-3 imply intrinsic signal pathway is involved.

Recent work by Zhang et al, (2020) identified an anti-tumor protein that inhibits malignant proliferation of MCF-y tumor xenografts, by activating the death receptor pathway. Immune modulation may indirectly inhibit tumor growth by shifting the balance of Th1/Th2 toward Th1.

Nameko may be useful in various auto-immune conditions such as multiple sclerosis, Crohn's disease, and rheumatoid arthritis.

The polysaccharides stimulate the production of more cytokine IL-10 and less IL-2 and TNF-alpha (Li et al, 2014).

The former inhibits synthesis of pro-inflammatory cytokines made by macrophages and Th1 T cells. Lower levels of IL-10 are found in patients diagnosed with multiple sclerosis, resulting in TNFalpha rising and creating inflammation. Brennan et al, (2008).

It also functions as an immune-modulator in the intestine. Patients suffering with Crohn's disease are helped by interleukin-10 producing bacteria in the gut. Bratt et al, (2006).

Polysaccharides from the edible mushroom may increase natural physical strength and endurance, based on a mice study (Zhang et al, 2022).

One of the advantages of medicinal mushrooms, in general, is the ability to modulate the immune system. An important part of this self-regulating system is dendritic cells. Note that this is different than dendrites, which play a role in nerve transmissions.

The formation of dendritic cells is fascinating. Their shape is perfect for what they do. When one looks at the various immune cells, only a dendritic cell can go from the outside of the colon to the inside.

It slips one of its tentacle-like arms in between two colon cells to start its exploratory adventure. When its arm reaches the layers of mucus, it dives through, like a periscope on a submarine, and surfaces inside the intestine. This arm then collects antigen from the colon lumen or mucus and leaves the way it entered.

Dendritic cells have a special molecule that resembles a flagpole rising out of the mucus membranes, or mesothelial surface. They run antigen up the pole for display and information purposes.

This explains how the two arms of the immune system communicate with each other, to address pathogens and inflammation.

Both T cells and dendritic cells have a common language called antigen.

We tend to think of dendritic cells in the colon, but they actually are found in any area of our bodies exposed to the environment, such as the skin, lungs, and vagina.

Dendritic cells are not just explorers, but cruise our body with antigen to show T cells, that are birthed in the thymus gland.

They cruise the body and in the spleen and lymph nodes meet up with dendritic cells and their antigen load.

When they find each other, a T cell is formed, usually in childhood, but anytime really, and stick around for life. This means they play a role in both innate and acquired immunity.

Two types of T cells, regulatory T cells (Tregs) and Th17 (named for the interleukin 17 cytokine they secrete) protect us in ways different from killer T cells, that are activated by dendritic cells. The latter attack pathogens and cancerous tumors.

Instead, they carry out the day-to-day duties of regulating inflammation in our body.

Tregs (including IL-10) reduce inflammation and Th17 cells increase inflammation.

In people with optimal immune function, these two play a perfect role of balance.

But if there is an imbalance of Th17, the pro-inflammatory cells, an auto-immune condition can result.

At one time, not that long ago, it was assumed that dendritic cells could only display antigen made from protein. This has been proven wrong!

Dendritic cells run polysaccharide antigens, suggesting the variety and shape of these carbohydrates play a key role in immune health.

This is the main reason water-soluble compounds, such as beta-glucans, in both mycelium and fruiting bodies, are of great influence and importance.

Healthy bacteria and fungi in our guts are commensals that help regulate inflammation. They help fine tune the inflammatory response to avoid the host developing chronic inflammation, and yet allow pro-inflammatory cells to be trigger-happy when pathogens appear.

Recent work by Ray et al, (2018) found evidence that the splenic anti-inflammatory pathway signals are transmitted via a novel neuronal-like function of the mesothelial cells. These cholinergic signals are disrupted by anti-cholinergic OTC medications, as mentioned in a previous article in Fungi magazine (10(3):36-40).

Li et al, (2018) identified a polysaccharide that down-regulates the NF-kappa B signaling pathway via the toll-like receptor 2. This helps to mediate the production of cytokines involved in efficient immunity.

Ethanol extracts showed significant inhibition of inflammation associated with a hyper-sensitive immune system. Sano et al, (2002).

The mushrooms are an excellent source of extractable bioactive compounds, including potential pre-biotic activity. Rodrigues et al, (2017).

A case control study (1998-2002) on the reduced risk of stomach cancer in people eating Nameko mushrooms found a significant benefit. Those eating no mushrooms less than once a week were given an odds ratio (OR) of 1.0. Those individuals eating Nameko more than once a week had an OR of 0.56 Ikekawa (2005), suggesting a nearly 50% reduction in cancer risk.

It is certain Nameko mushroom will soon take its rightful place in the Fungal Pharmacy, as a choice edible, with added medicinal benefit.

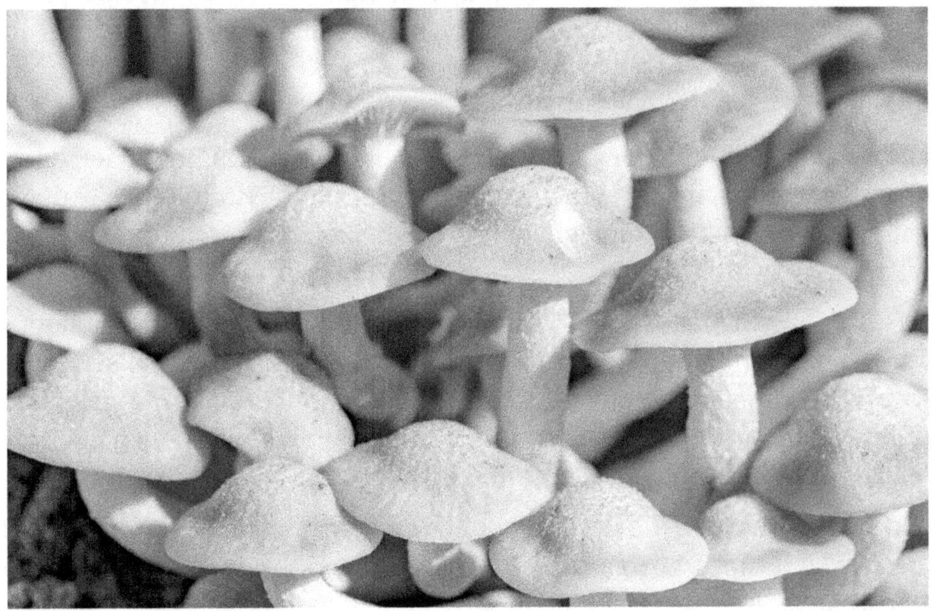

Pholiota nameko

PARASOL
(*Macrolepiota procera* (Scop.) Singer)

Parasol mushroom are a choice edible; commonly found on lawns and pastures in early fall. The immature mushrooms are known as drumsticks and are battered or sautéed. The whole open mature cap makes a delicious barbeque dish.

Shaggy Parasol (*Chlorophyllum rachodes*), formerly known as *M. rachodes* looks similar, but is smaller, and dislikes open pastures. It also lacks the brown, double-edged moveable veil ring. It is also edible, but some people react to undercooked caps, or suffer strong allergic reaction, even after cooking. Caution is advised.

In Northwestern Himalaya, India, the Parasol is known as flower of the earth (*dkarti ka phool*).

It has a sweet taste, and contains cinnamic acid (21.5 mg/kg dry wt.). In TCM, the mushroom is eaten to promote digestion.

The fruiting body is rich in 5-hydroxytryptophan (5-HTP), a precursor to serotonin and melatonin.

The mushroom is both edible and medicinal. Work by Secme et al, (2018) identified inhibition of A549 human lung cancer cell lines. It reduced invasion of cancer cells, and induced apoptosis via various pathways.

The mushroom contains novel trypsin inhibitors, including macrospin. They are resistant to high temperatures and extreme pH values, suggesting benefit in biotechnology, medicine and agriculture (Lukanc et al, 2017).

It also contains lanostane triterpenoids that possess anti-inflammatory and anti-proliferative activity. Identified as lepiotaprocerins A-L, the twelve compounds were studied for inhibition of nitric oxide, and lepiotaprocerins A-F displayed more significant inhibition than positive control L-N^{G}-monomethyl arginine.

Lepiotaprocerins G-L, showed cytotoxicity against a number of human cancer cell lines. Compound I was active against *Mycobacterium tuberculosis* H37Ra (Chen et al, 2018).

Other work suggests the mushroom possesses potent free radical scavenging activity. Cytotoxic activity was noted for human epithelial HeLa, human lung carcinoma A549, and human colon carcinoma LS174 cell lines (Kosanic et al, 2016).

Recent work by Zara et al, (2022) identified a novel G6PD inhibitor, suggesting benefit in the treatment of A549 and other lung cancers.

Arora et al. (2013) found ethanol extracts cytotoxic against breast (MCF-7), colon (COLO-205) and kidney (ACHN) cancer cell lines. Significant activity was observed especially against the colon cancer cell line.

A lectin, isolated from the fruiting body, does not provoke cancer cell cytotoxicity, but binds to aminopeptidase N (CD13) and integrin alpha3beta1. These are two glycoproteins that are overexpressed on the membrane of cancer cells.

The lectin, upon binding is endocytosed in a clathrin-dependent manner and accumulates initially in the Golgi apparatus, and then in the lysosomes.

This suggests a lectin that may enable protein drugs, or other cytotoxic compounds to enter cancer cells, and enhance their activity (Urga et al, 2017).

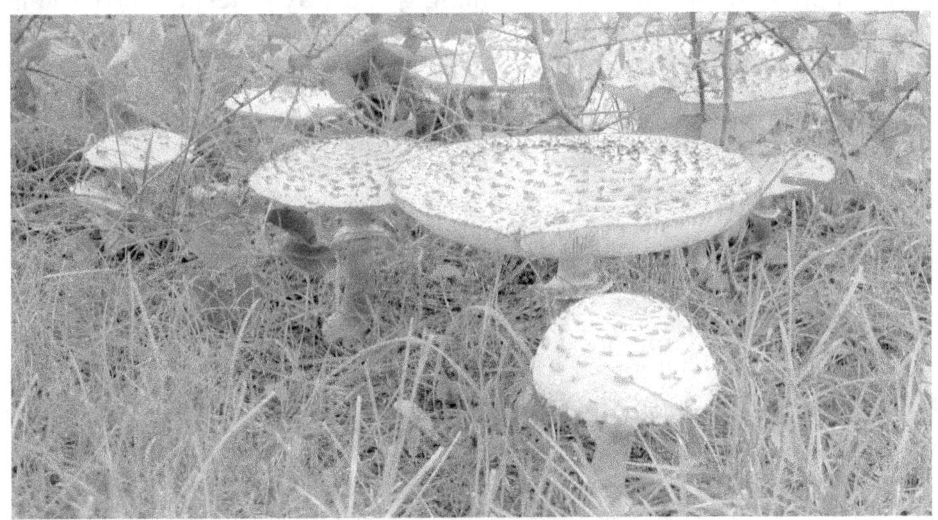

Macrolepiota procera

The relative safety of this and other medicinal mushrooms was compared to the chemotherapy drug 5-Fluorouracil (5-FU). Work by Arora et al, (2014) examined the anti-proliferative and cytotoxic effect on normal, kidney epithelial cells. The mushroom extracts led to minimum cell damage compared to chemotherapy drug 5-FU. No surprise there!

Like many medicinal mushrooms, the lipids of this species help increase erythrocyte membrane fluidity, suggesting benefit in treating hypertension and other cardiovascular disease related to decreased fluidity (Mujic et al., 2011).

Water soluble polysaccharides possess immune-modulating effects, stimulate probiotic co-cultures, and inhibit growth and biofilm development of *E. coli*, *Streptococcus mutans*, and *Salmonella enterica*. Georgiev et al, 2022.

Exposure to the toxin nonylphenol significantly affects male reproductive disorders and is found in human breast milk, urine and blood. These detergent-like substances are highly toxic to aquatic life, and are used in large volumes in laundry detergents, personal hygiene products, automotive, latex paint and lawn care.

A polysaccharide, derived from mycelium, remarkably improved oxidative stress, apoptosis, autophagy and inflammatory responses, and suppressed the Akt/mTOR signaling pathway in testicular tissue in mice. This suggests a possible treatment strategy for ameliorating the chemical exposure (Wang et al, 2002).

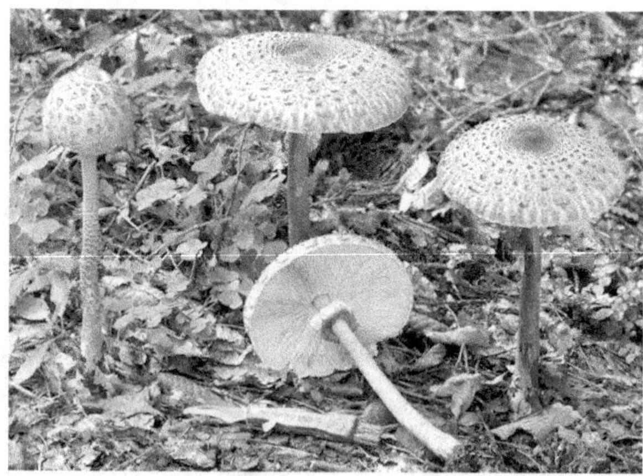

Macrolepiota procera courtesy of Daniel Winkler

PHELLINUS IGNIARIUS

(*Phellinus igniarius*)- Another Medicinal Mushroom Associated with Birch.

The birch tree attracts a number of important medicinal mushrooms including Chaga, or True Tinder Conk (*Inonotus obliquus*), False Tinder Conk (*Fomes fomentarius*), Birch Polypore (*Fomitopsis betulina*), and the oxymoronic Gilled Polypore (*Trametes betulina*).

The False Tinder Polypore (*P. igniarius*) may be added to this list, albeit the fungi also enjoy consuming willow and alder, hence another common name, Willow Bracket mushroom.

Various Arctic peoples decocted the fruiting body for stomachache and as a laxative, but it is better known as an ash, combined with tobacco, and known as Iqmik, meaning "thing to put in the mouth."

It is estimated that over 50% of First Nations adults in Yukon and Alaska mix the burnt fruiting body ash with finely cut tobacco to form pellets or quids, held in the mouth. The nicotine is delivered more rapidly to the brain.

Beautiful wood, bone, leather and ivory boxes were traditionally carved to hold the ash, which is widely available for purchase in the north.

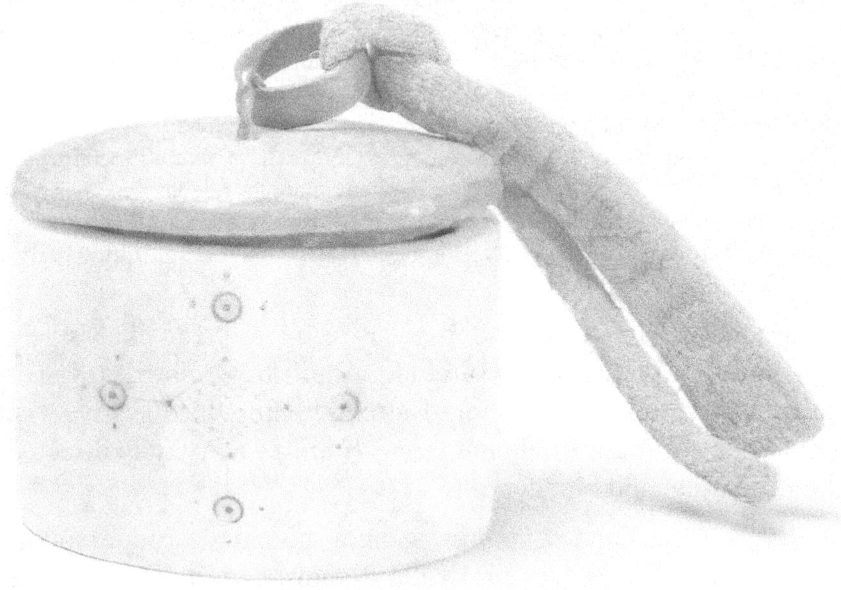

The work iqmik is derived from the Yupik people of western Yukon.

The pH of an iqmik mixture with tobacco is 10.9. The alkalinity delivers the tobacco alkaloids more readily to the brain. It may be prepared by drying the conk, and then incinerating to ash, in a tin can on a wood fire. The ash is mixed with finely cut or shredded tobacco, placed in mouth and chewed. It is often used by pregnant women, as a replacement for smoking tobacco, who believe it is safer, but in fact is worse, for both mother and fetus. It is definitely a concern for oral health, and mouth and throat cancers. The retail price in Alaska, as of May 2017 of the ash was $288 US per pound.

A good ethnomycology article on Iqmik by Pleninger (2009) is found in an early edition of *Fungi* magazine.

Recent work by Zhou LW et al, (2016) suggests that the *Phellinus igniarius* complex may include ten species in eastern Asia, eight in Europe, and six in North America, or fifteen species in the complex worldwide.

CONSTITUENTS-fruitingbody-3,4-dihydroxybenzaldehyde,4-(3,4-dihydrophenyl-3-buten-2 one, inonoblin C, phelligridin C-G, inoscavin C, interfungin A-C, hispolon, styrylpyrone-type polyphenols, inoscavin A-D, hypholomine B, naringenin, sakuranetin, aromadendrin, folerogenin, eriodictyol, coumarin, scopoletin, igniarius A-D, igiarens A-D, igniarine (tirucallane-type triterpenoid), meshimakobnol A & B, cyclophellitol, davallialactone, phelligridimers, syringic, caffeic and protocatehuic acids, iso-ergosterone, ergosterol, ergosterol peroxice, glutamic acid (1.2%). Mycelium culture- sesquiterpenoids 12-hydroxy-alpha-cadinol, 3alpha, 12-dihydroxy-delta-cadinol, 3alpha, 6alpha-dihydroxyspiroax-4-ene; steroids 3alpha, 17 alpha, 19,20-tetrahydroxy-4alpha-methylpregn-8-ene and 3alpha, 12alpha,17alpha,20-tetrahydroxy-4alpha-methylpregn-8-ene; fourteen cyclo-dipeptides, three sesquiterpenes, three steroids, N-acetyl-phenylalanine, adenosine, phenyldiethanol, o-hydroxy-phenyl ethanol, benzoic acid, p-methoxybenzoic acid, hexacanoic acid and 3-pyridinecarboxylic acid. Galactosamine is present, but not in fruiting body. Zeng H et al, (2016).

Traditionally, the fruiting body was used to treat excessive uterine bleeding, invigorate blood circulation and treat diarrhea. It is said to quench an appetite for alcohol by strengthening the digestive system. In Traditional Chinese Medicine, *Sang Huang*'s activity is directed to the liver meridian and bladder.

Both *Phellinus* and *Inonotus* genera contain large amounts of a styrylpyrone-type polyphenol yellow-colored pigment, thought to have a role similar to flavonoids in plants. They display anti-oxidant, anti-inflammatory, cytotoxic, anti-platelet aggregation, anti-diabetic, anti-dementia and anti-viral activity. Work by Lee & Yun (2011) looked in depth into their medicinal importance.

The decocted fruiting body shows activity against influenza A and B viruses, including 2009 pandemic H1N1, human H3N2, avian H9N2 and oseltamivir-resistant H1N1 viruses. It is suggested the extracts may interfere with early replication cycle, including attachment to the target cell. (Lee S et al, 2013).

Water extracts of the fruiting body show considerable anti-herpetic (herpes simplex virus 1) activity. (Dogan H.H. et al, 2018).

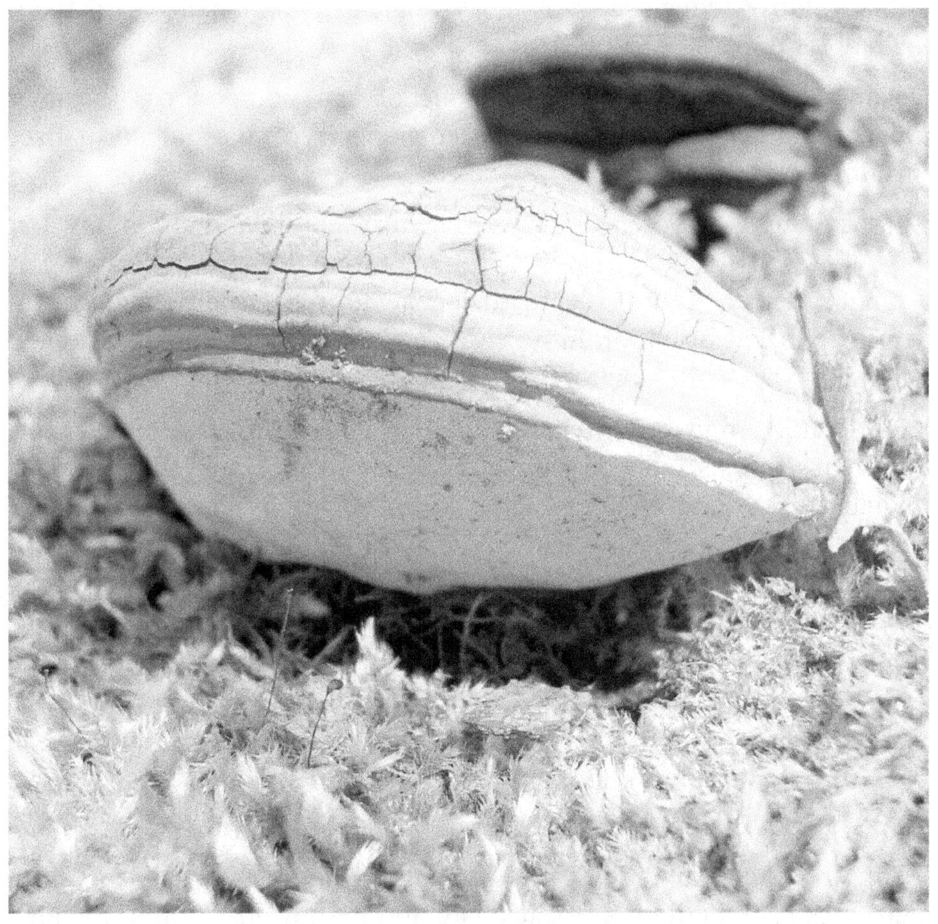

Phellinus igniarius

Work by Kim JY et al, (2016) looked at neuraminidase inhibitors from medicinal mushrooms. They found the fruiting bodies of *Phellinus igniarius* exhibit significant activity against neuraminidase from H3N2 influenza viruses. Phelligridins E & G, isolated from the fruiting body, were found to inhibit neuramindases from H1N1, H3N2, and H5N1 influenza viruses.

Various *Phellinus igniarius* strains were cultured, by submerged fermentation, in work by Zhu H et al, (2102). Inhibition of gram negative bacteria and Borellia species, associated with Lyme disease, was disrupted via anti-quorum sensing activity; inhibiting bacterial communication.

Hypholomine B, isolated from the fruiting body, has been found to inhibit aldose reductase, a pathway related to retinopathy in diabetic patients (Lee YS et al, 2008).

Zheng et al, (2017) found polyphenol-rich compounds, in mice, improved glucose tolerance, reduced hyperglycemia and normalized insulin levels.

Inoscavin A is a potent anti-inflammatory compound. Work by Lee SW et al, (2014) found significant, potent lipoxygenase inhibition, and Wang GJ et al, (2009) identified lanostanol-type triterpenoids in the fruiting body, that inhibit nitric oxide production. Both studies suggest significant anti-inflammatory activity.

One exciting find by Li et al, (2014) found a tincture injected into multiple sclerosis-induced female mice, profoundly decreased the daily incidence rate and clinical scores of encephalomyelitis. The authors suggest there is high therapeutic potential for ameliorating progression of this auto-immune disease. It may combine well with Hericium species for this condition.

Work by Suabjakyong P et al, (2015a) suggests polysaccharides of the fruiting body may help restore interleukin-6/interleukin-10 balance in the body. This disturbance is thought related to chronic inflammatory disease, obesity, type 2 diabetes, as well as mania and depression.

Polysaccharides from the mycelium were found by Li SC et al, (2015) to inhibit the growth of colon (SW480) and liver (HepG2) cancer cell lines. The authors suggest this could be developed into a natural carcinoma preventative agent and/or functional food.

The compound hispolon exhibits anti-tumor activity on lung cancer cell lines A549 and H661, through apoptosis (self-programmed death), inducing G0/G1 cell cycle arrest and other pathways. Hispolon enhanced expression of p53, an important gateway in the prevention and treatment of cancer. (Wu Q et al, 2014).

Hispolon may be useful to treat acute myeloid leukemia. In work by Hsiao PC et al, (2013), hispolon suppressed cell proliferation in various cell lines, including HL-60 leukemia cell lines.

A mouse study by Zhou et al, (2014) looked at the activity of a fruiting body extract on liver (H22) and melanoma (B16) cancer cell lines. Inhibition of cancer cell growth was noted, but the regulation appeared to occur in different pathways and antibody profiles.

In work by Rouhana-Toubi et al, (2009) the mycelium was subjected to ethyl acetate in order to extract low molecular weight compounds. Inhibition of human ovarian (ES-2) cancer cell growth was noted.

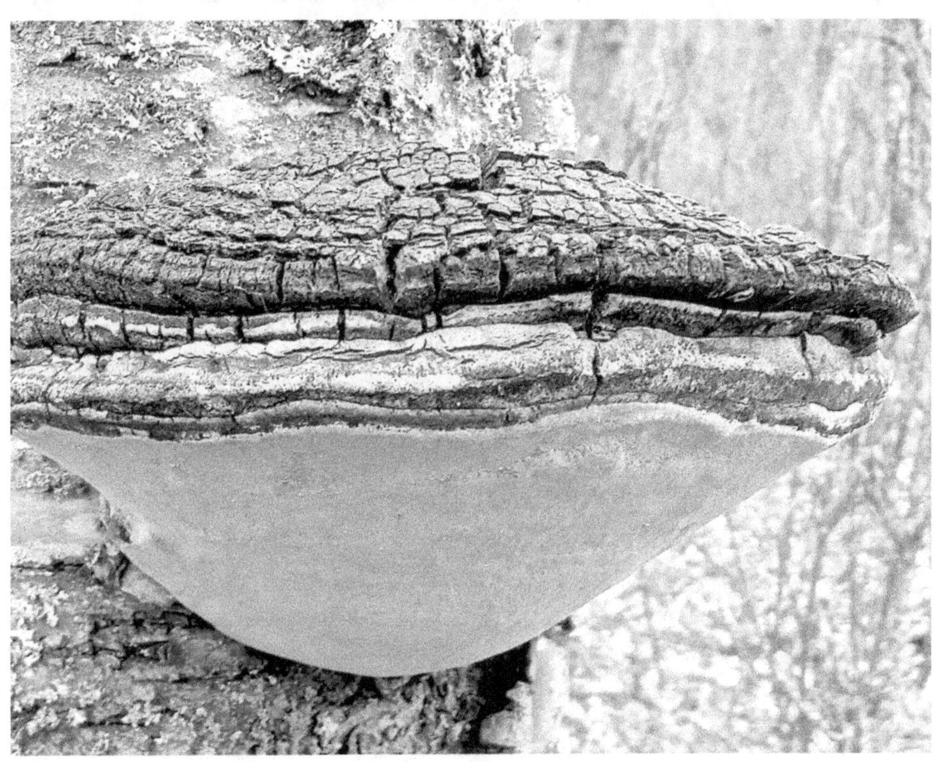

Phellinus igniarius

The same fraction showed strong inhibition of MGC-803 (gastric), BEL-7402 (hepatic), and MCF-7 (breast) cancer cell lines. The extract induced S-phase cell cycle arrest in the gastric cells, and apoptosis. (Wang et al, 2017)

Recent work by Smith et al, (2017) found potent inhibition of human cervix cancer cell lines from ethanol extracts.

Several sesquiterpenes, isolated from cultured mycelium, exhibit relaxing effects on phenylephrine-induced vasoconstriction. (Yin RH et al, 2015).

A tincture of the fruiting body was found, in another study, to inhibit hippocampal neuronal brain death following ischemia, suggesting use for ameliorating stroke induced neuron death in a clinical setting. (Kim JH et al, 2015).

A study by Suabjakyong et al, (2015b) looked at acrolein, produced by polyamines, as a major cause of cell damage. Ethanol extracts of the fruiting body prevent acrolein toxicity in mouse neuroblastoma cell lines. Various polyphenols in the fruiting body were identified.

Song TY et al, (2008) found ethanol extracts of the fruiting body inhibit the migration and invasion of hepatocarcinoma cell lines, and decreased vascular endothelial growth factor. Synergy with oxaliplatin or 5-flurouracil was noted, suggesting adjuvant possibilities with chemotherapy.

A recent study by Dong Y et al, (2016) found decoctions of the fruiting body increase both the production, and secretion of bile. In medical terms, the mushroom is both a choloretic and cholagogue.

Recent work by Jiang et al, (2018) identified new constituents from the fruiting body possessing anti-inflammatory activity.

The ash is prepared into a vibrational medicine and written about in *Mushroom Essences: Vibrational Healing from the Kingdom Fungi.* (Rogers 2016). Iqmak essence is associated with patterns of self-deprecation and fear of success. You can find out more at www.mushroomessences.com.

CAUTION - Do not use in patients with organ transplants, or combine with drugs that suppress the immune system. *Phellinus igniarius* MAY inhibit P450 enzymes, so caution with medications is advised.

PIOPINNO
VELVET PIOPINNO
BLACK POPLAR MUSHROOM
POPLAR FIELD CAP
(*Agrocybe aegerita* [Brig.] Singer)
(*Cyclocybe aegerita* Vizzini)

Piopinno is a very popular edible (nutty and crunchy) mushroom enjoyed around the world. It is easy to grow on hardwood chips and sawdust and commands a good price, especially when produced organically. In the suitable climate it grows on logs, generally fruiting in spring.

Piopinno is given name in Italy, where it is also called "fungus on a stick". Pliny the Elder, in Naturalis Historia Libri XIII, mentions its "cultivation."

In Japan it is known as Yanagi-matsutake, and in China, Tea Tree Mushroom. It is used in TCM for diuretic benefit.

This delicious mushroom is rich in compounds with health benefit.

A lectin identified by Zhao et al, (2003) exerts anti-tumor effect via apoptosis (self-programmed death) and DNase activity. Inhibition of human HeLa (cervical), SW480 (colon), three gastric (SGC-7901, MGC80-3, BGC-823), and HL-60 (leukemia) cancer cell lines were noted.

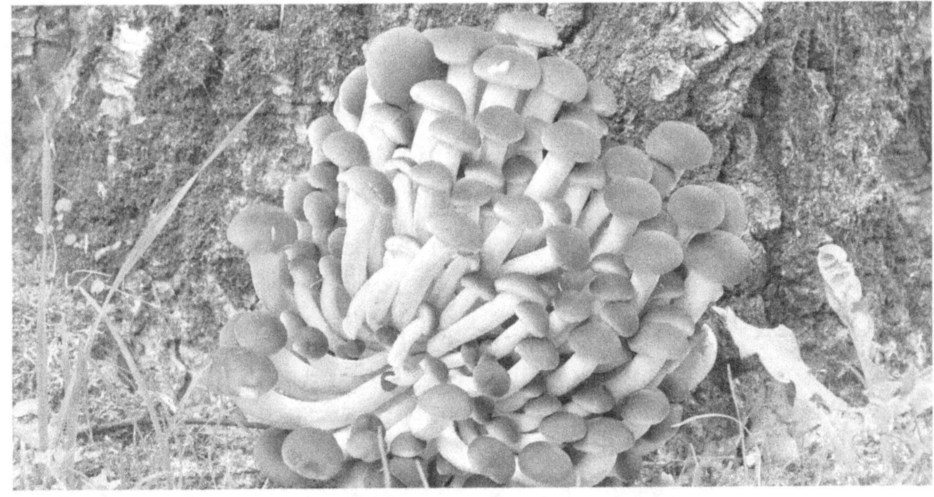

Agrocybe aegerita

Work by Liu et al, (2017) looked at the relationship between apoptosis and autophagy induced by lectins. They found inhibition of autophagy exerts a synergistic effect on the anti-tumor activity of the lectin, and may help reduce the dosage of lectin used in anti-tumor therapy. The autophagy inhibitor may also be synergistic with certain chemotherapy drugs that induce both apoptosis and autophagy.

A protein with deoxyribonuclease activity, derived from the fruiting body, possesses antitumor activity against various cancer cell lines (Chen et al, 2012).

A galectin alone, or in combination with anti-PD-1 (programmed cell death protein) significantly inhibited the growth of liver tumors. Increased expression of multiple cytokines and chemokines, and activation of T cells and macrophages was noted in work by Ye et al, (2021) on tumor-bearing mouse livers.

Galectin appears to recognize the 3'-sulfo-TF antigen in tumor cells, and may serve as a reagent for cancer diagnosis and targeted therapy for the antigen (Li et al, 2021).

Water-soluble fractions inhibit tumor growth, via different mechanisms. One fraction upregulated the mRNA level of Th2 cytokine interleukin-10, while another increased the mRNA level of granulocyte-macrophage colony-stimulating factor, and anti-inflammatory cytokine transforming growth factor-beta (Liang et al, 2014).

The mushroom contains a ribotoxin-like protein named ageritin, which has a prominent effect on cancer cell viability and no effects on eukaryotic and bacterial cells (Lampitella et al, 2021).

Ageritin exhibits cytotoxicity to COLO 320 (colon), HeLa (cervical) and Raji (lymphoma) cells by promoting apoptosis (Citores et al, 2019).

Ageritin shows promising anti-cancer properties vs. aggressive brain tumours (Landi et al, 2017).

When a polysaccharide from the fruiting body was combined with chemotherapy, it regulated immune function in rat esophageal carcinoma. Work by Ji et al, (2013) suggests this may be due to modulating cytokine activity, specifically down-regulation of TNF-alpha and upregulation of IFN-gamma.

Various peptides from the fruiting body exert hypotensive effect of 54% on angiotensin 1-converting enzyme (ACE-1). Optimal extraction was noted for 40:1 extract for three hours, at 30ºC and pH of 8 (Wu et al, 2010).

A novel serine protease shows anti-coagulation and fibrinolytic activity. Work by Li et al, (2021a) suggests the enzyme may be therapeutic for humans, in treating thrombosis, or as a functional food. The enzyme is both a plasmin-like fibrinolytic and plasminogen activator.

An alcohol extract inhibits *Pseudomonas aeruginosa* biofilm, and may be useful in other drug-resistant bacteria (Petrovic et al, 2014).

A lectin, isolated from the fruiting body, exhibits anti-viral activity in a mouse study. Inactivated virulent avian influenza (H9N2) was introduced alone, or with lectin at different levels. The IgG, IgG1 and IgG2a antibody levels were significantly increased in mice receiving both, compared to inactivated H9N2 alone. It appears the lectin adhered to the surface of the virus (Ma et al, 2017).

A follow-up study by Ma et al, (2018) suggests the lectin exerts immune adjuvant effects by promoting chemotaxis and phagotrophy activity of neutrophil leucocyte and macrophage, to improve innate immunity.

Both ethanol and water extracts reduce serum levels of uric acid, suggesting benefit in treating gout. A study on hyperuricemia mice found a significant reduction on xanthine oxidase (Yong et al, 2018). Due to the purine content of mushrooms in general, they are often recommended to be restricted in conditions of gout. But not piopinno!

Some work involves polysaccharides derived from mycelium. Water-soluble polysaccharides improve anti-oxidation, anti-aging and organ protection in mice, by decreasing lipid peroxidation and remitting lipid metabolism. Jing et al, (2018) suggest the polysaccharides be used in functional foods for the prevention and alleviation of aging and its complications.

Submerged culture has also revealed several terpenoids, including bovistol, bovistol derivatives B & C, and pasteurestin C. Bovistol B is cytotoxic, and was originally derived from Bovista (puffball) species (Surup et al, 2019).

PUFFBALL

> I found a giant puffball, weighing twenty pounds
> I took it home, sliced it into perfect juicy rounds,
> I fried each slice with ginger, and spices that I knew
> Served it up, gulped it down, it tasted like tofu.

> RDR (Rogers, 2011).

True story. I came upon a Giant Western Puffball (*Calvatia booniana*) in an open pasture, and the next morning took it down to a local television breakfast show contest, *Humungous Fungus*! And for that, I won a mushroom dinner for ten at an excellent Italian restaurant.

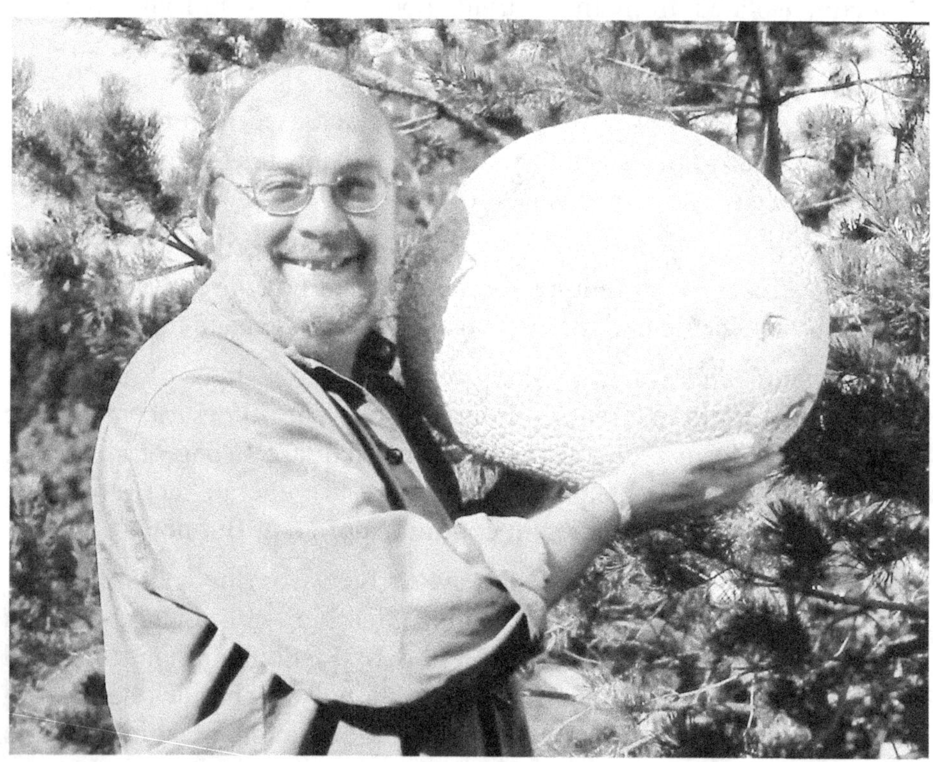

There are three main genera of puffballs, Calvatia, Bovista and Lycoperdon. The latter is amusing, as it translates roughly to "wolf fart", or "wolf breaking wind." In France, *pet de loup,* means "fart of the wolf", and from the Gaelic *puca* derives puckfist, meaning "fairy fart", a less noisy release of gas.

Calvatia is derived from the Latin *calvus,* meaning "bald."

Throughout the world, and in North America, various indigenous peoples used the dry immature centres, or mixed the spores with spider webs to staunch external bleeding, including cut umbilical cords. Other groups used the spores for assorted issues, including diaper rash, neck rashes, and mixed with grease for hemorrhoids and ringworm.

Members of the Blackfoot Confederacy consumed spore infusions for internal hemorrhage and bleeding. An interesting paper by William R. Burk (1983) recorded puffball usage among North American Indians.

Giant Puffball (*Calvatia gigantea*) was studied over 70 years ago for its content of clavacin, that inhibited sarcoma 180, mammary adenocarcinoma 755, leukemia L-1210 and HeLa cancer cell lines (Lucas et al. 1957). Research was discontinued due to toxicity against normal human cell lines.

This species is rich in protein (34.37%), but also contains gentisic acid, and trehalose (9.78g/100g), a unique sugar found in mushrooms, seaweed and condensed on Douglas Fir needles (Kivrak et al. 2016).

Work by Eroglu et al, (2016) found an extract from this species inhibits proliferation of A549 human lung cancer cell lines.

Methanol extracts were found, in vivo, to reduce blood glucose levels by 29.3%. (Ogbole et al, 2019).

Calvatia craniiformis is an edible, grapefruit-sized puffball, with a bright yellow gleba. Both water and methanol extracts reduced tumor mass in mice with transected hepatocellular carcinoma cell line on legs (Jameel et al, 2018). Immune modulation, induction of apoptosis, and anti-tumor activity was shown for both extracts.

The widespread Mosaic Puffball, *C. caelata* (*C. bovista/. C. utriformis*) contains a ubiquitin-like peptide that potently inhibited proliferation of spleen cells, but reduced by half the viability of breast cancer cell lines (Lam et al, 2001).

Extracts show inhibition of various bacteria including *Bacillus subtilis, E. coli, Klebsiella pneumoniae, Pseudomonas aeruginosa, Salmonella typhimurium, Staphylococcus aureus, Streptococcus pyogenes,* and *Mycobacteria smegmatis.*

Work by Dulger, (2005) found a 60% methanol extract exhibits inhibition similar to the antibiotic gentamycin.

Calcaelin, a protein isolated from this species, exhibits antimitogenic activity to mouse splenocytes, and reduced the viability of breast cancer cells (Ng et al. 2003).

Lilac-Spored Puffball (*C. lilacina*) contains protein extracts with efficacy against human colorectal adenocarcinoma (SW480) cells and human monocytic leukemia (THP-1) cell lines (Wu et al, 2011).

Earlier work by Tsay et al, (2009) identified a protein extract that induced cell programmed death in four human colorectal cancer cells. Glutathione depletion was found responsible for inducing apoptosis, rather than the ROS-mediated pathway.

Recent work by Zeng et al, (2021) found various extracts, from this species, inhibit the proliferation of lung (A549), colorectal (Caco-2), and breast (MDA-MB-231) cancer cell lines. Isolated fractions triggered severe cell death in the latter cell lines, by activating the apoptotic pathway dependent on mitochondrial reactive oxygen species and caspase activation.

The rare puffball, *C. nipponica* has been found to inhibit antiogenesis, via downregulation of VEGF, p38 and ERK signaling pathways. (Lee et al, 2017).

The same research team (Lee et al, 2020) identified cyathisterol, that suppressed cell viability induced by 17beta estradiol in MCF-7 breast cancer cell lines.

This puffball is reputed to possess aphrodisiac properties. Two compounds, isolated from the fruiting body, were evaluated for relaxation responses to precontracted penile corpus smooth muscle. The results suggest possible benefit in treating erectile dysfunction (Lee et al, 2020a).

Western Giant Puffball (*C. booniana*) mushroom essence relates to the development of ego and its relationship to bodily functions.

The oral stage, represented by sucking, drinking, and kissing, expresses receptivity and yielding. Any distortion of this early dependent reaction can lead to frustration. Biting, for example, expresses clinging, grasping and greed. Nail biting is one manifestation of this inner lack of comfort.

The anal phase was referred to as the sadistic phase by Freud and associated with aggression and self-assertion. There is an unconscious desire to turn an automatic response of the intestines into an accomplishment and increased independence.

Exposing the buttocks, known as mooning, is typically a masculine pursuit reflecting ego assertion against the feminine. It is an outward expression of fear associated with owning one's feminine.

As a reaction to early or harsh toilet training, a young child may hold back in rebellion. This later forms an adult who hates a mess, is obsessively tidy and punctual and respects authority. The anal character exhibits eight diagnostic features of the obsessive-compulsive personality disorder. Coprolalia (shit speech) is a prominent feature of Tourette's syndrome. Irritable bowel syndrome, for example, is associated with a high level of neuroticism, problems with self-assertion and reported history of abuse.

Urination represents yielding or controlling an outgoing libido stream. Golden showers, and chronic bladder infections may signal imbalance on this level.

The genital stage relates to initial self-arousal, and masturbation. It is the final stage of creating "I," and the original primitive magical all-identity is overcome.

Whitmont (1969) notes, "Masturbation expresses the final point of transition from narcissistic nondualistic participation to the relative freedom of dualistic consciousness." (Rogers, 2016: 176-178).

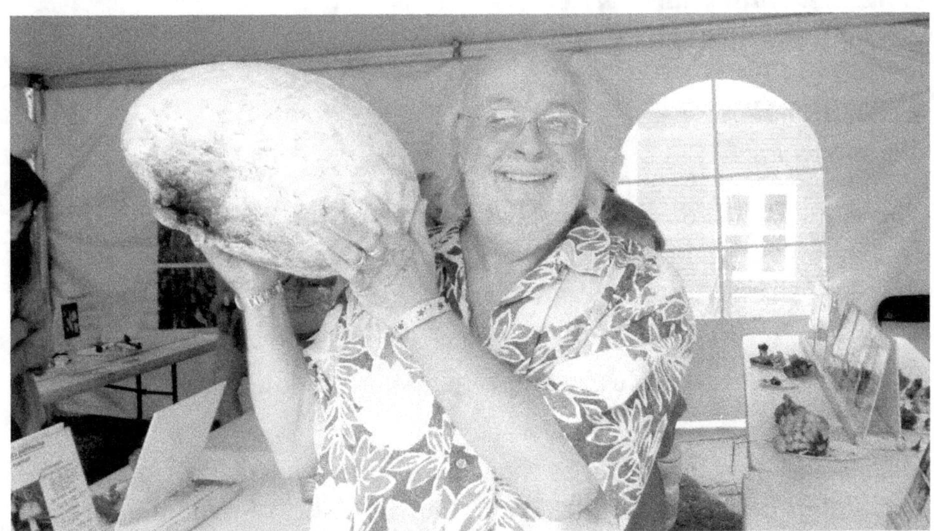

RAMARIA

Clumps of pink ramaria that weave
like coral ridges of convoluted brains
Sending messages through a
rooted intercom to tanoak, bay and fir.

Ruth Gunn Mota, from *The Forest Speaks*

CLUSTERED CORAL
CAULIFLOWER CORAL
PINK-TIPPED CORAL
(***Ramaria botrytis***)
FUZZY-FOOTED CORAL
(***R. cystidiophora***)
GOAT'S BEARD
CHANGLE
(***R. flava***)
SALMON CORAL
YELLOW-TIPPED CORAL
(***R. formosa***)
YELLOW-BROWN CORAL
(***R. flavo-brunnescens***)
FLACCID CORAL
(***R. flaccida***)
(***Phaeoclavulina flaccida***)
ORANGE CORAL
(***R. largentii***)
ACRID CORAL
(***R. botrytoides***)

The Coral, or Ramaria species, are some of the most beautiful fungi in the forest. At first glance they remind one of undersea creatures. Ramaria derives from the Latin, *ramus*, meaning "branch". Today, they are taxonomically clumped into *Gomphaceae* family.

Some are choice edibles, while others can be quite bitter, and others poisonous.

One of the most beautiful is the pink Cauliflower Coral, found under hardwoods and conifers throughout much of North America.

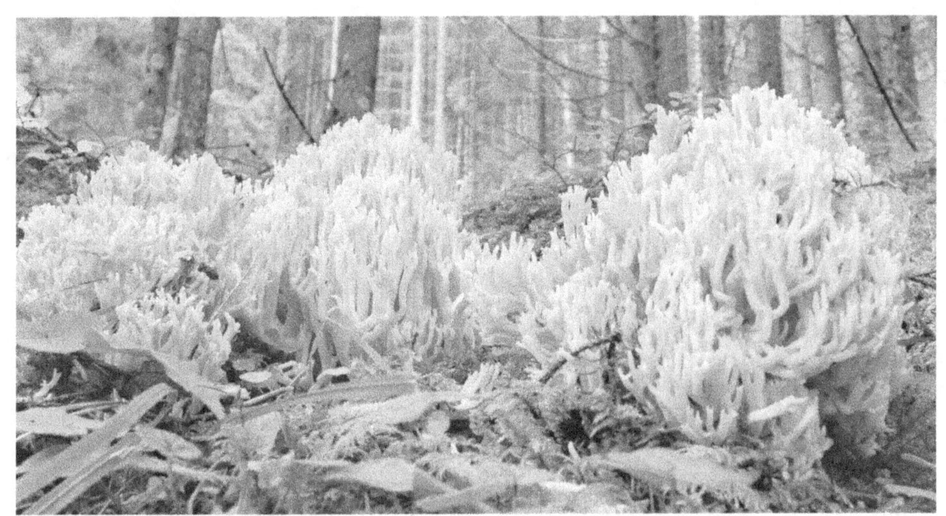

Ramaria aurea

Cauliflower Coral (*R. botrytis*) extracts exhibit activity against *Enterococcus faecalis* and *Listeria monocytogenes*; and show bactericidal effect on *Pasteurella multocida, Streptococcus agalactiae,* and *S. pyogenes* (Alves et al, 2012).

Clustered Coral shows inhibition of a number of human pathogenic bacteria, including *Escherichia coli, Klebsiella pneumoniae, Vivrio cholerae, V. alginolyticus, Pseudomonas aeruginosa* and *Streptococcus aureus*.

The fruiting body contains nicotianamine, a polyamine that inhibits angiotensin 1-converting enzyme (ACE), suggesting benefit in hypertension and other cardiovascular conditions. The water-soluble compound increases bioavailability of iron utilization (Rogers & Sept, 2020:81).

Polysaccharides show strong anti-oxidant and radical scavenging activity (Li, 2017).

A unique and novel anti-tumor protein has been isolated from the fruiting body in work by Zhou et al, (2017), and exhibits strong activity against A549 (lung) cancer cell lines. Both apoptosis, and hemagglutinating and Dnase activity are thought to be involved. Early work by Chung (1979) found inhibition of proliferation of HeLa (cervical carcinoma) cell lines, *in vitro*.

It contains a unique compound, pistillarin, that possesses significant lipid anti-oxidant activity (Sakemi et al, 2022).

Salmon Coral (*R. formosa*) contains a ribonuclease with HIV-1 reverse transcriptase inhibitory activity. The optimal extraction is at 60 degrees Celsius with a pH 5 (Zhang et al, 2015).

The fruiting body may have some application in acute respiratory distress and inflammation. Ramarin A and B, and other compounds inhibit human elastase, in vitro. It exhibits about 50% of activity from a compound in green tea, epigallocatechin gallate (EGCG). Kim et al, (2015).

Fuzzy-Footed Coral (*R. cystidiophora*) fruiting body contains four butenolides (ramariolides A-D). Ramariolide A, an unusual spiro oxiranebutenolide shows in vitro activity against *Mycobacterium tuberculosis*, and *M. smegmatis* (Centko et al, 2012). According to MacKinnon & Luther (2021:374) the "thick white mass of basal mycelium, may have a strong citrus or strong anise odor."

Work by Deo et al, (2019) on 17 mushrooms collected from Haida Gwaii, British Columbia, examined its anti-proliferative, immune stimulating and anti-inflammatory properties. Work at the University of Northern British Columbia, led by Dr. Chow Lee, continues to impress with their emphasis on bioregional mushroom medicine.

Goat's Beard is another choice edible mushroom. Work by Liu et al, (2013) found ethanol extracts moderately antibiotic, and highly anti-oxidant. The extracts exhibit very strong inhibition, in vitro, against breast cancer (MDA-MB-231) cell lines.

Goat's Beard (*R. flava*) possesses significant anti-oxidant and free radical scavenging effect, far greater than alpha tocopherol or synthetic preservatives BHA and BHT (Ozen et al, 2011).

Water extracts of the fruiting body show potential cytotoxic effects on HepG2 cancer cell lines, and some anti-bacterial activity (Sadi et al, 2016).

The polysaccharides act as prebiotic, stimulating *Lactobacillus rhamnosus*, and improving the production of short chain fatty acids (Zhou et al, 2022).

Orange Coral (*Ramaria largentii*) fruiting body not only possesses antioxidant activity, but is devoid of genotoxicity, and has a remarkable

DNA protective ability against hydrogen peroxide induced damage (Aprotosoale et al, 2017).

Flaccid Coral (*R. flaccida*) polysaccharides inhibit the growth of sarcoma 180 tumors, in vivo (Dong et al, 2020).

Acrid Coral (*R. botrytoides*) appears at first glance, like Cauliflower Coral, with a white color and pink/purple tips. Arora (1986:656) notes it is inedible, with an "exceedingly acrid taste that can linger in one's mouth for up to twelve hours after tasting it!"

Like other Ramaria species, it is anti-oxidant and shows activity against human HCC (hepatic) cancer cell lines (Rogers & Sept 2020:81).

Yellow-Brown Coral is found throughout North and South America. In my province of Alberta, the mushroom is listed as imperiled, and I have yet to find a specimen on my own, or on the tables at regional forays.

Scheid et al, (2022) published a review of mushroom poisoning of cattle and sheep from this mushroom growing under Eucalyptus trees in South America. It causes ulcerative lesions on the skin, tongue and esophagus, and loss of hair on the tip of tail. Sheep exhibit nervous symptoms on occasion.

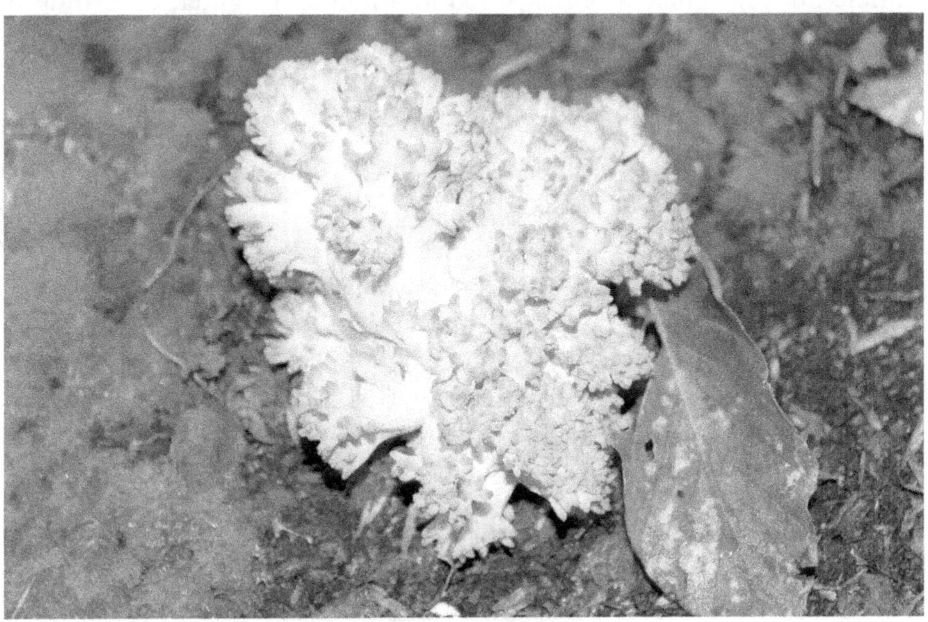

Ramaria botrytis

RED-BELTED CONK
(*Fomitopsis mounceae/F. ochracea*)

This beautiful, varnished red brown shelf fungus is one of the most common polypores in the world. It is often noted for its guttation drops, which taste salty and bitter. Licking the fruiting body is a ritual for both rookie and veteran medicinal mushroom foragers.

There are a few things to know about the name and confusing taxonomy of this fungus. *Fomitopsis* is derived from *fomes*, meaning "tinder, to burn, or heat up," as in foment; *pinicola* means "inhabiting pine." But I have observed it living with every deciduous and coniferous tree imaginable, so it is not really that picky, and associated with 83 softwood and 42 hardwood trees.

Here is the confusing part. *Fomitopsis pinicola* is very likely a European polypore, according to work by Haight et al, (2019). *Fomitopsis mounceae* and *F. ochracea* are found across North America. *Fomitopsis schrenkii* is found in the southwest regions of North America, and readily differentiated by DNA sequencing. *Fomitopsis mounceae* looks very similar to *F. ochracea*, but the latter lacks red coloration, and the cuticle does not melt when exposed to a flame of lighter, according to mushroom guru Daniel Winkler.

The Blackfoot of Alberta put the dried polypore in a buffalo horn, along with a live coal from the fire when moving camp. They used a piece of the fungus as a purgative and thought that too large a dose would turn the hair gray, hence the name *APOPIKATISS* ("makes your hair gray") (Johnston, 1987). Red-belted Conk is known as *MECH QUAH TOO* (Red Touchwood) by the Cree of eastern Canada. The fruiting body was traditionally dried and powdered to stop wounds and bleeding. A half teaspoonful of the powder was put in water and steeped, then swallowed as an emetic for purification (Hobbs, 1995). Traditionally, a decoction was ingested as a daily tonic to reduce inflammation of the digestive tract, and increase general resistance.

The Northern Dene cut the fungus into small chunks and smoked it with tobacco to treat headaches. The Iroquois differentiated polypores, according to the tree upon which they grow. As a group they were called *UNÄ'SA* preceded by the tree name.

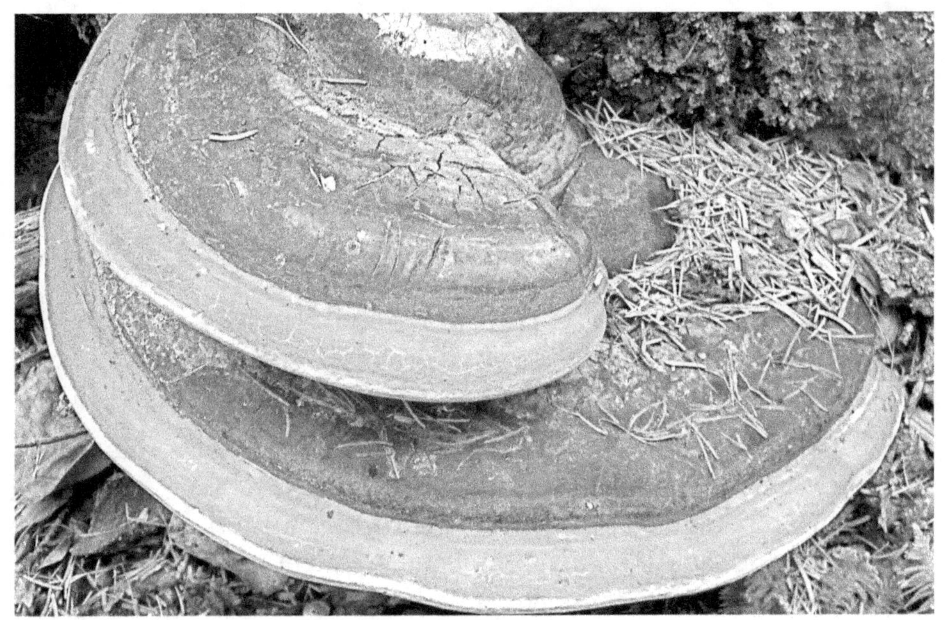

Red Belted Conk

Various polypores including Red-belted Conk, *Grifola frondosa*, and *Laetiporus sulphureus* were boiled and used to flavor soups. There are isolated reports of boiling the conks until edible, but that would be a tough chew—at least with mature specimens. It was probably a case of an alternative to stone soup, with other ingredients providing the nourishment. Or more likely, the polypore acts as an anti-bacterial that preserves the soup from spoilage, and gives everyone an immune boost, especially in winter.

CONSTITUENTS - ergosterol, 3 compounds related to trametenolic acid, polyporenic acid C, ergosta-7, 22-dien-3beta-ol, fungisterol, eburicoic acid, lanosterol, inotodiol, 21-hydroxylanosta-7, 9(11)-24-trien-3-on, 21-hydroxylanosta-7, 9(11)-24-trien-3b,21-diol, 3a-oxylanosta-8,24-dien-21-oleic acid, 5, 6-dihydroergosterol and pinicolic acid.

Other constituents include pachymic acid, pinicolol B, polycarpol, six nucleoside-type compounds including cytidine, adenosine monophosphate (AMP), adenosine diphosphate (ADP), adenosine, inosine, and thymidine. In the top layer of the fruiting bodies: lanostane derivatives and triterpenes, including (+)-pinicolic acid A, and (+)-trametenolic acid. Concentration of these compounds in the surface layer of fruiting body is higher than the rest of fungus, and lower in young fungus compared to more mature.

In Japan, the mushroom is known as TSUGASA RUNO KOSHIKAKE. The conk is considered a cancer preventative, albeit not supported by any human clinical trials.

There has been quite a bit of research on this fungus, under the name *F. pinicola.*

Solid state fermentation of *F. pinicola* on wheat bran increased the antioxidant capacity by 5.7 times, reduced phytic acid content, and increased its protein, total phenols and alkylresorcinols content. This suggests a novel way to convert wheat bran into a more nutritious cereal food ingredient (Tu et al, 2020).

The polypore contains a number of anti-histamine vegetable sterols with application in skin preparations. The oils exhibit circulatory stimulating properties and contain C14–C18 fatty acids with moisturizing properties. Various amino acids regulate moisture content and octadecanoate exhibits surface cell immune stimulation. Various capric/caprylic triglycerides may be useful in day and night creams, cleansing milks and liquid soaps.

An oil-soluble red dye can be extracted as well.

Red-belted Conk contains polysaccharides with moderate tumor inhibition, and immune modulating properties. A 30 mg daily dosage showed, in vivo prevention rate of 51.2% against sarcoma 180 solid cancer cells (Shibata et al, 1968). It can be used daily as a tonic to reduce inflammation of the digestive tract, and increase resistance to disease. The polypore has been widely used for persistent, intermittent fevers, chronic diarrhea, periodic neuralgia, nervous headaches, excessive urination, jaundice as well as chills and fevers. During the 1800s, the polypore was soaked in whiskey as a remedy for shivering chills and fevers associated with colds and flu (Vermeulen, 2007). Austrian studies, by Dresch et al, (2015) found anti-bacterial activity against *Bacillus subtilis* and *Staphylococcus aureus.*

Alkaline extracts of the fruiting body show regulation of blood sugar via increased insulin secretion, or prevention of STZ-induced pancreatic damage (Sang Il-Lee et al, 2008).

Work by Wol-Suk Cha et al, (2009) found extracts may be useful for preventing and treating liver and kidney problems associated with diabetes and hyperlipidemia. A recent study by Zahid et al. (2020) fed different doses of water and ethanol extracts (EE) to streptozotocin-induced diabetic rats. Results concluded EE at 300 mg/kg was more hypoglycemic, hyper-insulinemic, anti-oxidant, and anti-hyperlipidemic than control, diabetes mellitus control and metformin. Increased insulin secretion helped regulate high blood sugar. Human implications are as yet unknown.

The fruiting bodies may be useful as a functional food or treatment for diabetes, due in part to glucose uptake in insulin-resistant HepG2 cells (Zhang et al, 2020). Various lanostane triterpenoids and their glycosides were investigated for COX-1 and COX-2 inhibition, suggesting potent anti-inflammatory benefit. (Yoshikawa et al, 2005). Extracts reduce IP-10 inflammatory process, and show anti-tumor potential (Cheng et al, 2008). The ethanol extract induces cell apoptosis, suggesting anti-tumor activity in vivo and in vitro.

Red-belted Conk extracts show activity, both in vitro and in vivo, against various cancer cell lines, significantly greater than *Ganoderma sinense* and Agarikon (*Laricifomes officinalis*) (Wu et al, 2014). A methanol extract inhibits human leukemia (THP-1) and colon adenocarcinoma (HT29) cell lines, and varying degrees of effects against a variety of pathogenic fungi (Angelini et al, 2018). A triterpenoid extracted from fruiting body induces HeLa (cervical) cancer cell apoptosis through a caspase-mediated pathway (Li et al, 2018).

Work by Ren et al. (2006) found ether and ethyl acetate extracts of this polypore exhibit significant cytotoxic effect against human cervical and hepatoma cancer cell lines.

Various triterpenoids and triterpene sugar esters exhibit in vitro cytotoxic effects against five human cell lines, including apoptosis of HL-60 cells (Peng et al, 2019). A study of thirty various polypores by Macáková et al. (2010) found Red-belted Conk exhibited the highest free radical scavenging activity of all. The results were not correlated, as is the usual case, with phenolic content of the extracts. This suggests significant anti-oxidant potential.

All or some of the above research may be invalid, as *F. pinicola* is now considered a European, or perhaps Asian species. Some in vitro work involved wild-harvested fruiting bodies derived from North America. A review by Bishop (2020) found only three in vivo studies, with two finding inhibition of tumor growth and prolonged survival rates in mice.

The conk has a slightly bitter, sweet, moistening and warming nature. It is contraindicated for menopausal flushing, or choleric constitutions with liver heat, gall bladder irritation, or inflammation. Avoid its use in the early phases of feverish states. It works well as a daily warm tea for chronic arthritis or bone-deep coldness, helping move circulation and restore vitality and lubrication to affected areas. In clinical practice I found both tea and tinctures useful for various autoimmune conditions, including Sjögren's syndrome, and rheumatoid arthritis. Red-belted Conk is useful in intermittent, remittent and bilious fevers, with headache, yellow tongue, constant nausea, faintness at epigastrium, and constipation. *Fomitopsis pinicola* is indicated for an impaired immune system, and prostate adenoma.

The fungus contains several volatiles including (R)- and (S)-oct-1-en-3-ol (49%) octan-3-one and various sesquiterpene hydrocarbons including beta barbatene, alpha pinene, camphene, gamma cadinene, trans calamenene, and aromatic compounds including furfural, benzaldehyde, phenyl acetaldehyde, and 2-pentylfurane, in studies by Rosecke et al, (2000) and Fäldt et al, (1999).

Cosmetic oils, derived from the fruiting body help restore skin health in the form of creams, salves and lotions. See recipe below. Noted herbalist, Darcy Williamson, steam-distills the conks and produces a wonderful hydrosol. She suggests it is useful for liver and bowel conditions, stating "Red-belted Conk hydrosol acts as a tonic to reduce inflammation of the digestive tract and has proven effective in some cases of Irritable Bowel Syndrome. This fungus has also been used to treat jaundice and liver dysfunctions."

Red-belted Conk mushroom essence is associated with responsibility and flexibility. Being responsible for our actions is the cornerstone of a life filled with integrity. Flexibility exhibits the virtue of discernment Rogers (2016).

Preparations

For tinctures, thinly slice the fresh polypores and make a 1:5 tincture with 95% alcohol. Let sit for two weeks, shaken daily. Remove the alcohol and squeeze the marc dry. Take this dry material and make a 1:10 decoction. Slowly simmer (70°C) to one-third, cool, strain and combine the two. Dosage is 2–4 ml daily or more for chronic conditions.

For cosmetic oil, combine thinly sliced polypores at 1:5 with a good monosaturated vegetable oil in crock pot. Set at lowest heat and simmer slowly for 4–6 hours. Remove from heat, squeeze well in cheesecloth and preserve with contents of one 800 IU natural vitamin E capsule for each liter of oil. This is a fantastic skin conditioner.

For decoctions, larger pieces can be chopped into half inch slices, so that more surface area is exposed. I use an electric planer to slice paper-thin strips. Freshly harvested fruiting bodies can be carefully sliced with sharp knife. It must be simmered for at least one-half hour to extract the active constituents. twenty to thirty grams twice daily in soup or tea.

For cultivation, work by Du et al. (2020) found optimal culture of mycelium at 31°C and pH 6. A substrate combination of 20% corn cob, 30% sawdust, 20% wheat bran, etc., produced highest yield of fruiting bodies, which take about seven months to develop.

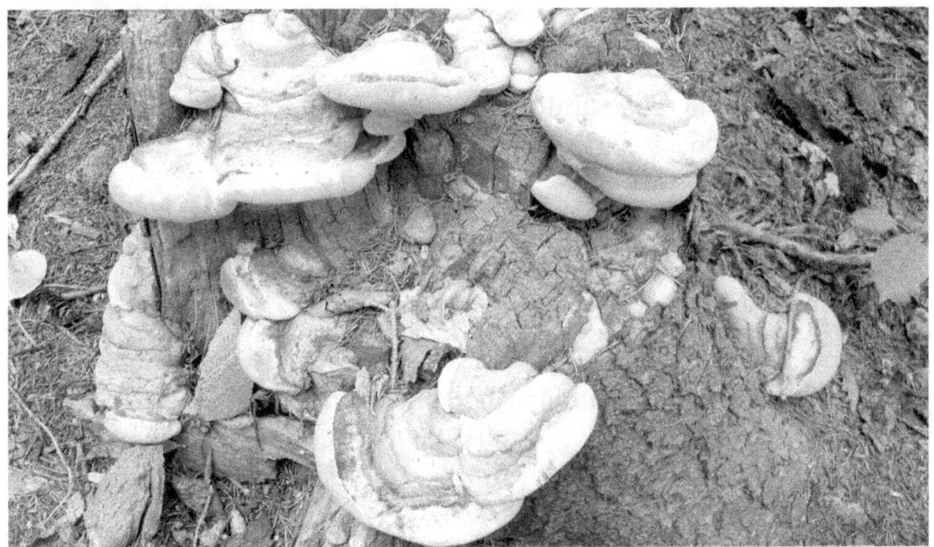

Fomitopsis mounceae

RED POLYPORE
(*Pycnoporus sanguineus*)
(*P. cinnabarina var. sanquinea*)
(*Trametes sanguinea*)
CINNABAR RED POLYPORE
(*P. cinnabarinus*)
(*T. cinnabarina*)

Back in 2005, I was invited to southern Alberta as a plant identification expert. The trip was replete with excessive rain and numerous other challenges. But I did find and photograph a Cinnabar Red Polypore growing on an alder. I used the photo for the front cover of my self-published (now out of print) *The Fungal Pharmacy: Medicinal Mushrooms of Western Canada*, the following year. Nothing like limiting your reader audience!

Both are hardwood white rot saprophytes. Blood Red polypore is tropical, while Cinnabar is widespread and found worldwide.

Both polypores are used in TCM to reduce fevers, swellings and dampness. A decoction is recommended for arthritis, rheumatism and gout, and well as various fungal infections, both internal and external.

In Malaysia, where known as Chendawan Merah, the fruiting body is taken internally for dysentery, and powder applied to staunch bleeding and prevent infections.

Indigenous people of Australia sucked on the polypore for sore mouth, and rubbed it in baby's mouth for thrush and painful teething (Rogers, 2011:403).

Red Polypore is cytotoxic to Caco-2 and HT-29 colon epithelial cancer cell lines, with IC_{50} values of 81 and 31 µg/ml, respectively (Doskocil et al, 2016).

Earlier work by Ren et al, (2006) found various extracts cytotoxic to HeLa (human cervical epitheloid) and SMMC-7721 (human hepatoma) cancer cell lines.

Submerged cultures produce an extracellular fluid with anti-oxidant and anti-bacterial activity, including *Vibrio fischeri*, and *Staphylococcus aureus* (Jascek et al, 2015).

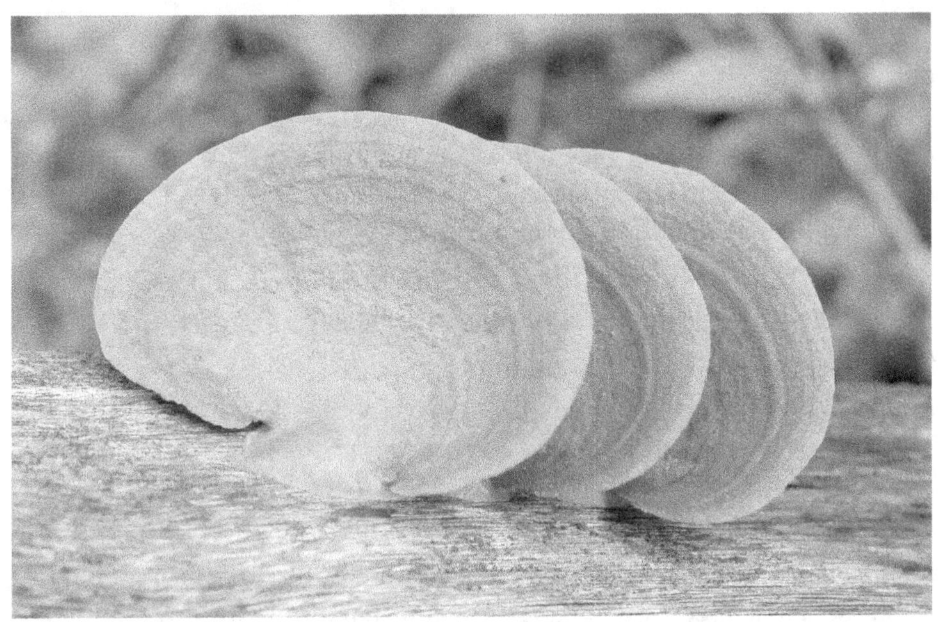

Pycnoporus sanguineus

One compound, lambertellin, significantly inhibited the expression of inducible nitric oxide synthase, and cyclooxygenase 2 (COX-2), suggesting anti-inflammatory properties. It also decreased expression of pro-inflammatory cytokines IL-6 and IL-1B. Lambertellin modulates mitogen activated protein kinase (MAPK), and nuclear factor kappaB signaling pathways (Jouda et al, 2018).

A polysaccharide from Blood Red Polypore shows promise for alleviation of inflammatory bowel disease (IBD) including colitis. A study by Li et al, (2020) looked at the potential in a murine colitis model, and found a polysaccharide upregulated the expressions of Zonula occludens, E-cadherin and proliferating cell nuclear antigen. Most interesting is that it inhibited the helper T cells mediated immune response by decreasing the proportions of Th cells, including Th2, Th17 and regulatory T cells. It also inhibited autophagy to help restore epithelial tissue.

In a double dip of research papers, the same team found ethanol extracts displayed remission of colitis-related inflammation by suppressing Th cells via induction of self-programmed death (apoptosis). (Chen et al, 2020).

When cultured in cow milk, extracts induced apoptosis in HT-29, LS180 and SW948 colon cancer cell lines (Piet et al, 2021).

A water, and then, ethanol extraction of polysaccharides from *Trametes sanguinea*, exhibited strong inhibition on migration, invasion and tube formation of human umbilical vein endothelial cells. This suggest possible benefit in tumor therapy (Yan et al, 2022).

Laccase, from Cinnabar Red polypore produces cinnabarinic acid, which shows inhibition of Gram-positive bacteria (Eggert, 1997).

Polyporin, derived from cultured Blood Red and Cinnabar Red mycelium, and water extracts of fruiting bodies show activity against *Staphylococcus aureus, S. albus, Streptococcus salivarius, Pseudomonas aeruginosa, Salmonella paratyphi, E. coli, Klebsiella pneumoniae, Vibrio cholerae* and *Shigella paradysenteriae.*

Cinnabarin acid is active against Gram-positive bacteria including *Streptococcus* species. Cinnabarin is anti-bacterial, anti-viral and anti-fungal, and possess a basic ring-like structure similar to acitomycin D, an antibiotic used in cancer treatment. At very low dose it reduced rabies virus levels, four-fold (Smania et al, 2003).

The Blood Red Polypore contains significant amount of organic germanium (800-2000 ppm). In fact, this valuable micro-mineral is found in various medicinal mushrooms, including shiitake.

When first introduced in the late 1980s as a supplement, it was reported nephrotoxic, based on several studies with germanium dioxide and germanium lactate citrate (both inorganic). During this time frame Goodman (1988), published a paper on its efficacy in treating arthritis, osteoporosis and cancer. Studies found anti-viral, and immune benefit, including induction of interferon, macrophages, T-suppressor cells and augmentation of natural killer cell activity.

Recent work by Reddeman et al, (2020) found pure germanium sesquioxide, an organic form of the naturally occurring trace element, non-toxic in several studies.

A randomized, DB PC eight-week trial of 130 subjects found increased natural killer cell activity, and activation of immunoglobulin, B cells and tumor necrosis factor-alpha. Control group showed no change. (Cho et al, 2020).

Fans of *Cordyceps militaris* will be pleased to note the benefit of germanium enriched cultivation of the fruiting body (Wang et al, 2015).

MYCO-REMEDIATION

Fungal laccases are increasingly useful to remove harmful organic compounds from water systems.

For example. Laccases from Blood Red polypore myco-transform endocrine-disruptor compounds such as bisphenol A, 4-nonylphenol, 17-a-ethynylestradiiol and triclosan from ground water (Garcia-Morales et al, 2015). In comparison to purified laccases, the fungal enzyme cocktail is highly efficient, without requiring any additional purification steps.

Enzyme cultures of this mushroom remove 98.5% ciprofloxacin, 96.4% norfloxacin, and 100% sulfamethoxazole within two days (Gao et al, 2018).

The waste water discharged from pharmaceutical production of antibiotics is a major, largely unregulated, environmental and ecological concern.

Prozac, a SSRI anti-depressant drug has been found in west coast salmon.

These are just two examples of this one mushroom's ability to help clean up industrial contamination of our planet.

Blood Red polypore has been used in the alkaloid transformation of thebaine to 14-hydroxy-codeinone, obtaining a 40% yield

Thebaine is derived from modified poppies that cannot yield heroin or morphine, but can lead to production of codeine, oxycodone, and hydromorphone.

Although Purdue Pharma and others have been widely blamed, shamed and fined for the present opiate crises, the story goes back much further.

Johnson & Johnson (The Family Company) were looking for a source of codeine for their Tylenol Codeine product. They incentified farmers in Tasmania, off the south coast of Australia to begin production of the so-called Norman Poppy. Through two subsidiaries, Tasmanian Alkaloids and Noramco, they controlled 85% of the world's production of thebaine that is easily converted to oxycodone.

Between 1994 and 2015, the DEA allowed the amount of oxycodone into the country to increase by 3600%.

In 2016, J & J, sold off their two subsidiaries, but an Oklahoma court found them responsible for the opioid epidemic in the state and fined the company $575 million. Peanuts, as the company shares rose the following day.

Thebaine is still used for the production of hydromorphone for the relief of chronic pain, as well as naloxone to treat opioid addiction. It reminds one of the nicotine patch, and gum produced, and sold, to help wean consumers of smoking tobacco. Profits either way, as long as market share is maintained.

Deaths, related to addiction in the United States, now top 100,000 persons annually, or 274 individuals a day.

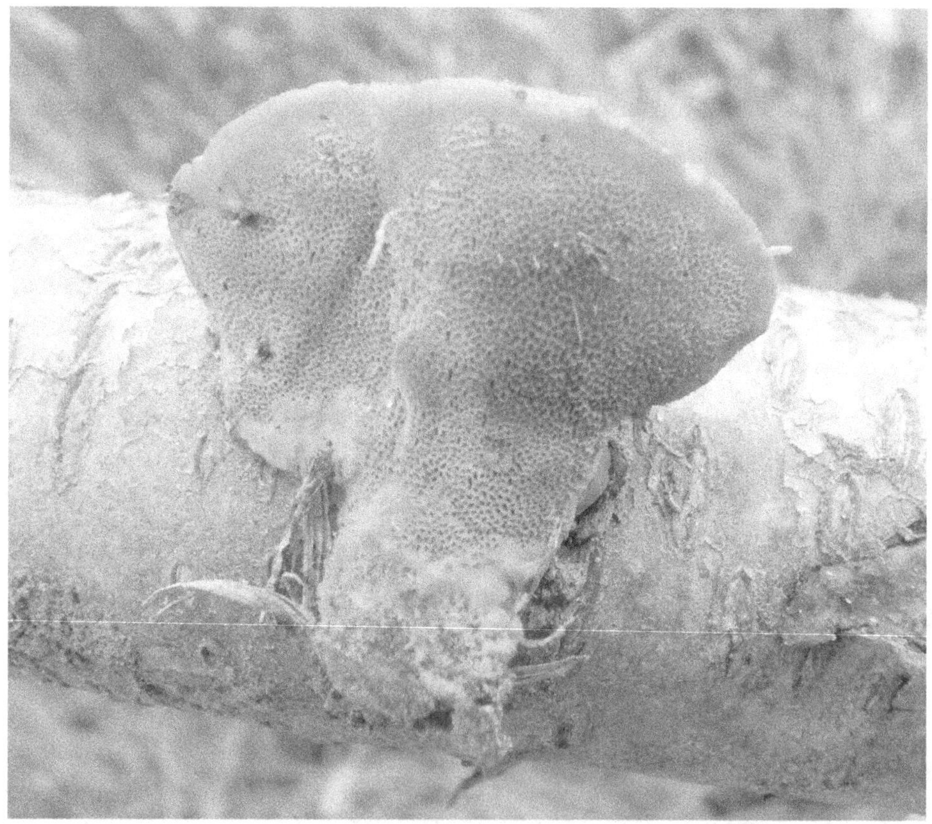

Pycnoporus cinnabarinus

RUSSULA

The mention of the genus Russula to mycologists will either produce a smile or a frown. Two sides of the edibility coin.

Identification of North American species is ongoing and ever changing due to DNA sequencing. Michael Kuo suggests sorting out the species, "is a joke."

There are several species I particularly enjoy eating, including The Shrimp (*R. xerampelina*), and Green Quilted (*R. virescens*).

The Shrimp Russula has demonstrated, in vitro, activity against malaria-inducing *Plasmodium falciparum* (Lovy et al, 1999).

The latter contains polysaccharides which inhibit alpha-glucosidase and alpha-amylase, suggesting hypoglycemic activity. They also suppress HepG2 (hepatic), A549 (non-small cell lung), and MCF-7 (breast) cancer cell lines, and mediate cellular immune response, in vitro (Li et al, 2021).

Chrome Yellow Russula, also known as Yellow Swamp Brittlegill (*R. claroflava/R. flava*) is edible, with a pleasant vanilla or coumarin-like odor. Studies have found gold levels of 136 nanograms per gram in fruiting body. Organic gold may be useful in depression and rheumatoid arthritis (Rogers, 2011:375).

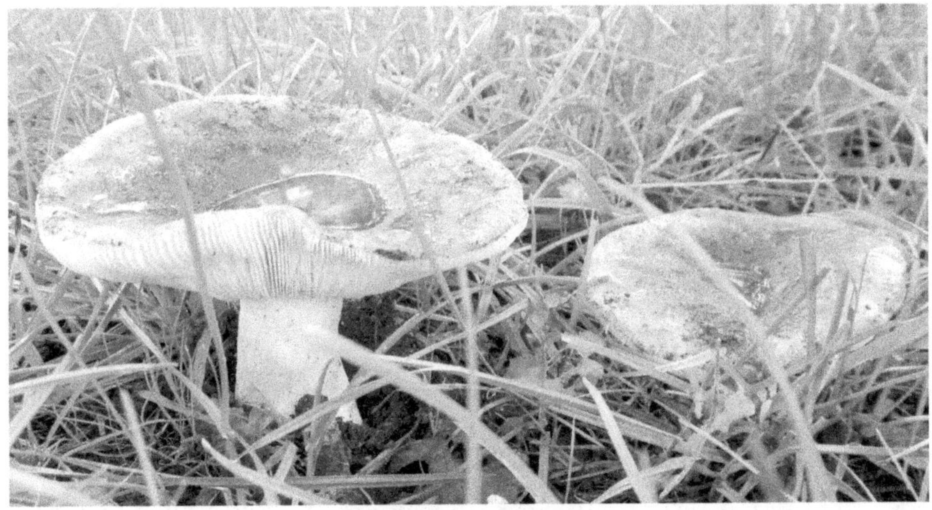

Russula xerampelina

I avoid several species, including The Sickener (*R. emetica*), Blackening Russula (*R. nigricans*), and the deadly Rank Russula (*R. subnigricans*). David Arora (1986:90) suggests the latter is "better trampled than sampled", and contains an unstable toxin only recently identified. Work by Matsuura et al, (2016) suggests cyclopropylacetyl-(R)-carnitine may be the culprit. This is an Asian species, known in Japan as Nisekurohatsu, and responsible for rhabdomyolysis, which breaks down skeletal muscle. The mycoglobin released results in kidney failure and death within twenty-four hours. The COVID pill from Pfizer, Paxlovid contains ritonavir, which combined with anti-cholesterol medications such as lovastatin, can lead to the same life-threatening breakdown of muscle fibres.

Rank Russula poisoning was treated with a Reishi (*Ganoderma lucidum*) 1:6 decoction in one human study (Xiao et al, 2003). Fourteen patients given the tea improved clinically at an improved rate over the eleven control patients. Kidney, liver and cardiovascular markers, as well as blood in urine, all improved significantly in treated group. Note: This is not recommended, simply noted, as there is presently no antidote for this toxin.

Rank Russula was once believed in California, but this mushroom turns out to be *R. cantharellicola*, which reddens but does not turn black. It is also not recommended as edible, for it may contain similar toxins, but no one knows.

Emetic Russula (*R. emetica*) polysaccharides, extracted by ultrasound, exhibit high antidiabetic (56.3%) and anti-hypertensive (70.5%) inhibition (Kaewnarin et al, 2020). It smells fruit-like, and in Hungary and Slovakia the skin is removed, dried and flavors goulash. The rest of mushroom is discarded.

Blackening Russula contains a most unusual compound, dichloroacetic acid. This is generally considered a pollutant due to water disinfection (Lajin et al, 2021). The fruiting body contains 80% ergosterols, and nigricanin, an ellagic acid generally found in strawberries and raspberries. I find it commonly in northern Alberta, and is eaten by some members of my mycology group. Not me.

I have sampled Short-Stalked Russula (*R. brevipes*)- noted by Arora as "better kicked than picked," but much prefer it when parasitized by

Hypomyces lactifluorum DNA, and transformed into the choice edible Lobster Mushroom (Lapierriere et al, 2018).

This is not to say Short-Stalked Russula is without merit. Ethanol extracts inhibit *Bacillus subtilis* (Niazi et al, 2021). In the same study, the edible Green Russula (*R. aeruginea* exhibited enhanced anti-fungal activity.

My true fascination with mycology extends to health and medicinal benefits.

Russula delica shows 53.1% inhibition on *Proteus mirabilis* biofilm formation. This drug-resistant bacterium is a leading cause of difficult to treat urinary infection, and death in nursing homes. It also inhibits *Acinetobacter baumannii* biofilm, but with only 29% efficacy (Alves et al., 2014).

This species also inhibits the growth of gram-negative bacteria, such as *Escherichia coli*, *Morgaella morganni*, and *Pasteurella multocida*; and gram-postive species such as *Staphylococcus aureus*, methicillin-resistant SA, *Enterococcus faecalis*, *Listeria moncytogenes*, *Streptococcus agalactiae* and *S. pyogenes* (Alves et al, 2021).

Work by Zhao et al, (2010) found the fruiting body contains an anti-proliferative ribonuclease, inhibiting both HepG2 and MCF-7 cancer cell lines.

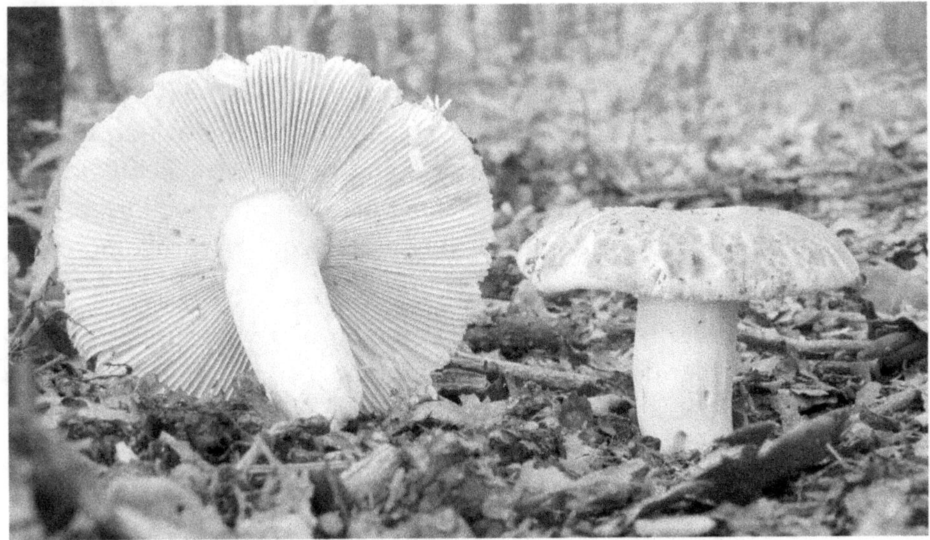

Russula virescens

Water extracts of *Russula delica*, *R. laurocerasi*, and Blackening Russula (*R. albonigra*), in work by Mallick et al, (2014) inhibit *Leishmania donovani*, a parasitic protozoan. Although edible, the latter is "better punted than hunted", according to Arora (1986).

Water soluble heteroglycans from this mushroom show in vitro macrophage activation, as well as splenocyte and thymocyte proliferation (Nandi et al, 2013).

Russula nobilis, formerly *R. mairei*, and the bitter Geranium-scented Russula (*R. fellea*) exhibit anti-inflammatory effects, decreasing production of nitric oxide and IL-6, in vitro (O'Callaghan et al, 2015). Both are poisonous, but not deadly.

Do not confuse *M. mairei* with Powdered Russula (*R. mariae*), a commonly found, but mediocre edible found in hardwood forests of eastern North America.

Hot water decoctions of the bitter, Red-Capped, or Bog Russula (*R. paludosa*) inhibit HIV-reverse transcriptase activity by 97.6% (Wang et al, 2007).

A lectin from *R. delica* also exhibited similar activity with an IC50 of 0.26 microM; and potently inhibited HepG2 hepatoma and MCF-7 breast cancers, in vitro (Zhao et al, 2010a).

Leathery-looking Russula (*R. alutacea*) is considered a tasty edible in parts of the world. A purified polysaccharide has been found to protect against inflammatory and oxidative damage in an in vivo study by Li et al, (2020). In TCM, it is part of Tendon Easing Powder, to treat lumbago, painful, numb limbs and discomfort in bones. The edible *R. integra* (*R. polychroma*) is used in same powder; but as well to remove heat from the liver and with ginger root, as a decoction for women with poor energy circulation.

Darkening Brittlegill (*R. vinosa*) is common and widespread. Water-soluble polysaccharides show potential immune stimulating activity, by promoting macrophage proliferation, phagocytosis, and release of nitric oxide and cytokines (TNF-alpha and IL-1beta). Zhang et al, 2021).

SHAGGY MANE
LAWYER'S WIG
INKY CAP
CHICKEN DRUMSTICK
(*Coprinus comatus*)

Shaggy Mane is easily identified, in the wild, and has a mild but delicious flavor. Coprinus derives from the Greek, *kopros*, meaning "dung", while comatus is from the Latin *coma*, meaning "shaggy".

The mushroom, known as *maotouguisan*, has long been cultivated in China, but the maturing spores quickly trigger deliquescence into a black, gooey mass.

The biggest challenge to widespread cultivation is keeping the fruiting bodies fresh. High humidity and low temperatures (under 4 degrees Celsius) reduced the browning, cap opening and black juice, but after ten days storage they were unacceptable for commercial sales (Peng et al, 2020).

In North America, it is often gathered in autumn as a choice, but time-sensitive edible.

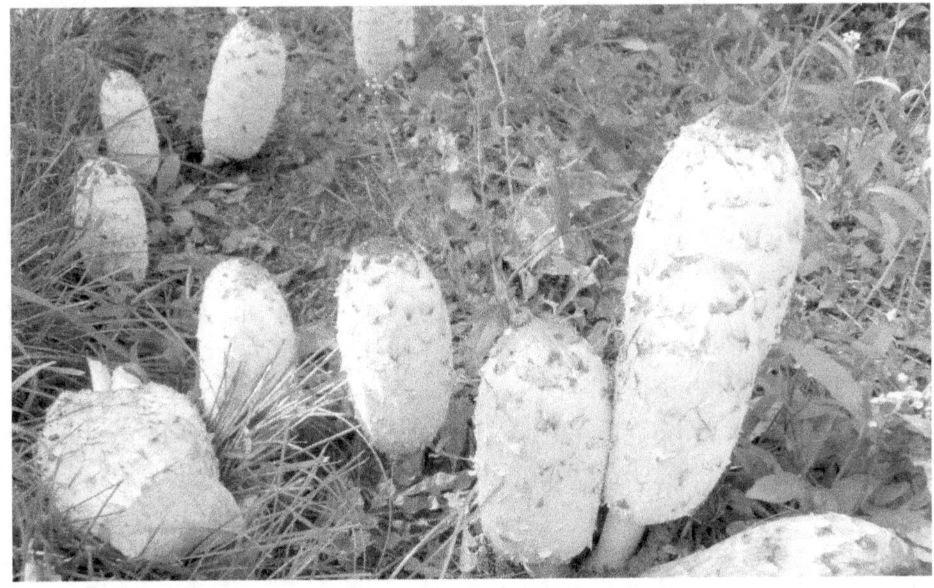

Coprinus comatus

This "ink" with its microscopic spores, was formally used to identify the veracity of written messages between allies during wartime. A more permanent "ink" can be obtained by adding a few iron filings to the liquid.

It is estimated to release 1.6 million spores per minute, or over 5.25 billion spores during its short lifetime.

Various compounds have been derived from the fruiting bodies, mycelium or fermentation liquor.

One study by Zaidman et al, (2008) found ethanol extracts inhibited dihydrotestosterone-induced LNCaP prostate cancer cell viability, suppressed prostate-specific antigen (PSA), and G1 phase arrest.

I devoted an entire chapter in an earlier book (Rogers, 2011) to its health benefits, and thus there is no need to rehash previous in vitro studies on pathogens.

However, there are several new and exciting studies over the last decade that suggest Inky Cap be once again revisited for its potential medicinal benefits.

Work by Dotan et al, (2011) followed up the work by Zaidman (2008) and found the mushroom extract is a natural anti-androgenic modulator, and inhibits proliferation and viability of prostate cancer cell lines.

Shaggy Mane liquid cultures, extracted with ethyl acetate, contain potent compounds that inhibit NF-kappaB function and MCF-7 breast cancer cells (Asatiani et al, 2011).

A few years later, Rouhana-Toubi et al, (2013) found the same extract reduced the viability of three lines of human ovarian cancer. A follow-up study by Rouhana-Toubi et al, (2015) suggests the extract induced apoptosis in ovarian cancer cells, via both intrinsic and extrinsic pathways.

Inky Cap has additional compounds of interest. The fruiting body, like all mushrooms, contains ergothioneine (762.35µg/g), an anti-oxidant more stable and powerful than L-glutathione. It contains significant levels of gamma amino butyric acid (GABA), (1092.45 µg/g), a neurotransmitter with relaxing and calmative benefit.

A unique 130-amino-acid, glycan binding protein exhibits selective and potent cytotoxicity to human T-cell leukemia Jurkat cells. This suggests potential use in cancer diagnosis and treatment (Zhang et al, 2017).

An unusual co-culture of Morel (*Morchella esculenta*) and Inky Cap in a fermentation broth resulted in an extract that inhibited proliferation and promoted apoptosis of human glioma U251 cells. Work by Zhong et al, (2020) suggests the induction of self-programmed death may be via the mitochondrial intrinsic pathway.

Recent work, and review of the literature, has focused on the hypoglycemic benefit of the mushroom, as well as alcohol liver protection, cancer inhibition, anti-androgenic and anti-inflammatory effects (Cao et al, 2020).

Polysaccharides ameliorate induced liver fibrosis by mediating inflammation and apoptosis (Zhao et al, 2022).

A gut microbiome study on mice, found an Inky Cap protein increased gut bacteria stability, and attenuated acute alcohol liver damage (Li et al, 2021).

The Smooth Inky Cap (*Coprinopsis atramentaria*), on the other hand, contains coprine, which shuts down the ability of the liver to detoxify alcohol, resulting in unpleasant effects.

The compound comatin, found in the fruiting body, shows possible benefit in diabetes and obesity, by modulating either cellular function, or influencing biochemical pathways (Dubey et al, 2019).

Quinic acid also possesses anti-diabetic and anti-oxidant activity (Karaman, M et al, 2021).

Mycelium polysaccharides, in mice trials, improved insulin resistance and energy metabolism, and significantly suppressed kidney oxidative stress, and inflammation. Kidney damage was prevented via two important pathways, suggesting benefit in preventing diabetic nephropathy (Gao et al, 2021).

Like all mushrooms, Lawyer's Wig possesses both functional properties and potential hazards. Work by Nowakowski et al, (2020) reviews the anti-oxidant, anti-cancer, anti-androgenic, hepatoprotective, acetylcholinesterase inhibition, anti-inflammatory, anti-diabetic, anti-obesity, anti-bacterial, anti-viral and anti-fungal properties.

A rat study by Ratnaningtyas et al, (2022) found ethanol extracts reduced fasting blood glucose levels by nearly 27%; HbA1c by 4-4.30%, and increased insulin levels by 13.8.

Some of the more negative aspects include dermatitis and atopic predisposition, accumulation or contamination of heavy metals or toxins, and possible confusion with poisonous mushrooms. The latter is highly unlikely.

A sample of the fruiting body, mycelia and filtrate from submerged cultivation was tested, in vitro, and shows rather potent inhibition of acetylcholinesterase, comparable to the pharmaceutical drug donepezil (Karaman et al, 2020). Various edible and/or medicinal mushrooms show promise for neuro-degenerative conditions. These include *Agaricus bisporus, Hericium erinaceus, Ganoderma lucidum, Grifola frondosa, Amanita muscaria, A. caesarea, Armillaria ssp., Boletus edulis, Cordyceps militaris, Flammulina velutipes, Fomitopsis betulina, Inonotus obliquus, Pleurotus ssp., Macrolepidota procera, Trametes versicolor, Wolfiporia cocos, Auricularia polytricha,* and Psilocybin-containing mushrooms (Rogers, 2019:315-328.)

Synthetic psilocybin has proven beneficial in over 100 human, DB, PC clinical trials to date, for the treatment of anxiety, depression, addiction, PTSD, OCD and other mental health conditions (Rogers, 2021).

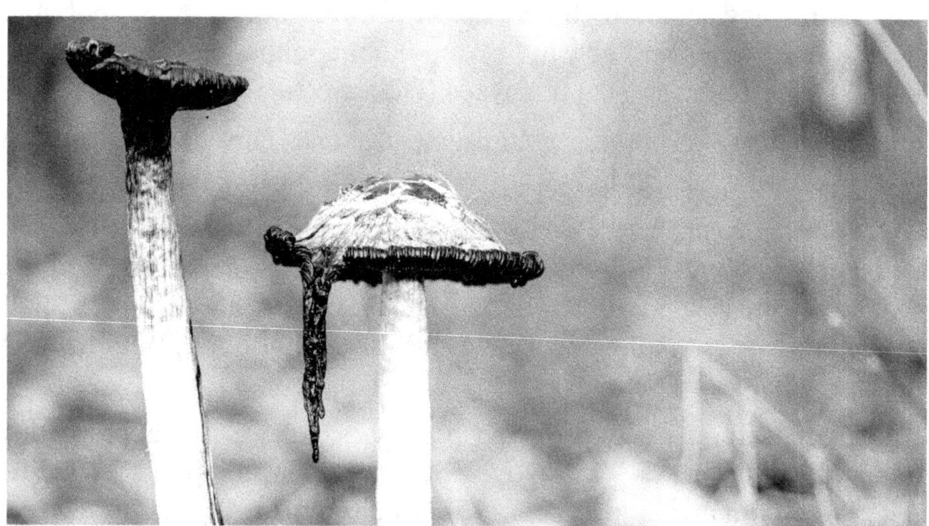

Coprinus comatus

SUILLUS

Suillus is derived from the Latin, meaning "little pig or swine."

They are considered edible, but the slimy caps are removed as they can cause intestinal distress in some individuals.

The genus has a long history of use, from ancient Rome to several TCM formulas, including Tendon Easing Powder, and Pine Mushroom Elixir.

Slippery Jack (*S. luteus*) is a northern hemisphere mushroom that has managed to hitchhike around the world. It has a relationship with pine (*Pinus radiata*) plantations in Ecuador, and its abundant fruiting is one of the reasons for this particular timber choice. The Saraguros, an indigenous people from southern Ecuador use the introduced mushroom for gastrointestinal disorders and headaches (Andrade et al, 2022).

In northern Alberta, I find large amounts nearly every autumn, but am not that excited. They are excellent protein, but the slimy caps, and spongy, lacy network make them a less desired edible. If you look carefully, you will note that instead of gills, there is an intermediate stage toward pores. They are a favorite of squirrels that pick them fresh and dry them under conifer branches, for food. Various fungi comprise up to 25% of their winter stores of food.

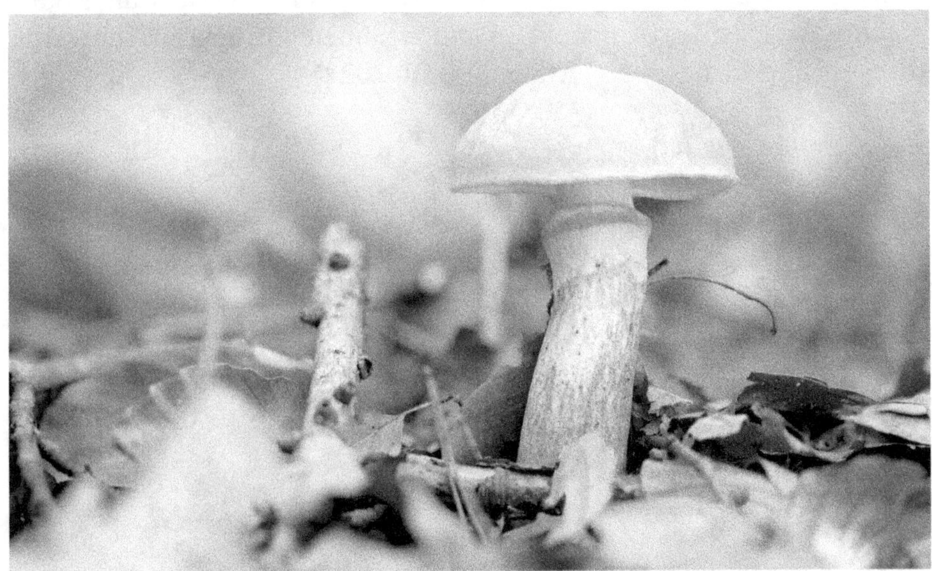

Suillus grevillei (S. clintonianus)

The use of blue light and hot-air drying at 60 degrees Celsius, improve the umani and aroma of the dried mushrooms (Feng et al, 2022; Hou et al., 2022).

However, the genera offer a wide variety of medicinal benefits.

Work by Tomasi et al, (2004) looked at 58 species and found four species, including Milk Bolete (*Suillus granulatus*) and Slippery Jack (*S. luteus*) active against at least one of two cancer cell lines. Both are common in pine forests.

Milk Bolete contains a beta-carboline compound, flazinamide, that exhibits weak anti-HIV-1 activity, that might interfere in early stages of viral life cycle (Wang et al, 2007).

The fruiting body contains water-soluble heteropolysaccharides that exert immune modulation by interacting with toll-like receptor 2, and activating various signaling pathways (Gao et al, 2022).

Suillin, shows both in vitro, and in vivo, activity against p-388 leukemia cell lines. (Tringali et al, 1989).

The same team (Tringali et al, 1989a) isolated five tetraprenyl phenols and found two exhibited anti-microbial properties.

Suillin, isolated from *S. luteus* possesses anti-acetylcholinesterase activity, suggestive of benefit in the treatment of neurodegenerative diseases like Alzheimer's (Andrade et al, 2022).

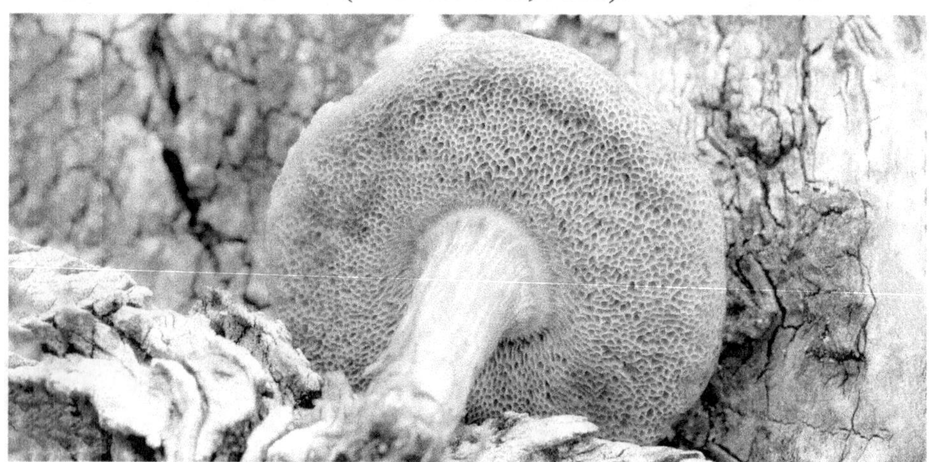

Suillus granulatus

Another unique benzofuran, suillusin, appears generated from polyporic acid (Yun et al, 2001). Thank goodness, as polyporic acid is a deadly toxin.

Polysaccharides derived from the fruiting body show anti-oxidant and increased splenocyte proliferation (Zhou et al, 2016).

Ethanol extracts of Slippery Jack (*S. luteus*) exhibit potent anti-tubercular activity (Gordien et al, 2010).

Work by Morel et al, (2018), found various extracts active against the HCT116 colon adenocarcinoma cell line.

Iso-suillin, isolated from the fruiting body, inhibited proliferation and induced apoptosis (self-programmed death) in human hepatoma (SMMC-7721) cell lines, without any toxicity to normal human lymphocytes (Jia et al, 2014). This suggest possible benefit as adjuvant in liver cancer treatment.

León et al, (2008) isolated a phytosphingosine-type ceramide, named suillumide, from a tincture of the fruiting body.

The compound exhibited cytotoxicity against the human melanoma (SK-MEL-1) cell line.

Flavonoids isolated from Slippery Jack exhibit hypoglycemic activity in insulin resistance mice. It effectively reduced blood sugar, HDL cholesterol, LDL, total cholesterol, triglycerides, as well as alanine and aspartate aminotransferase levels. Damage to liver, kidney and pancreas in diabetic mice was mitigated, suggesting a possible functional food for type two diabetes (Zhang et al, 2021).

Mushrooms are generally considered a contributing dietary risk to gout. One study, however, found Tamarack Jack (*Suillus grevilli*) inhibits xanthine oxidase. (Ványolós et al, 2014).

It contains nearly 17g/100grams of beta-glucans (Mironczuk-Chodakowska & Witkowska, 2020).

Iso-suillin, isolated from *S. flavus* increased apoptosis, mitochondrial membrane potential depolarization and G0/G1 arrest against human chronic myeloid leukemia (K562) cell lines. Two anti-apoptosis proteins, NF-kappaB, and Bcl-2 were also down-regulated, suggesting possible benefit in treating this form of cancer (Wang et al, 2014).

This compound was found to induce apoptosis in human small lung cancer (H446) cell lines (Zhao et al, 2016). At a higher concentration it promoted lymphtocyte proliferation.

Recent work by Yan et al, (2021) found iso-suillin potently inhibited A549 lung carcinoma cell line proliferation through early G_1 arrest and induced apoptosis. A A549 xenograft model also found inhibition of tumor growth and progression. Induction of p53 phosphorylation is involved.

White Suillus (*S. placidus*), commonly associated with white pine in eastern North America, also contains suillin.

The compound induced apoptosis in three human liver cancer cell lines, both through death receptor and mitochondrial pathways (Liu et al, 2009).

Ringless Yellow Boletus (*Suillus collinitus*) is found under pine in southern Europe. The ethanol extracts of fruiting body possess high anti-oxidant activity, while the methanol extracts were most potent against MCF-7 breast cancer cell lines. It appears to have a p53-mediated effect on normal cell cycle distribution and apoptosis induction in the breast tumor line (Vaz et al, 2021).

The Euro Cow Bolete (*S. bovinus*) was introduced into eastern North America in Scots Pine plantations. The mushroom is edible but not great. Linnaeus, the father of binomials, originally named it *Boletus bovinus*.

It contains variegatic, atromentic and xerocomic acids.

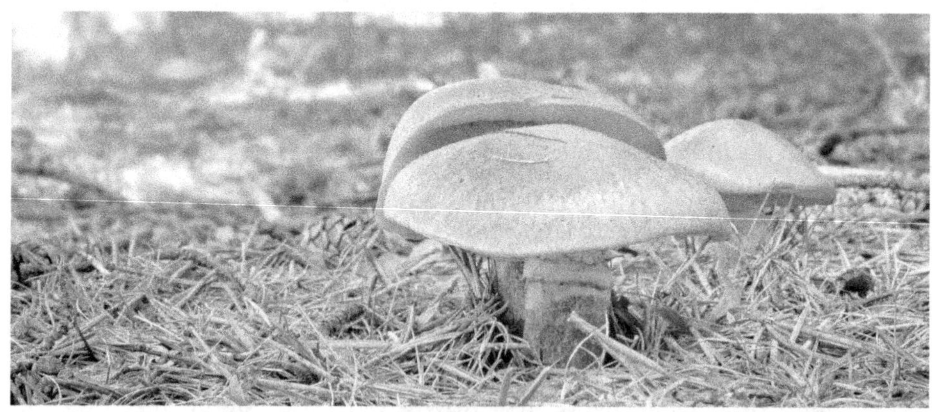

Suillus grevillei

TIGER MILK MUSHROOM

PUT A TIGER IN YOUR (FERMENTATION) TANK

Tiger Milk Mushroom (*Lignosus rhinocerotis*) is a polypore found in Malaysia and other parts of Southeast Asia. The common name refers to where a tigress drips milk while feeding. I first became familiar with another tiger's milk in the early 1980s, when introduced to Peruvian ceviche, and drinking the delicious remaining lime juice.

Rhinocerotis ungulates were prehistoric relatives of rhinoceros and other horned mammals.

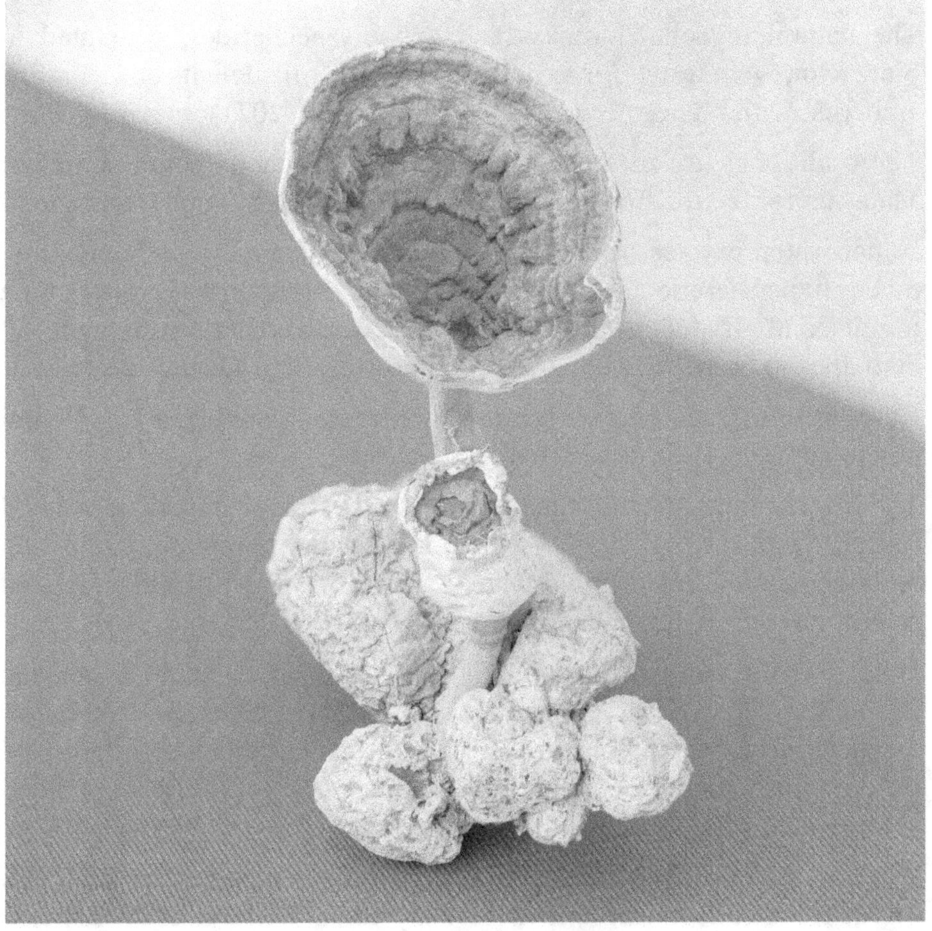

Lignosus rhinocerotis

The underground sclerotium is harvested, and traditionally used for stamina, mental alertness and respiratory conditions; but recent work suggests benefit in numerous human health conditions.

These include cognitive function, neuro-protection, immune modulation, anti-asthmatic, anti-coagulation, anti-inflammatory, anti-microbial, anti-viral, anti-cancer and antioxidant properties (Nallathamby et al, 2018).

The sclerotia is not widely available in North America, but mycelial biomass, exopolysaccharides, and culture broth fermentation is an alternative source and potential substitute (Lau et al, 2014).

Electrical stimulation increases the growth of mycelium by 10.3% over first eight and sixteen days (Jamil et al, 2020).

The natural mycelial biomass and exopolysaccharides, generated in bioreactor, were tested for toxicity and teratogenic defects on Zebrafish embryos; with no negative results (Usuldin et al, 2021).

The traditional use of the mushroom, by indigenous communities in Malaysia for the treatment of asthma, is confirmed by modern research.

A hot-water extract using Soxhlet, alleviated airway inflammation, mucus hypersecretion and hyper-responsiveness against allergic asthma in mice and rat studies (Johnathan et al, 2021). IgE in serum, and Th2 cytokines in bronchoalveolar lavage fluid were significantly decreased.

Cold water extracts show a bronchodilator effect mediated by calcium down-signaling (Lee et al, 2018).

The significance of cold versus hot water extracts should be studied further. Work by Rashid et al, (2022) looked at differential toxicity and teratogenicity of hot and cold-water extracts of both wild and cultivated sclerotium on zebrafish embryos.

Hot water extracts were nontoxic, and cold-water extracts delayed hatching by up to 48 hours, and shows slight toxicity, as well as minor tachycardia in zebrafish larvae. Of interest is that wild sclerotium cold water extracts induced curved trunk and bent tail, an ill-effect not noted in cultivated sclerotium. Human implication is presently unknown.

A recent study by Tan et al, (2021) involved 50 volunteers taking 300 mg of tiger milk mushroom twice daily for three months. Significant suppression of IL-1beta, IL-8, malondialdehyde and respiratory symptoms was noted. There was also significant reduction of IgA, total antioxidant capacity, pulmonary function, and improved immunity.

The traditional use of decoctions for increasing mental alertness during hunting, led to an interesting study (Seow et al, 2015). Hot water, ethanol and crude polysaccharides were tested on rat PC-12 cells. The hot water extract exhibited neuritogenic activity comparable to neuron growth factor (NGF), while the extracts and crude polysaccharides stimulated neuritogenesis without stimulating the production of NGF.

Recent research by Tan et al, (2021a) found neuritin modulation is involved in neurite outgrowth induced by mushroom extracts.

Lion's Mane (*Hericium erinaceus*) is highly touted for neuronal health, albeit with only a few human trials. Work by Samberkar et al, (2015) investigated the potential of Lion's Mane and Tiger Milk to stimulate neurite growth in dissociated cells of brain, spinal cord and retina, when compared to brain derived neurotrophic factor. Lion's mane extract at 50µg/mL triggered neurite outgrowth at 20.47%, 22.47%, and 21.7% on respective cells, while Tiger Milk induced outgrowth of 20.77% and 24.73% in brain and spinal cord; and 20.77% in retinal cells at only 25µg/mL respectively.

The mushroom sclerotia is used in TCM for liver cancer, chronic hepatitis and gastric ulcers.

Like Reishi (*Ganoderma lucidum*) the tiger mushroom modulates the C-terminal domain of angiotensin-converting enzyme, which regulates blood pressure, and is implicated in lung injury, fibrosis and Alzheimer's disease (Goh et al, 2022).

Animal studies suggest benefit from the mushroom powder on gastric mucosa, including anti-ulcer activity (Nyam et al, 2016). Beta glucans (8%) extracted from the dry sclerotia promoted mucosal wound healing and accelerated intestinal epithelial cell proliferation. This suggests possible benefit in the treatment of peptic ulcers and inflammatory bowel disease (Veeraperumal et al, 2021).

The sclerotial powder was tested against a number of oral cancer cell lines (Yap et al, 2022). Cold water extracts induced apoptosis in gingiva, tongue and buccal mucosa cells, probably via the TNF pathway.

Hot water extracts, and water soluble after ethanol extracts suppress cytokine production in dengue-infected monocytes, suggesting a possible reduction in inflammation associated with viral disease. The extracts were least toxic to Vero cells, and yet showed very prominent anti-Dengue virus activity. No virucidal effect was noted (Ellan et al, 2019, 2019a).

A serine protease, isolated from a cold-water extract, showed cytotoxicity against human breast (MCF-7) cancer cell lines (Yap et al, 2015).

(+)-Torreyol and alpha cadinol, cloned from sesquiterpene synthase genes in the sclerotium, were found to exhibit selective potent cytotoxicity against the same cancer cell line (Yap et al, 2017).

Tiger Milk mushrooms contain an immune modulating protein, with cytotoxic effect on MCF-7, HeLa and A549 cancer cell lines (Pushparajah et al, 2016).

Freeze-dried powder exhibits significant benefit in streptozotocin-induced diabetic rats over a two-month period (Nyam et al, 2017).

A medium molecular weight fraction, derived from cold water extraction, potently inhibits glycation, and may be of possible benefit in preventing diabetic complications (Yap et al, 2018).

Tiger Milk Mushrooms! As Tony says "They're GGGRRRREEEAAATT!"

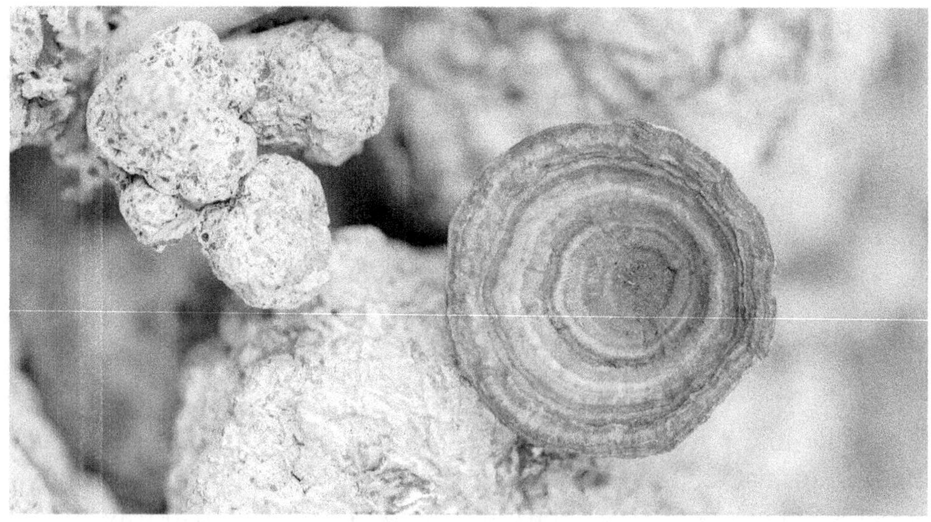

Lignosus rhinocerotis

TRICHOLOMA

Trich or Treatment

It is no dream!
Matsutake are growing
On the belly of the mountain

SHIGETAKA

When I first began my journey into mushroom identification, various genera stumped me time and again. But none were trickier for me than the various species of *Tricholoma*. White spores, central fleshy stipe, gills adnexed-to-sinuate and no ring or volva, I would repeat to myself. Of course, over the years, they became much easier to spot, but I am still stumped at times. There are over 100 species in North America, many of them inedible, or downright poisonous.

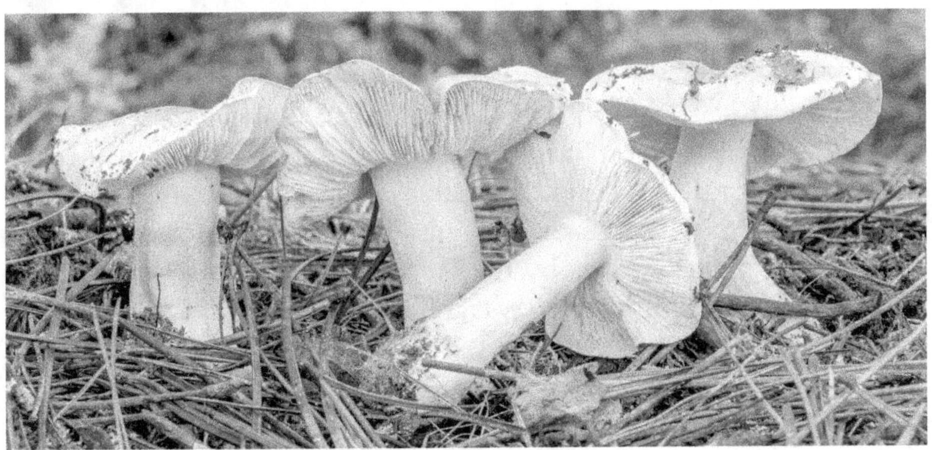

Tricholoma equestre

Tricholoma is from the Greek, meaning "with hair on the edge or lump," helping confuse one further. The largest specimen of *Tricholoma* in the world is found an hour or so northeast of my home in the town of Vilna, Alberta. Weighing more than 17,000 pounds and standing nearly twenty feet high, the "Burnt Tricholoma" sculpture was built in 1993. Its namesake (*Tricholoma ustale*) is a mushroom that's no more edible than the sculpture. Though this mushroom has an odor of anise or licorice, ingestion results from a gastric irritant containing ustalic acid.

In fact, 86 cases (affecting 347 patients) of poisoning from this mushroom were reported from 1989 to 2010.

My first firm identification of an edible member of the genus was *Tricholoma flavovirens*, also known as Man on Horseback. It has bright yellow gills and stipe, and when found in mossy areas is a choice consumable. Or so I thought. Soon after enjoying my first meal, there was news out of Europe that the same or similar *T. equestre* may be poisonous and fatal. One Polish study tracked all *T. equestre* patients admitted to poison centers in Gdansk and Biala Podlaska between 2001 and 2010 (Sein and Chwaluk, 2010).

A mortality rate of 20% was observed, and included acute respiratory failure, myocarditis with arrhythmia and cardiovascular collapse. Known as rhabdomyolysis, the condition can progress to kidney failure and death. After consuming 100-400 grams of mushrooms for three to four days, four patients developed fatigue, muscle weakness, myalgia and in two cases, respiratory failure. One patient, aged 72 years, died on the second day of hospitalization. In others, the symptoms disappeared in two or three weeks (Anand et al, 2009).

Various authors suggest the European and North American species are not the same. Deng and Yao (2005) suggest the correct name for *T. flavovirens* is *T. equestre*. And just to add to confusion, Massart (2003) refer to the species by the synonym *T. auratum*, suggesting a morphologically similar species may be the culprit.

But the news of Man on Horseback is not all bad. Many mushrooms possess anti-bacterial activity and Man on Horseback is no exception, with strong activity against *Bacillus subtilis*. Weaker activity against *E. coli*, *Staphylococcus aureus*, *S. epidermidis*, and *Pseudomonas aeruginosa* was noted (Yamac and Bilgili, 2006). A mice study with freshly frozen (not cooked) mushrooms found myo-, cardio- and hepatoxic effects (Nieminen et al, 2008). An interesting compound, flavomannin-6,6'di-methyl ether, has been found, in vitro, to inhibit growth of human adenocarcinoma colorectal cancer cell lines (Pachón-Peña et al, 2009). Work by Hata et al, (2002) found a sterol in this mushroom that stimulates the enzyme alkaline phosphatase in mouse osteoblasts. High levels of this enzyme are associated with increased proliferation and differentiation of osteoblasts and prevention of osteoporosis.

One of my favorite mushrooms is the Pine Mushroom (*T. murrillianum*) formerly known as *Armillaria ponderosa*. This is a widely prized, commercial mushroom found throughout western North America but most abundant in the Pacific Northwest. The species is named in honor of William Alphonso Murrill.

The eastern NA mushroom is now known as *T. magnivelare.* "Magnivelare" is from the Latin, meaning "with big veil."

Tom Volk suggests the taste is "an incredible and complex flavor you won't ever forget—even though you won't be able to adequately describe it to anyone." David Arora (of *Mushrooms Demystified*) describes the odor as "an provocative compromise between 'red hots' and dirty socks." Indeed, the cinnamon and slight valerian/garden cress scent combined with firm texture lends itself to delicious thin slices toasted on the barbeque or added to miso soup. This fall, I attended the Fungi Festival in Sicamous, British Columbia, and although it was unseasonably dry, I picked many Pine Mushrooms, along with lots of White Chanterelles (*Cantharellus subalbidus*) and numerous Lobster mushrooms (*Hypomyces lactifluorum*).

The Thompson or Ntlakyapamuk people of southern British Columbia know this mushroom well. They call it */q'ám'es*, as well as wood or mountain mushroom. It was said that eating them raw would cut your tongue. Dried specimens were later added to soups and stews. Work by Nancy Turner and others (1990) recorded that a woman was named */q'é[-q'a]m'∂s* after the pine mushroom. She was washed in a broth as an infant to make her strong. In turn, Turner's own daughter was given this name, because she was washed in the juice from a jar of mushroom a Thompson woman had given her.

A choice edible, St. George's Mushroom is known to the Thompson people as thunder storm, *(s)/kí?[-ki?x*, or thunderstorm head. It is known as *Tricholoma gambosa* or *Calocybe gambosa*. The common name is derived from England, where it pops out of the ground around the time of St. George's Day (April 23). Thunderstorm is interesting, as cultures around the world have long associated mushrooms with thunder and lightning. It was believed the vibration or sound triggered mushrooms appearing from nowhere. The beating of oak logs in a drumming manner was long practiced in Japan with shiitake cultivation. The rain accompanying these heavenly displays of force is the more probable science based source of fruiting. In China, the dried mushroom is used as a tea to treat measles and sick children feeling agitated and upset. Inhibition rates against both sarcoma 180 and Ehrlich carcinoma are 90% (Ohtsuka et al, 1973).

Another pop[u]lar mushroom of the Thompson is /m∂λqi?/ (*meaqi*), also known as The Sandy, or Cottonwood Mushroom (*T. populinum*). The neighboring Shuswap call it *semtl'aka*, the Okanagan-Colville, *petl'kin*, and the Lillooet, *meix qin*. It grows in sandy soil beneath large poplar trees and has a sweet, mealy scent like sweet bedstraw (*Galium* species) or cucumber. Both the Sandy and Thunderstorm are widely picked, dried and stored for winter. Formerly, the fruiting bodies were strung on strings and hung to dry. Some people freeze them, but others prefer to can various *Tricholoma* species, because they are not as tough.

The Shingled Trich (*T. imbricatum*) is a very common species found under conifers. It has a dry, dull brown cap with a solid stem; firm, white flesh and a faintly farinaceous scent. Studies have found high levels of anti-oxidant activity in the fruiting body based on five complementary free radical scavenging tests. More exciting was the moderate inhibition activity against both acetylcholinesterase and butyrylcholinesterase enzymes (Gülsen et al, 2012). This suggests possible use in the treatment of Alzheimer's or Parkinson's disease.

Isocyathisterol, chaxine C and volemolide show cytotoxicity against A549 (lung), and five other human cancer cell lines (Zhang et al, 2020).

Streaked Tricholoma (*T. portentosum*) is found under pine, and has gills and stalked tinged with greenish-yellow. It is commonly found around the world, and known in Japan as *shimo-furishimeji*, in Poland as *siwki*, and in Sweden, *streckmusseron*. It is a choice edible with strong earthy flavor, but care must be taken in identification. The poisonous *T. pardinum* and *T. virgatum* are similar in appearance, so care is advised.

The small Mouse Tricholoma (*T. terreum*) methanol extract is cytotoxic against the HT-29 human colon cancer cell line, and possesses anti-oxidant and free radical scavenging ability (Yuvali & Onbasil, 2022).

Another inedible, probably poisonous, species is the Soapy Tricholoma (*T. saponaceum*). David Arora notes that a fairly infallible feature is the pinkish-orange color of the flesh at or near the base. It lacks the fibrillose scales of *T. virgatum* and *T. pardinum* mentioned above. During the 1950s and 60s in Switzerland, Tricholoma poisonings accounted for 20-50% of all reported intoxications, with Tiger Trich (*T. pardinum*) most notable. Soapy Trich is quite abundant in the Rocky Mountains just west of my home. Lab work has led to the discovery of two strong fibrinolytic enzymes in the fruiting body. The activity is via direct cleavage of fibrin clotting and not as a plasminogen activator (Kim and Kim, 2001).

Many members of genus *Tricholoma*, contain tricolomic acid, a flavor enhancer that excites brain neurons. In large doses, it is lethal to flies. Jonathan Ott, in his wonderful book, *Pharmacotheon*, writes a "single fly even squeezed through the tiny opening of the screw-cap vial in which the small amount of tricolomic acid solution was kept, and there met his death!" Ott detected tricholomic acid in *Pleurotus* species, and "probable that it occurs in the shiitake." Tricholomic acid is a likely candidate for the neurotoxin used by Oyster mushroom to immobilize nematodes. The structural analog, glutamic acid, in the form of monosodium glutamate is a neurotoxin, associated with headaches, numbness, tingling, dizziness, nausea and other uncomfortable symptoms, especially in people deficient in B6. The book *Excitotoxins* by Russel L. Blaylock is a thorough exposé of this widespread additive, disguised on food labels with names like hydrolyzed yeast or protein, seasonings, broth, protein isolate or twenty other names that are permitted by FDA. Due to possible damage to immature brain tissue, it was removed from baby food in 1970.

The *Tricholoma* genus, as you can see, is full of tricks and treats!

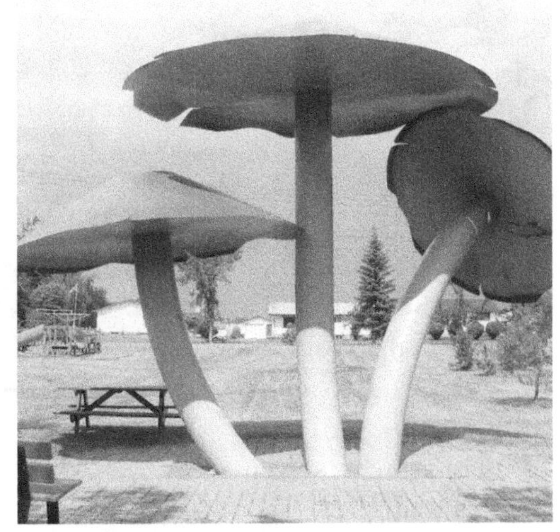

Giant Tricholoma in Vilna, Alberta

TRUFFLES

We don't care to eat toadstools that think they are truffles. Mark Twain

Truffles (*Tuber* spp.) numbered 140 species at last count, and are ectomycorrhizal with angiosperm and gymnosperm trees.

Some are highly valued due to their aroma and taste, with The White Truffle (*T. magnatum*) commanding from 1200 to 4000 euros per kilogram, depending upon the annual harvest. In 2007 a White truffle weighing 1.5 kilograms sold for a record $330,000 US.

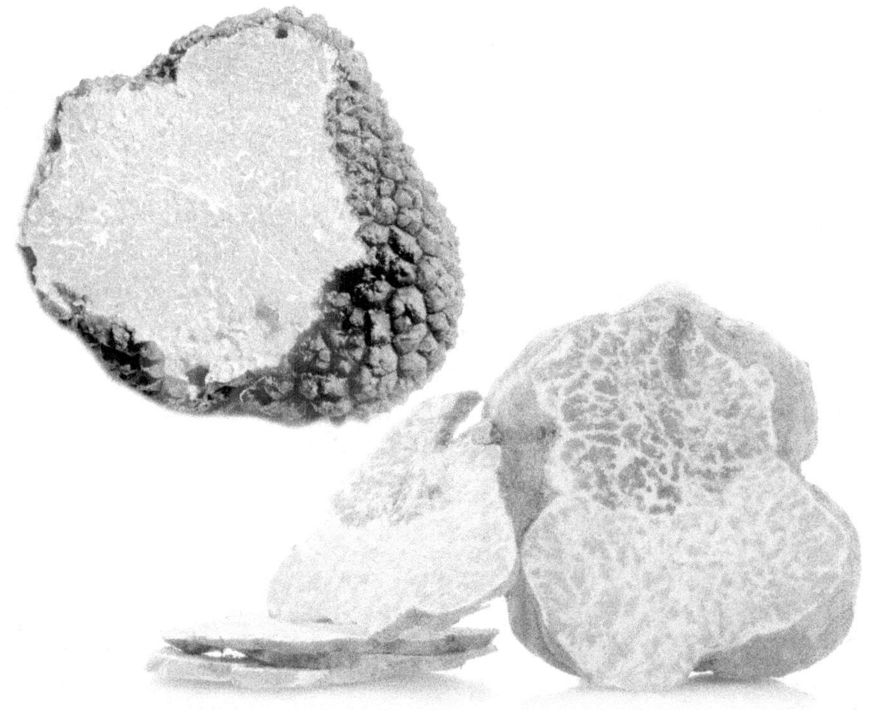

Adulteration is difficult to detect by novice olfactory senses. Recent work by Segelke et al, (2020) looked at five commercially relevant truffle species using Fourier transform near-infrared (FT-NIR) spectroscopy. White truffle (*T. magnatum*) could be differentiated from *T. borchii* with accuracy of 100%. The Black Truffle (*T. melanosporum*) could be distinguished from *T. aestivum* and various less-desirable Chinese truffles with accuracy of 99%.

Truffles have a short shelf life, even under ideal 4 degrees Celsius storage. A *Lactobacillus plantarum* strain has been found to inhibit growth of eleven Penicillium, including *P. digitatum* DSM 2750, a green mold involved in truffle spoilage (Sorrentino et al, 2013). Consumers may prefer this approach, compared to the increasingly common use of irradiation.

Cultivation of White truffle still lacks a good method, with distribution limited to Italy, Hungary, Slovenia and Croatia. A trip to the latter country to gather and dine on this delicacy is on my bucket list. My wife possesses Croatian ancestry, so she may even consider coming as well.

Other aromatic truffles such as Black Truffle (*T. melanosporum*), *T. brumale* and Black Summer Truffle (*T. aestivum*) have been successful in plantation. Inoculation of oak and hazelnut saplings may result in fungi development up to a decade later. Yields of up to 200 kilograms a year may be obtained from one hectare, and up to ten kilograms from a mature tree. The first seedling inoculated with Black Truffle hit the market nearly fifty years ago. Today, truffle orchards are found around the world, including Australia, New Zealand, Canada and the United States. Climate change is sure to encourage more truffle cultivation.

The history of culinary use goes back to the Bronze Age on the east coast of the Mediterranean. Various hypogeous fungi were gathered and eaten by ancient Babylonians, Etruscans, Egyptians, Greeks and Romans.

Plutarch (46-120 A.D.) believed they were produced by lightning, warmth and damp soil (Rosa-Gruszecka et al, 2017).

Several Truffles possess not only potent olfactory and gustatory prowess, but health benefits beyond their musky androstanol content. This excitatory porcine chemical is part of masculine sexual appeal.

Truffles are a traditional aphrodisiac due to this steroidal pheromone. It is found in the underarm perspiration of men, and urine of women; helping increase sexual attraction.

Alcohol extracts of related Desert Truffle (*Terfezia boudieri*) increased levels of luteinizing hormone and testosterone significantly in a rat study (Khojasteh et al, 2013).

Studies in this direction with Tuber species have yet to be conducted.

Black Truffle (*T. melanosporum*) has long been considered a medicinal mushroom. It attenuates oxidative stress, reducing vascular complications associated with type 2 diabetes.

Work by Wu et al, (2022) found black truffles possess strong hyperlipedemic and anti-inflammatory effect comparable to glibenclamide and medications prescribed for type-2 diabetes.

A rat study by Zhang et al. (2018;2020) found benefit from water extracts of black truffle on STZ-induced hyperglycemia via Nrf2 and NF-kappaB pathways. The authors suggest future clinical studies can warrant a potential anti-diabetic drug in the form of diet. Great! Where do I get a prescription?

White Truffles (*T. magnatum*) and Black Summer Truffles (*T. aestivum*) have been studied for their anti-oxidant, anti-inflammatory and cytotoxic activity (Beara et al, 2014).

Both species showed moderate antioxidant activity. White truffles exhibit anti-inflammatory activity by inhibiting COX-1 and 12-LOX pathways. Alcohol extracts showed cytotoxicity against various human cancer cell lines, including HeLA (cervical), MCF-7 (breast) and HT-29 (colorectal). Water extracts also showed activity against breast cancer cell lines.

Over fifty polysaccharides have been identified in four Tuber species including *T. melanosporum* and *T. aestivum* fruiting bodies and fermentation systems by Zhao et al, (2014). Cytotoxic activity was found against human lung (A-549), colo-rectal (HCT-116), liver (HepG2), leukemia (HL-60) and breast (SK-BR-3) cancer cell lines. Fractions containing Beta-D-glucan with triple helix conformation showed significantly higher inhibition, and heteropolysaccharides with lower molecular weight exhibited higher anti-tumor activity than higher weight.

A water soluble heteroglycan in *T. rufum* was studied by Pattanayak et al. (2017) on human blood lymphocytes. Positive immune response was observed due, in part, to maintenance of redox balance.

Black truffles (*T. melanosporum*) contain endocannabinoid metabolic enzymes and anandamide, two compounds also present in cannabis. Anandamide is responsible for melanin synthesis in normal human epidermal melanocytes, and a key fatty acid neurotransmitter derived from arachidonic acid, with anti-cancer activity.

It is possible that anandamide and endocannabinoid systems enzyme evolved earlier than endocannabinoid-binding receptors, and may have been ancient attractants to truffle eaters that possess these receptors (Pacioni et al, 2015).

Other endocannabinoid metabolic enzymes identified were N-acylphosphatidyl-ethanol-amine-specific phospholipase D, fatty acid amide hydrolase, diacylglycerol lipase and monoacylglycerol.

Work by Picardi et al. (2014) found anandamide inhibited angiogenesis of highly invasive and metastatic breast cancer cells. Earlier work by Patsos et al. (2005) found metabolites of anandamide induce apoptosis of colorectal cancer cells and stimulated non-apoptotic cell death in COX-2 overexpressed colorectal cancer cells.

Anandamide decreased EGFR-overexpressed prostate cancer cells by interacting with cannabinoid CB1 receptor, inhibiting cancer cell proliferation (Mimeault et al, 2003). Cannabis and truffle infused chocolates sound like a winning combination! And superior to the numerous Cannabis Truffle recipes on line.

Magic Truffles are legally sold in Smart Shops in The Netherlands, and are a milder version of psilocybin (similar to a microdose), derived from the mycelium/sclerotia.

Truffles are indigenous and commercially grown as far north as Quebec and Ontario. Both Appalachian (*T. canaliculatum*) and Burgundy (*T. uncinatum*), mycorhizzal with oak and hazel, are available. You can contact info@truffesquebec.com for more information. *Mycorrhiza Biotech*, in North Carolina, have developed a method to cultivate *T. borchii* truffles with Loblolly pine.

Oregon White Truffle (*T. oregonense*) mushroom essence helps us understand the complexities of the human psyche and the many masks used to cover insecurity and feelings of aloneness. It helps us rediscover our primal spark, and helps one to discern the conceit, deceit, pretense and hypocrisy widespread in modern society (Rogers, 2016).

TYLOPILUS
BITTER BOLETE
(*Tylopilus felleus*)
BURNT-ORANGE BOLETE
(*T. ballouii*)
(*Rubinoboletus ballouii*)
(*Gyroporus ballouii*)
VIOLET GREY BOLETE
(*T. plumbeoviolaceus*)
(*Boletus plumbeoviolaceus*)

The Tylopilus species are bitter and largely inedible. Some are acceptable after cooking, depending upon one's individual taste buds.

They possess small pores, that turn pink as the spores mature, ranging from pink-brown, to red-brown.

Tylopilus derives from the Greek *tylo* meaning, "bump" and *pilo*s, "hat". Ballouii is named in honor of Dr. W.H. Ballou. Felleus is from the Latin *fel*, meaning bile or bitter. Plumeoviolaceus derives from the Latin *plumbeus* meaning "lead-colored", and *violaceus*, for purple. The former genus Gyroporus suggests "having round spores."

Caution should be observed when purchasing commercial, possibly adulterated, dried porcini from China (Casale et al, 2016).

Bitter Bolete has a reticulate network over the whole stipe. Ethanol extracts of the fruiting body are selectively cytotoxic to NIH-3T3 (sarcoma & leukemia virus) and MCF-7 (breast) cancer cell lines (Susaniková et al, 2018).

Slanc et al. (2004) examined sixty species of macrofungi. They found *T. felleus* fruiting body exhibited pancreatic lipase inhibitory activity of 96%.

The related *T. neofelleus* looks similar but has smaller spores. It is restricted to Asian countries, including India, China, Taiwan and New Guinea.

Tylopeptins A & B have been identified and shown active against a few Gram-positive bacteria (Lee et al, 1999).

Burnt-Orange Bolete (*T. ballouii*) is considered a non-poisonous edible.

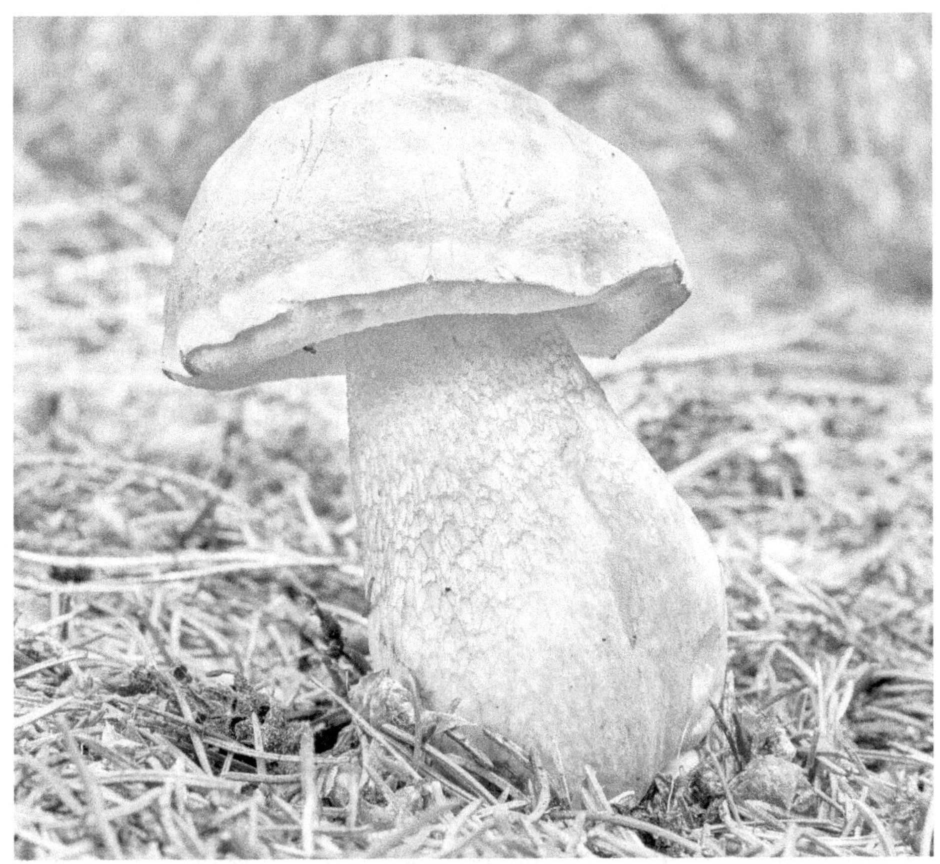

Tylopilus felleus

The dried fruiting body contains variegatic acid, responsible for the blueing reaction in Boletes, Suillus and related genera.

Variegatic acid is an inhibitor of Beta-hexosaminidase release and tumor necrosis factor (TNF)-alpha secretion from rat basophilic leukemia (RBL-2H3) cells.

On the other hand, variegatic acid inhibits PKCbeta1 activity (Sugaya et al, 2020). The latter is important in curtailing diabetic complications, or disordered fatty acid metabolism. Hyperglycemia and microvascular complications are reduced.

Fucogalactomannan is a non-sulphated polysaccharide, derived from this mushroom. Work by Lima et al, (2016) found this compound to possess anti-oxidant and anti-inflammatory activity.

Burnt-Orange Bolete polysaccharides were found in mice studies, to stimulate the immune system through toll-like receptor-4, via NFkappaB pathway. The same study found the water-soluble compounds promoted maturity of human monocyte-derived dendritic cells (Li et al, 2021).

Other work by Li et al, (2021a) examined the immune modulating effect of an ethanol extract, which was fractionated. Two compounds, pistillarin and 1-ribofuranosyl-s-triazin-2(1H)-one exhibited significant immune suppressive effect on human peripheral blood mononuclear cells. They reduced inflammatory cytokine production, including tumor necrosis factor-alpha, interleukin-10, interferon (IFN)-gamma and IL-1beta. Pistillarin was identified in the family Boletaceae, for the first time.

Violet-Grey Bolete is common in oak forests of eastern North America, and Korea.

It contains tylopiol A & B, uridine, alllitol, uracil and ergothioneine; as well as two novel secoergosterols.

Uracil is usually associated with cancer drugs. A recent review by Ramesh et al, (2020) looked at the potential of uracil and its derivates in a number of pathogenic and physiological disorders.

Uridine is a pyrimidine nucleoside involved in the regulation of a number of biological systems, with likely targets including the respiratory, circulatory, reproductive and nervous systems; as well as treatment of cancer and HIV (Connolly & Duley, 1999).

More precisely, uridine plays a crucial role in synthesis of RNA, glycogen and the biomembrane in humans, and is present in blood plasma in considerably higher amounts than other purine and pyrimidine nucleosides. It also helps protect against the ravages of the chemotherapy drug 5-fluououracil (5-FU). Some of the factors associated with an increase include enhanced ATP consumption, enhanced uridine diphosphate-glucose consumption via glycogenesis; and inhibited uridine uptake by cells via the nucleoside transport pathway.

Other factors include increased intestinal absorption, and increased 5-phosphribosyl-1-pyrophosphate and urea synthesis. On the other hand, factors that decrease uridine in blood plasma are associated with increased uptake by cells via the nucleoside transport pathway and decreased pyrimidine synthesis (Yamamoto et al, 2011).

Uridine natural products show benefit as enzyme inhibitors and antibiotics (Arbour & Imperiali, 2020).

Allitol is a rare sugar alcohol, also found in other mushrooms, including Oyster (Pleurotus species). A 9:1 ratio of allitol and a terpene shows significant inhibition against *Haemonchus contortus*, a major parasite infecting sheep (González-Cortázar et al, 2021).

According to McIlvaine, who consumed numerous mushrooms during his lifetime, the fruiting body of *T. chromapes* is edible. This may be true, but it is a hyper-accumulator of the toxic heavy metal mercury, and attention to the terrain is critical.

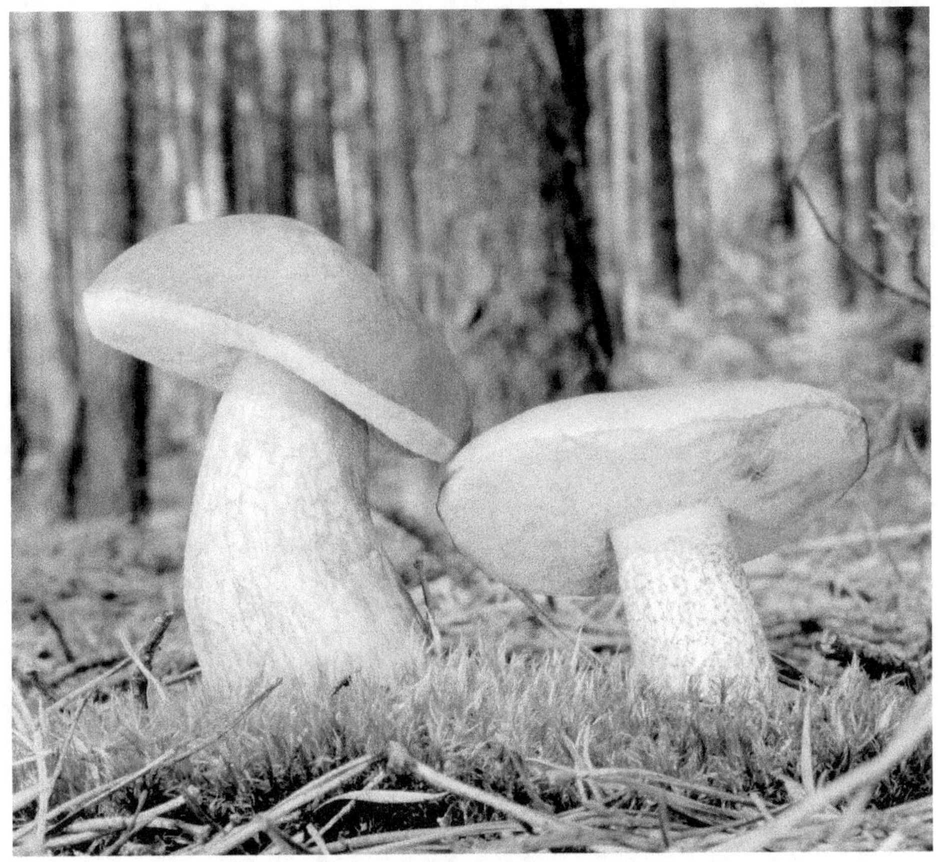

Tylopilus felleus

UMBRELLA POLYPORE
(*Dendropolyporus umbellata*)
(*Polyporus umbellatus*)

The Mind is like an Umbrella. It's most useful when open.
Walter Gropins

CONSTITUENTS - Fruiting body- ergosterol, beta-glucans, alpha-hydroxy-tetraconsanoic acid, biotin, polysaccharides, Gu1-4, Ap1-10, 3,4-dihyroxybenzaldehyde, aceto-syringone, polyporusterones A-G, ergone (<10µ/g). Sclerotia- polysaccharides, makisterone derivatives, silica, ergosterols, D-mannose, D-galactose, D-glucose, triterpenoids, steroidal compounds, long chain fatty acids, ceramides, phenols, thaumatin-like protein genes, uronic acid, ergosterol, ergosta-4,6,8(14), 22-tetraen-3-one (ergone).

Mycorrhizal bacteria- 21 strains, including 5 *Pseudomonas*.

About two decades ago, while biking through a local ravine, I spotted a large mushroom. As I got closer, I became excited that perhaps I had found Maitake (*Grifola frondosa*). That evening I took the fruiting body to our mycological society meeting and found out it was the closely related and similar-looking Umbrella Polypore (previously named *Grifola umbellata*).

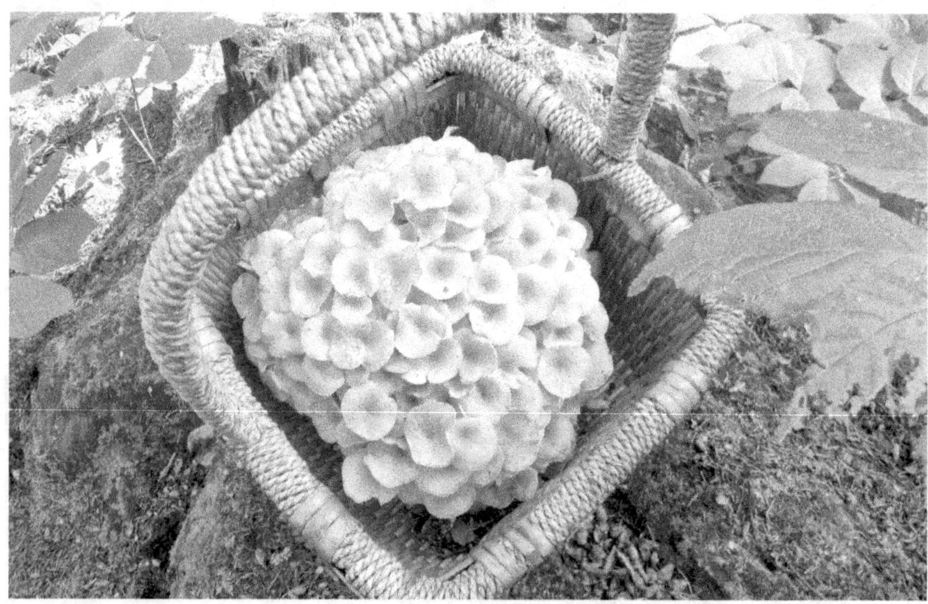

Polyporus umbellatus

Maitake is considered an eastern North American species although I was introduced, by Willoughby Arevalo, to a large specimen under a red oak in downtown Vancouver, British Columbia.

The fruiting body I found (Chorei) was delicious, and I return most summers to the same spot for further gustatory delights.

Later I learned the underground sclerotia, Zhu Ling, is highly prized in Traditional Chinese Medicine (TCM).

In *Ben Cao Gang Mu* Materia Medica, written by Li Shi Zhen in 1578, the mushroom helps in "dispersing invading vicious factors and facilitating urination. Long term use makes one feel happy and vigorous and look younger."

The sclerotia has been used for thousands of years for edema, scanty urine, jaundice and vaginal discharge.

The sclerotia is a strong anti-aldosterone diuretic. An eight-gram decoction increases six-hour output of urine by 62%, with a 53% increase in chloride removal.

It may surprise some readers of the symbiotic relationship between the saprophytic Umbrella, and Honey mushrooms.

The invading rhizomorphs of the latter invade, or infect the Umbrella sclerotia and create unique secondary compounds (Huang et al, 2017). The relationship is more than simply symbiotic, as the sclerotia requires Honey rhizomorphs to supply nutrition. Or perhaps, the Honey mushroom consumes the rhizomorphs for food. The entire mechanism is not yet fully understood (Xing et al, 2020).

At the same time, a defense response to invasion creates unique thaumatin-like proteins (Liu et al, 2017).

Research by Lee et al. (2007) cultured umbrella and honey mycelia together, and greatly increased production of ergone (86.9μ/g) and growth of mycelium.

Ergone is an anti-aldosteronic diuretic, with *in vitro* cytotoxicity against human HepG2, Hep-2 and Hela cancer cell lines, but sparing normal human cells (Zhao et al, 2010).

The fruiting body contains polyporusterones A-G, which show cytotoxic effect on leukemia 1210 cell lines (Ohsawa et al, 1992). The fruiting body also contains novel beta-glucans that potently activate B cells, macrophages and dendritic cells, as well as IgM production, in vivo (Dai et al, 2012).

Polyporusterones A and B, as well as acetosyringone, promote hair growth (Ishida et al, 1999).

But it is the underground sclerotia that has been most widely studied.

Perhaps the greatest benefit of umbrella polypore sclerotia polysaccharides (PUPS) are their immune-enhancing, anti-tumor, anti-inflammatory and hepatoprotective activity.

PUPS induce activation and maturation of bone-derived dendritic cells via toll-like receptor 4, including enhanced production of interleukin-12 and IL-10; as well as increased T cells. (Li et al, 2010).

Bladder cancer is one of the most malignant tumors associated with macrophage immune dysfunction. A newly identified water-soluble polysaccharide shows increased immune modulation as well as increased IL-6, IL-1beta, and IL-23 (Liu et al, 2020).

Twenty-two patients with recurrent bladder cancer benefited from decoctions of the sclerotia (Yang et al, 1999). In this first study, the sclerotia prevented recurrence post-operatively.

By regulating intrarenal fatty acyl metabolites, the polysaccharides prevent kidney damage, measured by creatinine levels, and subsequent kidney fibrosis (Wang et al, 2021).

Bladder cancer models, found PUPS activated macrophages of M1 type and inhibited proliferation, regulated apoptosis and inhibited migration (Jia et al, 2021).

Ergosterol and D-mannitol increase urinary output, with significant excretion of sodium and chloride, but spare potassium (Zhao et al, 2009). Uronic acid (8.5%) has been identified in some branched polysaccharides, indicating higher anti-oxidant activity (He et al, 2016).

A significant review of efficacy in treating hepatitis B in China has been recently published by Guo et al, (2019). Nearly 400 million people, worldwide, suffer hepatitis B, making these clinical trials of great importance.

A total of 11,703 clinical reported cases from over 100 publications during the past 27 years were evaluated. More importantly for me, they were translated in English. The bottom line is that most studies showed the effectiveness of PUPS for treating hepatitis B virus (HBV), in most reported cases.

PUPS was originally named *Polyporus umbellatus* extract 757 in 1979 and renamed in 1983. Both injection and capsule form are approved by the Chinese FDA for mono or combination therapy.

Only twenty cases (0.17%) of adverse reactions were associated with the PUPS injections, none with capsules.

PUPS maintain relatively stable C-AMP/C-GMP ratio in liver cells, reduce serum transaminase activity, promote glycogenesis and help regenerate and repair the hepatocytes. It also enhances immunity by inhibiting hepatitis B replication by increasing phagocytic ability of macrophages, activating T lymphocytes, and thus antibody production of B lymphocytes.

Chronic hepatitis B infection can lead to fibrosis, cirrhosis and carcinoma.

Liu et al, (1993) treated 156 cases of chronic hepatitis B infected patients with PUPS injection. After three months, levels of HBV-DNA decreased by 58.8%.

Capsules also help. In a study by Chen & Luo (2001), 28 patients with HBV showed positive liver markers, with anti-HBeAb positive in 53% of patients.

Combined therapies, including hepatitis B vaccine, or interferon, acyclovir or IRNA (immunoglobulin ribonucleic acid) are all better than when treated with drug alone.

Over 5570 cases of chronic hepatitis B infection from 44 studies were treated with a combination of hepatitis B vaccine and PUPS.

All parameters, including normalization of alanine transaminase, was significantly better than control taking only vaccine.

Interferon is sometimes used in chronic cases, but has low response time and significant side effects.

Nineteen studies involving 710 patients treated with PUPS and interferon, clearly showed improved efficacy over interferon therapy alone.

In 120 liver cancer patients, this combination reported an overall 66% response, with efficacy better than the 400 hepatectomy cases in control group with rate of 41%.

In the cases of combined therapy with the anti-viral drug acyclovir, as well as IRNA, combining treatment with PUPS was superior to the drug alone.

Four clinical trials on patients with lung cancer and treatment with chemotherapy and PUPS were conducted.

Gu, B. (1981; 1984) treated 150 lung cancer patients with PUPS and chemotherapy drugs (CTX, VCR, MTX, 5-FU). Results show that all PUPS treatment groups had better response rate and in addition, the improvement on six-month survival was significantly elevated.

In another clinical trial, 30 patients with small cell lung cancer were given chemotherapy alone, and 50 patients were given chemotherapy along with PUPS (Bian & Li, 1997). Short term curative rates were better for PUPS group.

Work by Tan et al, (2016) suggests possible benefit in breast cancer treatment, inducing apoptosis (self-programmed death) by AKT, an essential signaling pathway to regulate cell proliferation. A fusion of Umbrella and *Ganoderma lucidum* mycelium inhibited cell proliferation and induced apoptosis in MCF-7 breast cancer cell lines, with minimal effect on normal cells. The combination increased calcium signaling, that plays an important role in inducing apoptosis (Kim et al, 2016).

Red Sage (*Salvia miltiorrhizae*) is widely used in TCM for a wide range of health issues, particularly cardiovascular concerns.

A *Pseudomonas* bacterial strain, ZL8, isolated from mycorrhiza, inhibits fungal pathogens, and promotes the growth of Red Sage, and increased ability to dissolve phosphate (Han et al, 2022).

In a clinical trial of 90 patients with chronic hepatitis B, three groups were formed. One group received the herb only, the second group only PUP, and third group received combined treatment.

After three months, the follow up revealed the combined therapy was more potent than either on its own. ALT levels were normal in 83.3% of combined group, compared to 43.8% in herb group, and 56.3 in PUPS group (Xiong, 1993).

PUPs demonstrate pulmonary anti-fibrotic activity by suppressing extracellular matrix deposition, albeit an *in vivo* study (Jiang et al, 2020).

Bladder cancer ranks 6th and results in around sixteen thousand annual deaths in US. The tuberculosis vaccine Bacille Calmette-Guerin (BCG), which celebrated its 100th year anniversary last year, is often used for superficial bladder conditions with a short-term 67% efficacy. PUPs strongly reduce side-effects and are synergistic in rat bladder cancer cell models (Zhang et al, 2015).

Recruitment for 20 BCG human clinical trials involving BCG is presently ongoing, related to respiratory damage associated with COVID-19. Time will tell.

Perhaps Umbrella polypore, or reishi would give equally good results!

DOSAGE - Decoction of dried sclerotium, 6 to 15 grams daily.

Polysaccharide extracts-3 to 6 grams daily in divided doses.

CAUTION - avoid use in cold, dry conditions. Contraindicated for patients taking diuretic medication.

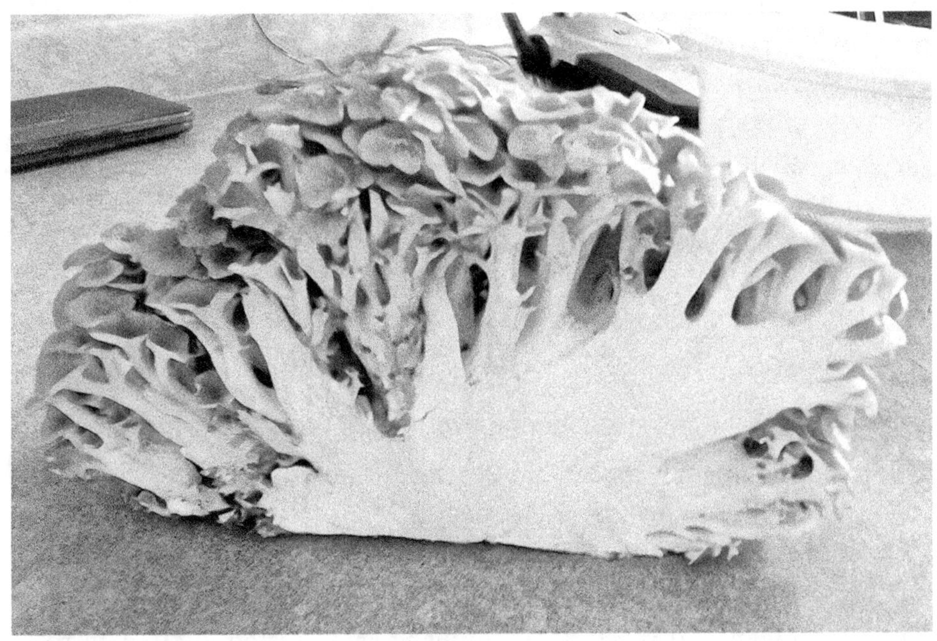

Polyporus umbellatus

WAX GILLS AND WAX CAPS
HYGROPHORUS AND HYGROCYBE
PINK MOTTLE WOODWAX
FALSE RUSSULA
RUSSULA-LIKE WAX CAP
(*Hygrophorus russula*)
GOLDEN TOOTH WAX CAP
GOLD FLECKED WOODWAX
(*H. chrysodon*)
EBONY WAX CAP
(*H. latitabundus*)
OLIVE WAX CAP
OLIVE HYGROPHORUS
SHEATHED WAX GILL
(*H. olivaceoalbus*)
IVORY WAXCAP
COWBOY'S HANKERCHIEF
(*H. ebureus*)
BLUSHING WAX CAP
TURPENTINE WAX CAP
(*H. abieticola*)
WITCH'S HAT
(*Hygrocybe singerii*)
(*H. conica*)
PERSISTANT WAXY CAP
(*H. acutoconica*)
BLACKENING WAXCAP
(*H. nigrescens*)

The family of waxy caps contains over 600 species.

Hygrophorus means "moisture-bearing", and hygrocybe, "moisture head." Gliophorus means, "glue-bearing." Abieticola means "dweller of the firs."

Singeri is named in honor of Rolf Singer, the German mycologist. Eburneus means "of ivory." Psittacinus means "pertaining to a parrot."

It is not the caps which are waxy, however, but the gills.

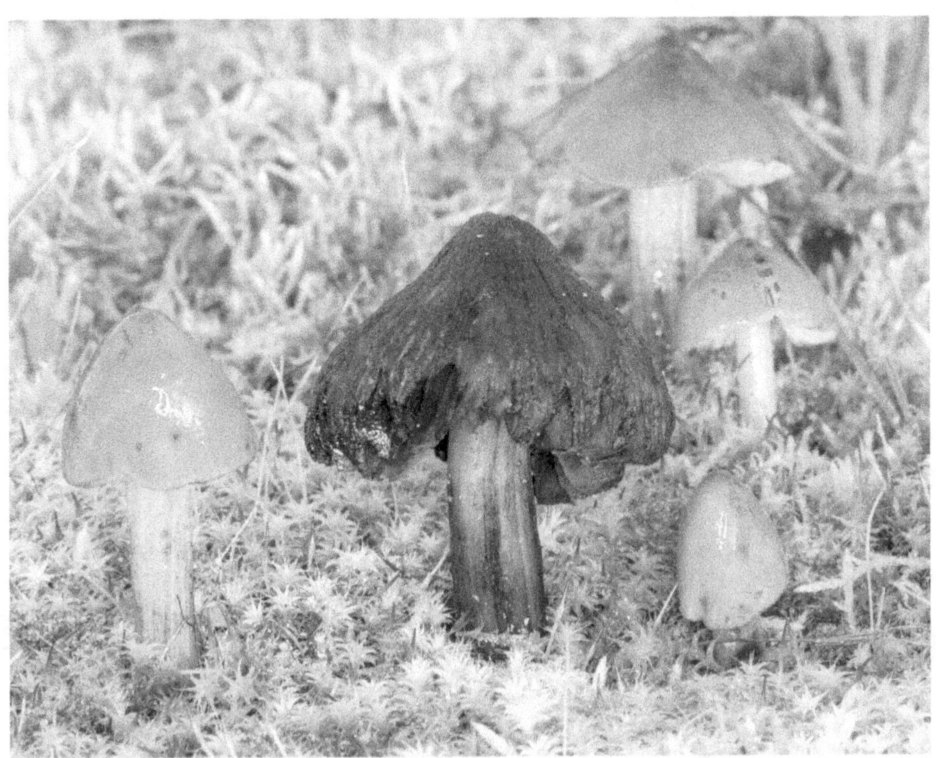

Hygrophorus conica

Hygrophorus species are thick and wide spaced, and ectomycorrhizal with trees.

Hygrocybe genus contains about one hundred species, and are often brightly colored, many staining black, after handling. Often found on grasslands, they were originally believed to be decomposers, but now considered symbionts with plants.

And large plants at that. The Giant Sequoia is an iconic conifer living on the western slopes of the California Sierra Nevada. *Hygrocybe* species have been found in relative mycorrhizal abundance beneath these long-lived trees (Carey et al, 2020). They can grow to 85 meters tall, with a circumference of 34 meters, and a lifespan of an estimated 3266 years.

In the 1950s, the genus Gliophorus was created to accommodate the Parrot Waxy Cap, and genetic work in the 2010s appears to justify the genus split (MacKinnon & Luther, 2021).

False Russula (*Hygrophorus russula*) initially appears at first glance to be Russula, but it has a non-brittle stipe. It is common under oak in eastern North America in late summer, and considered edible by a few authors.

A mannose-specific lectin isolated from the fruiting body showed homology with Hen of the Woods (*Grifola frondosa*) lectin. Work by Suzuki et al, (2012) found a mitogenic activity against spleen lymph cells of an F344 rat, and strong binding to human immunodeficiency virus type-1 gp120.

A novel ribonuclease isolated from the fruiting body at 58° C inhibits the activity of HIV-1 reverse transcriptase (Zhu et al, 2013).

Golden Tooth Waxcap (*H. chrysodon*) is easily identified by the golden granules or hairs on the cap, stipe and gills.

Chrysotriones isolated from the fruiting body, possess antifungal activity against *Fusarium verticillioides*, a common worldwide pathogen of cultivated plants. Chrysotriones are the first example of 2-acylcyclopentene-1,3-diones found in mushrooms (Gilardoni et al, 2007).

Another interesting group of fungicial compounds are hygrophorones, with a structural similarity to the antibiotic pentenomycin. Various species, including Ebony Waxcap (*H. latitabundus*), Olive Waxcap (*H. olivaceoalbus*), *H. persoonia*, and *H. pustulatus* were investigated, for these interesting compounds (Lubken et al, 2004).

Blushing Waxcap contains pseudohygrophorones, naturally occurring alkyl cyclohexenones that exhibit pronounced activity against phytopathogenic organisms (Otto et al, 2016).

Ivory Waxcap is also known by the colorful Cowboy's Hankerchief, in reference to its thick, slimy coating. MacKinnon (2021:84) remarks. "Edible but not for the myxophobic mycophagist (slime-hating mushroom eater)."

Work by Kosanic et al, (2020) looked at several possible health benefits from extracts of the fruiting body. The ability to inhibit acetylcholinesterase ranged from 13-46%, suggesting some possible neuroprotection.

Anti-bacterial and anti-fungal activity was moderate, while anti-oxidant activity was potent. Both human colorectal (HCT-116) and breast (MDA-MB-231) cancer cells lines were tested for cytotoxicity. The migration of former was significantly inhibited, while breast cancer cell lines were less sensitive to treatment.

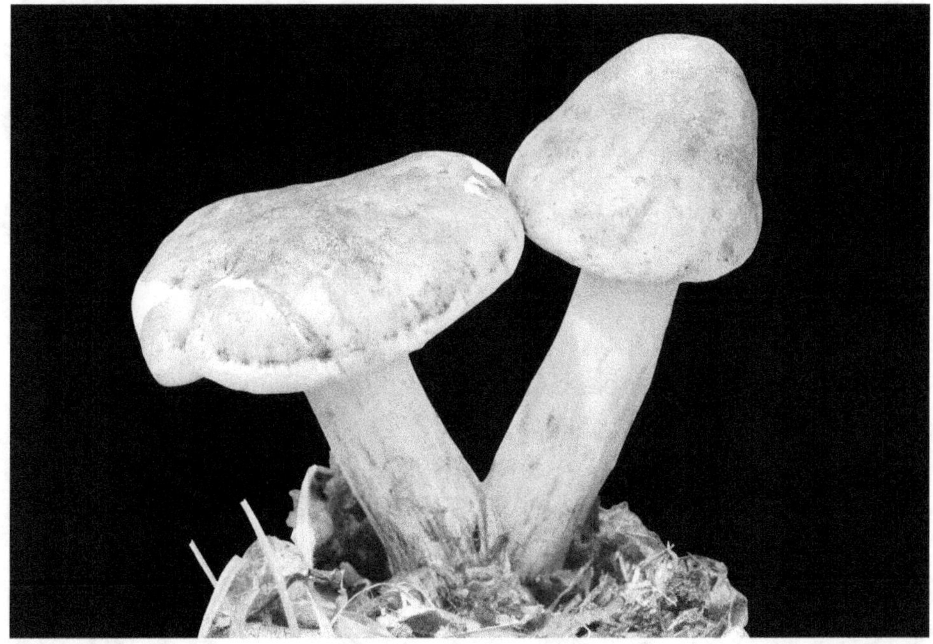

Hygrophorus russula

Ivory Cap contains the beta-carboline alkaloids harmane and norharmane (Teichert et al, 2008). These compounds are reversible competitive MAO inhibitors, helping increasing serotonin and its binding to receptors.

The related *H. hyacinthinus* contains the beta-carboline brunnein A, which weakly binds.

The most colorful, and a personal favorite, is Parrot Waxy Cap (*Glioporus psittacinus*). Formerly known as *Hygrocybe psittacina*, the bright green cap and yellow stipe always bring a smile.

Witch's Hat (*Hygrocybe. conica*) was at one time considered a mainly European species. In western North America it is best known as *H. singeri* complex. When handled the yellow-orange caps quickly blacken.

Slanc et al, (2004) examined extracts of sixty mushroom species, and found *H. conica* to exhibit lipase inhibition of 97% +/- 5%. Suppression of pancreatic lipase prevents the breakdown of fatty acids.

Persistent Waxy Cap, also known as Acute Conic Waxy Cap (*H. acutoconica*) looks very similar, but does not blacken when handled. It is found in southeastern United States, and although considered edible, is not very highly rated.

The fruiting body exhibits excellent antimutagenicity with a ratio of 97% for TA100, and a rate of 96% for TA98 strain against mutagens in the presence of metabolic activation system (Alkan et al, 2020). These are agar-based Ames tests, based on *Salmonella typhimurium* bacteria with a defective (mutant) gene unable to synthesize histidine. It is regularly used to screen for toxicity of new chemicals and drugs.

Blackening Waxcap (*H. nigrescens*) is confined to Europe and parts of Africa. Work by Millar et al, (2019) examined 23 mushrooms from the woodlands of Northern Ireland, for activity against the non-tuberculous *Mycobacterium abscessus*, isolated from cystic fibrosis patients. This species showed anti-mycobacterial activity against the isolates at 38.5 mg/ml.

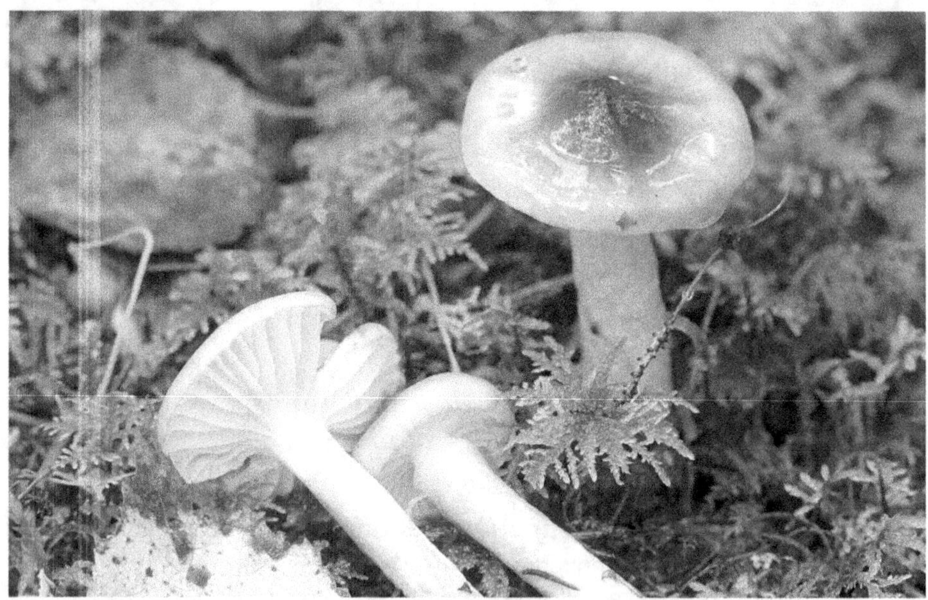

Hygrophorus olivaceoalbus

REFERENCES

AGARIKON References:

Altannavch, N., X. Zhou, A. Khan, A. Ahmed, S. Naranmandakh, J.J. Fu, H.C. Chen. 2022. Anti-oxidant and Anticancerous Effect of Fomitopsis officinalis (Vill. Ex Fr. Bond. Et Sing) Mushroom on Hepatocellular Carcinoma Cells in Vitro through NF-kB Pathway. *Anticancer Agents in Medicinal Chemistry* 22(8): 1561-1570.

Barbeau, M. 1929. Totem Poles of the Gitksan, Upper Skeena River, British Columbia. *National Museum of Canada Bulletin No. 61*, Ottawa.

Blanchette, R.A., D.T. Haynes, B.W. Held, J. Niemann, N. Wales 2021. Fungal mycelial mats used as textile by indigenous people of North America. *Mycologia* 113(2): 261-267.

Chen, Shiuan et al. 2005. Chemopreventative properties of mushrooms against breast cancer and prostate cancer. *International Journal of Medicinal Mushrooms* 2005 7 (3): 342-343.

Compton, Brian D. 1993. *Upper North Wakashan and Southern Tsimshian Ethnobotany: The Knowledge and Usage of Plants and Fungi among the Oweekeno, Hanaksiala (Kitlope and Kemano), Haisla, (Kitamaat) and Kitasoo Peoples of the Central and North Coasts of British Columbia.* Unpublished Ph.D. dissertation. University of British Columbia, Vancouver, BC.

Dugan, Frank M. 2011 *Conspectus of World Ethnomycology*. The American Phytopathological Society, St. Paul, Minnesota.

Fijalkowska, A., B. Muszynska, K. Sulkowska-Ziaja, K. Kaia, A. Pawlik, D. Stefaniuk et al. 2020. Medicinal potential of mycelium and fruiting bodies of an arboreal mushroom Fomitopsis officinalis in therapy of lifestyle diseases. *Scientific Reports* 10(1):20081.

Fijalkowska, A., A. Krakowska, J. Lazur, A. Wlodarczyk, P. Zieba et al. 2021. Fortified Mycelium of Fomitopsis officinalis (Agaricomycetes) as a Source of Biologically Active Substances Effective in the Prevention of Civilization Diseases. *International Journal of Medicinal Mushrooms* 23(9):29-44.

Golovchenko, V.V., S. Naranmandakh, J. Ganbaatar, A.Y. Prilepskii, G.L. Burygin, A.O. Chizhov, A.S. Shashkov. 2020. Structural investigation and comparative cytotoxic activity of water-soluble polysaccharides from fruit bodies of the medicinal fungus quinine conk. *Phytochemistry* 175:112313.

Graf, E. & H. J. J. Winckelmann. 1960. Versuche zum umbau der Hydroxy-Triterpencarbon-sauren von Fungus *Laricis* zu 11-Keto-Cortigosteroiden. *Planta Medica* 8(4) 403-410.

Grzywnowicz, Krzysztof. 2001. Medicinal mushrooms in Polish folk medicine. *International Journal of Medicinal Mushrooms.* 3(2-3):156

Hwang, C. H., B. U. Jaki, L. L. Klein, D. C. Lannkin, J. McAlpine, J. G. Naolitano, S. G. Franzblau, S. H. Cho, P. E. Stamets, G. F. Pauli. 2012. Biological and chemical evaluation of anti-TB coumarins from the polypore mushroom, *Fomitopsis officinalis*. *Planta Medica* 78.

Kroeger Paul, Kendrick B, Ceska O, Roberts C. 2012. *The Outer Spores: Mushrooms of Haida Gwaii*. Mycologue Pub. Sidney by the Sea, British Columbia.

Newcombe, C. F. 1897. *Unpublished notes on Haida plants*. C.F. Newcombe Accession 1897-47, Department of Anthropology, American Museum of Natural History. New York.

Newcombe, C. F. 1898-1913. *Unpublished papers*. Provincial Archives of British Columbia, Victoria, B.C.

Robbins, William J. et al. 1945. A survey of some wood-destroying and other fungi for antibacterial activity. *Bulletin of the Torrey Botanical Club* 72(2): 165-190.

Rogers, Robert D. 2011. *The Fungal Pharmacy: The Complete Guide to Medicinal Mushrooms and Lichens of North America*. North Atlantic Books, Berkeley CA

Sato, Mayumi et al. 2002. Dehydrotrametenolic acid induces preadipocyte differentiation and sensitizes animal models of noninsulin-dependent diabetes mellitus to insulin. *Biological and Pharmaceutical Bulletin* 25 (1): 81.

Stamets, Paul. 2005. Notes on nutritional properties of culinary-medicinal mushrooms. *International Journal of Medicinal Mushrooms* 7(3): 103-110.

Teplyakova, T. V, N.V. Purtseva, T. A. Kosogova, V. A. Khanin, V. A. Vlassenko. 2012. Antiviral activity of polyporoid mushrooms (higher Basidiomycetes) from Altal mountains from Russia. *International Journal of Medicinal Mushrooms*. 14(1): 37-45.

Turner, Nancy J. 2004. *Plants of Haida Gwaii*. Sononis Press. Winlaw, British Columbia.

Turner, Nancy J, L. C. Thompson, Terry Thompson, & Annie Z. York. 1990. Thompson Ethnobotany. *Knowledge and Usage of Plants by the Thompson Indians of British Columbia*. Memoir No. 3, Royal British Columbia Museum. Victoria, B.C.

Turner, Nancy J. *Plant Technology of First Peoples in British Columbia*. 1998. Published by UBC Press in collaboration with the Royal British Columbia Museum. Victoria, B.C.

Turner, Nancy J. 1979. *Plants in British Columbia Indian Technology, Handbook No. 38,* British Columbia Provincial Museum.

Vedenicheva, N.P., G.A. Al-Maali, N.A. Bisko, I.V. Kosakivska et al. 2021. Effect of Cytokinin-Containing Extracts from Some Medicinal Mushroom Mycelia on HepG2 Cells In Vitro. *International Journal of Medicinal Mushrooms* 23(3): 15-28.

Weaver, William Woys. 2001. *Sauer's Herbal Cures, America's First Book of Botanic Healing*. Routledge. New York.

ALBATRELLUS References:

Akiba, M, K. Kinoshita, Y. Kino, J.I. Sato, K. Koyama. 2020. Isolation of three new meroterpenoids and seven known compounds from *Albatrellus yasudae* and their AB-aggregation inhibitory activity. *Bioorganic Medicinal Chemistry Letters* 30(2): 126808.

Bycroft, B.W. 1987. *Dictionary of Antibiotic & Related Substances* CRC Press page 241.

Chen, Y., G.F. Peng, X.Z. Han, W. Wang, G.Q. Zhang, X. Li. 2015. Apoptosis prediction via inhibition of AKT signaling pathway by neogrifolin. *International Journal of Clinical and Experimental Pathology* 8(2): 1154-1164.

Deng, Q., X. Yu, L. Xiao, Z. Hu, X. Luo, Y. Tao, L. Yang, X. Liu, et al. 2013. Neoalbaconol induces energy depletion and multiple cell death in cancer cells by targeting PDK1-PI3-K/Akt signaling pathway. *Cell Death & Disease* 4, e804.

Dube, M., D. Llanes, M. Saoud, R. Rennert, P. Imming, C. Haberli, J. Kaiser, N. Arnold. 2022. *Albatrellus confluens* (Alb. & Schwein.) Kotl. & Pouz.: Natural Fungal Compounds and Synthetic Derivatives with In Vitro Anthelmintic Activities and Antiproliferative Effects against Two Human Cancer Cell Lines. *Molecules* 27(9):2950.

Hellwig, V., R. Nopper, F. Mauler, J. Freitag, L.J. Kai, D.Z. Hui, M. Stadler. 2003. Activities of prenylphenol derivatives from fruitbodies of *Albatrellus* spp. on the human and rat vanilloid receptor 1 (VR1) and characterisation of the novel natural product, confluentin. *Archiv der Pharmazie* (Weinheim) 336(2): 19-26.

Hettwer, S., S. Banziger, B. Sutter, B. Obermayer. 2017. Grifolin derivatives from *Albatrellus ovinus* as TRPV1 receptor blockers for cosmetic applications. *International Journal of Cosmetic Science* 39(4): 379-385.

Huang, I.C., H.Y. Chang, C.H. Hsu, W.H. Kuo et al. 2008. Targeting therapy for breast carcinoma by ATP synthase inhibitor aurovertin B. *Journal of Proteome Research* 7(4): 1433-1444.

Liu, L.Y., Z.H. Li, Z.H. Ding, Z.J. Dong, G.T. Li, Y. Li, J.K. Liu. 2013. Meroterpenoid pigments from the basidiomycete *Albatrellus ovinus*. *Journal of Natural Products* 76(1): 79-84.

Liu, L.Y., Z. H. Li, G.Q. Wang, K. Wei, Z.J. Dong et al. 2014. Nine new farnesylphols from the basidiomycete *Albatrellus caeruleoporus*. *Natural Products and Bioprospecting* 4(2): 119-128.

Liu, Q. Y., X.L. Shu, L. Wang, A. Sun, J.K. Liu, X.T. Cao. 2008. Albaconol, a plant-derived (sic) small molecule, inhibits macrophage function by suppressing NF-kappaB activation and enhancing SOCS1 expression. *Cellular and Molecular Immunology* 5(4): 271-278.

Luo, X.J., W. Li, L.F. Yang, X.F. Yu, et al. 2011. DAPK1 mediates the G1 phase arrest in human nasopharyngeal carcinoma cells induced by grifolin, a potential antitumor natural product. *European Journal of Pharmacology* 670(2-3): 427-434.

Luo, X. L., L.F. Yang, L.B. Xiao, X.F. Xia, X. Dong et al. 2015. Grifolin directly targets ERK1/2 to epigenetically suppress cancer cell metastasis. *Oncotarget* 6(40): 42704-42716.

Rogers, Robert. 2016. *Mushroom Essences: Vibrational Healing from the Kingdom Fungi*. North Atlantic Books. Berkeley, CA. page 82.

Szallasi, A., T. Biro, T. Szabo, S. Modarres, M. Petersen et al. 1999. A non-pungent triprenyl phenol of fungal origin, scutigeral, stimulates rat dorsal root ganglion neurons via interaction at vanilloid receptors. *British Journal of Pharmacology* 126(6): 1351-1358.

Wu, R., X. Yang, Q. Zhou, W.Y. Yu, M.W. Li et al. 2020. Aurovertin B exerts potent antitumor activity against triple-negative breast cancer in vivo and in vitro via regulating ATP synthase activity and DUSP1 expression. *Pharmazie* 75(6): 261-265.

Wu, Z.J.& Y. Li. 2017. Grifolin exhibits anti-cancer activity by inhibiting the development and invasion of gastric tumor cells. *Oncotarget* 8(13): 21454-21460.

Yan, H., X.X. Che, Q.T. Lv, L. Zhang, S. Gongol, et al. Grifolin induces apoptosis and promotes cell cycle arrest in the A2780 human ovarian cancer cell line via inactivation of the ERK1/2 and Akt pathways. *Oncology Letters* 13(6): 4806-4812.

Yang, X.L., C. Qin, F. Wang, Z.J. Dong, J.K. Liu. 2008. A new meroterpenoid pigment from the basidiomycete *Albatrellus confluens*. *Chemistry and Biodiversity* 5(3): 484-489.

Yaqoob, A., W.M. Li, V. Liu, C.Y. Wang, S. Mackedenski, L.E. Tackaberry, H. B. Massicotte, K.N. Egger, K. Reimer, C.H. Lee. 2020. Grifolin, neogrifolin and confluentin from the terricolous *Albatrellus flettii* suppress KRAS expression in human colon cancer cells. *PLoS One* 15(5): e0231948.

Ye, M., J.K. Liu, Z.X. Lu, Y. Zhao, S.F. Liu, L.L. Li, M. Tan, X.X. Weng, W. Li, Y. Cao. 2005. Grifolin, a potential antitumor natural product from the mushroom *Albatrellus confluens*, inhibits tumor cell growth by inducing apoptosis *in vitro*. *FEBS Letters* 579(16): 3437-3443.

Yu, X. F., W. Li, Q.P. Deng, S. You, H. Liu et al. 2017. Neoalbaconol inhibits angiogenesis and tumor growth by suppressing EGFR-mediated VEGF production. *Molecular Carcinogenesis* 56(5): 1414-1426.

Zhang, S., Y. Huang, S. He, H. Chen, B. Wu, S.Y. li et al. 2018. Heterocyclic compounds from the mushroom *Albatrellus confluens* and their inhibitions against lipopolysaccharides-induced B lymphocyte cell proliferation. *Journal of Organic Chemistry* 83(17): 10158-10165.

Zhao, Y.F., F. Jiang, X.Y. Liang, L.L. Wei, Y.Y. Zhao et al. 2018a. Grifolic acid causes osteosarcoma cell death *in vitro* and in tumor-bearing mice. *Biomedicine and Pharmacotherapy* 103: 1035-1042.

Zhao, Y.F. L. Zhang, A. Yan, D. Chen, R. Xie, Y.G. Liu et al. 2018b. Grifolic acid induces GH3 adenoma cell death by inhibiting ATP production through a GPR120 independent mechanism. *BMC Pharmacology and Toxicology* 19(1):26.

Zhou, G.Y., C.W. Pan, L.X. Jin, J.J. Zheng, Y.X. Yi. 2016. Neoalbaconol inhibits cell growth of human cholangiocarcinoma cells by up-regulating PTEN. *American Journal of Translational Research* 8(2): 496-505.

Zhu, H.F., F. Wang, X.M. Ju, L. M. Kong, T. An, et al. 2018. Aurovertin B sensitizes colorectal cancer cells to NK cell recognition and lysis. *Biochemical and Biophysical Research Communications* 503(4): 3057-3063.

ARMILLARIA References:

An, S., W.Q. Lu, Y.F. Zhang, Q.X. Yuan, D. Wang. 2017. Pharmalogical basis for the use of *Armillaria mellea* polysaccharides in Alzheimer's disease: Anti-apoptosis and antioxidation. *Oxidative Medicine and Cellular Longevity* Article ID 4184562.

Bohnert, M., S. Miethbauer, H.M. Dahse, J. Ziemen, M. Nett, D. Hoffmeister. 2011. In vitro cytotoxicity of melleolide antibiotics: structural and mechanistic aspects. *Bioorganic Medicinal Chemistry Letters* 21(7): 2003-2006.

Chang, W.H., H.L. Huang, W.P. Huang, C.C. Chen, Y.J. Chen. 2016. Armillaridin induces autophagy-associated cell death in human chronic myelogenous leukemia K562 cells. *Tumour Biology* 37(10): 14291-14300.

Chang, C.C., J.J. Cheng, I.J. Lee, M.K. Lu. 2018. Purification, structural elucidation, and anti-inflammatory activity of xylosyl galactofucan from Armillaria mellea. *International Journal of Biological Macromolecules* 114: 584-591.

Chen, R.Z., X. Ren, W. Yin, J. Lu, L. Tian, L. Zhao, R.P. Yang, S.J. Luo. 2020. Ultrasonic disruption extraction, characterization and bioactivities of polysaccharides from wild Armillaria mellea. *International Journal of Biological Macromolecules* 156: 1491-1502.

Chen, Y.J., S.Y. Wu, C.C. Chen Y.L. Tsao et al. 2004. *Armillaria mellea* component armillarikin induces apoptosis in human leukemia cells. *Journal of Functional Foods* 6(1): 196-204.

Chen, Y.J., C.C. Chen, H.L. Huang. 2016. Induction of apoptosis by *Armillaria mellea* constituent armillarkin in human hepatocellular carcinoma. *OncoTargets and Therapy* 9:4773-4783.

Chi, C.W., C.C. Chen, Y.J. Chen. 2013. Therapeutic and radiosensitizing effects of armillaridin on human esophageal cancer cells. *Evidence Based Complementary and Alternative Medicine* 2013: 459271.

Duan, Y.X. 2000. Observation on the clinical effect of Tian Xuan Qing (gastrodin) in treating vertigo and headache. *Chinese Traditional and Herbal Drugs* 31(4): 288, 303.

Feng, K., Q.H. Liu, T.B. Ng, H.Z. Liu, J.Q. Li, G. Chen, H.Y. Sheng, Z.L. Xie, H.X. Wang. 2006. Isolation and characterization of a novel lectin from the mushroom Armillaria luteo-virens. *Biochemical & Biophysical Research Communications* 345(4): 1573-1578.

Huang, J.W., C.J.S. Lai, Y. Yuan, M. Zhang, J.H. Zhou, L.Q. Huang. 2017. Correlative analysis advance of chemical constituents of *Polyporus umbellatus* and *Armillaria mellea* (in Chinese). *Zhongguo Zhong Yao Za Zhi* 42(15): 2905-2914.

Jiang, S. et al. 2002. Clinical study on Tian Xuan Qing (gastrodin) injection in treating blood supply insufficiency vertigo of the vertebra-basilar artery. *Chinese Traditional and Herbal Drugs* 33(5): 449-450.

Jiangsu Provincial Cooperation Research Group on Gastrodia Tuber. 1980. Curative effect of gastrodia tuber Armillaria fungus tablet in treating some diseases of the nervous system. *Jiangsu Journal of Traditional Chinese Medicine* 1: 35-37.

Koch, R.A. & J.R. Herr. 2021. Transcriptomics reveals the putative mycoparasitic strategy of the mushroom *Entoloma abortivum* on species of the mushroom genus *Armillaria. mSystems* doi: 10.1128.mSystems.00544-21.

König, S., E. Romp, V. Krauth, M. Rühl, M. Dörfer, S. Liening, B. Hofmann et al. 2019. Melleolides from Honey Mushroom Inhibit 5-Lipoxygenase via Cys159. *Cell Chemical Biology* 26(1): 60-70.

Kostic, M., M. Smiljkovic, J. Petrovic, J. Glamoclija, L. Barros, I. Ferreira, A. Ciric, M. Sokovic. 2017. Chemical, nutritive composition and a wide range of bioactive properties of honey mushroom Armillaria mellea (Vahl: Fr.) Kummer. *Food and Function* 8(9): 3239-3249.

Leu, Y.S. Y.J. Chen, C.C. Chen, H.L. Huang. 2019. Induction of autophagic death of human hepatocellular carcinoma cells by armillaridin from *Armillaria mellea. American Journal of Chinese Medicine* 47(6): 1365-1380.

Li, C.I., T.W. Lin, T.Y. Lee, Y. Lo, Y.M. Jiang, Y.H. Kuo, C.C. Chen, F.C. Chang. 2021. Oral Administration of *Armillaria mellea* Mycelia Promote Non-Rapid Eye Movement and Rapid Eye Movement Sleep in Rats. *Journal Fungi* (Basel) 7(5): 371.

Li, H.T., L.H. Tang, T. Liu, R.N. Yang, Y.B. Yang, H. Zhou, Z.T. Ding. 2020. Protoilludane-type sesquiterpenoids from Armillaria sp. by co-culture with the endophytic fungus Epicoccum sp. associated with Gastrodia elata. *Bioorganic Chemistry* 95: 103503.

Li, Z.J., Y.C. Wang, B. Jiang, M.L. Li et al. 2016. Structure, cytotoxic activity and mechanism of protoilludane sesquiterpene aryl esters from the mycelium of *Armillaria mellea. Journal of Ethnopharmacology* 184: 119-127.

Lin, Y.E., H.L. Wang, K.H, Lu, Y.J. Huang, S. Panyod, W.T. Liu et al. 2021. Water extract of *Armillaria mellea* (Vahl) P. Kumm. Alleviates the depression-like behaviors in acute-and chronic mild stress-induced rodent models via anti-inflammatory action. *Journal of Ethnopharmacology* 265: 113395.

Liu, T.P., C.C. Chen, P.Y. Shiao, H.R. Shieh, Y.Y. Chen, Y.J. Chen. 2015. Armillaridin, a honey medicinal mushroom, *Armillaria mellea* (higher basidiomycetes) component, inhibits differentiation and activation of human macrophages. *International Journal of Medicinal Mushrooms* 17(2): 161-168.

Mihail, J.D. 2015. Bioluminescence patterns among North American Armillaria species. *Fungal Biology* 119(6): 528-537.

Ojemann, L.M., W.L. Nelson, D.S. Shin, A.O. Rowe, R.A. Buchanan. 2006. Tian Ma, an ancient Chinese herb, offers new options for the treatment of epilepsy and other conditions. *Epilepsy Behavior* 8(2): 376-383.

Purtov, K.V., V.N. Petushkov, N.S. Rodionova, J. Gitelson. 2017. Why does the bioluminescent fungus *Armillaria mellea* have luminous mycelium but nonluminous fruiting body? *Doklady Biochemistry & Biophysics* 474(1): 217-219.

Rogers, R. 2016. *Mushroom Essences: Vibrational Healing from the Kingdom Fungi.* North Atlantic Books, Berkeley CA.

Ross-Davis, A.L. J.W. Hanna, N.B. Klopfenstein, M.S. Kim. 2012. Advances toward DNA-based identification and phylogeny of North American *Armillaria* species using elongation factor-1 alpha gene. *Mycoscience* 53(2): 161-165.

Stalpers, J.A, S.A. Redhead, T.W. May, A.Y. Rossman, J.A. Crouch, M.A. Cubeta, et al. 2021. Competing sexual-asexual generic names in *Agaricomycotina* (*Basidiomycota*) with recommendations for use. *IMA Fungus* 12:22 doi. org/10.1186/s43008-021-00061-3.

Watanabe, N., T. Obuchi, M. Tamai, H. Araki, S. Omura et al. 1990. A novel N6-substituted adenosine isolated from mi huan jun (*Armillaria mellea*) as a cerebral-protecting compound. *Planta Medica* 56(1): 48-52.

Xing, X., J.X. Men, L.L. Song, S.X. Guo. 2020. Do the main components of
the sclerotia of umbrella polypore mushroom, *Polyporus umbellatus*
(Agaricomycetes), correlate with Armillaria associates? *International
Journal of Medicinal Mushrooms* 22(5): 479-488).

Yao, L., J.H. Lv, C. Duan, X. An, C. Zhang, D. Li, C.T. Li, S.Y. Liu. 2022. Armillaria
mellea fermentation liquor ameliorates p-chlorophenylanine-induced
insomnia associated with the modulation of serotonergic system and gut
microbiota in rats. *Journal of Food Biochemistry* 46(2):e14075.

Yong, T.Q., S.D. Chen, Y.Z. Xie, D.L. Chen, J.Y. Su, O. Shuai, H.P. Hu, D. Zuo, D.L.
Liang. 2018. Hypouricemic Effects of Armillaria mellea on Hyperuricemic
Mice Regulated through OAT1 and CNT2. *American Journal of Chinese
Medicine* 46(3): 585-599.

Zhang, T.W. Y.H. Du, X.F. Liu, X.L. Sun, E. Cai, H.Y. Zhu, Y. Zhao. 2021. Study on
antidepressant-like effect of protoilludane sesquiterpenoid aromatic esters
from *Armillaria mellea. Natural Product Research* 35(6): 1042-2045.

Zhou, L.S. 1978. Observation on curative effects of *Armillaria mellea* fungus tablet
in treating 100 cases of neurasthenia and hypertension, etc. *Journal of New
Medicine* 10:13.

ARTIST'S CONK References

Donatini, B. 2014. Control of oral human papillomavirus (HPV) by medicinal
mushrooms, Trametes versicolor and Ganoderma lucidum: a preliminary
clinical trial. *International Journal of Medicinal Mushrooms* 16(5):497-498.

Elkhateeb, W.A., G.M. Zaghlol, I.M. El-Garawani, E.F. Ahmed, M.E. Rateb, A.E.A.
Moneim. 2018. Ganoderma applanatum secondary metabolites induced
apoptosis through different pathways: in vivo and in vitro anticancer studies.
Biomedicine and Pharmacotherapy 101:264-277.

Hanyu, X., L. Lanyue, D. Miao, F. Wentao, C. Cangran, S. Hui. 2020. Effect of
Ganoderma applanatum polysaccharides on MAPK/ERK pathway affecting
autophagy in breast cancer MCF-7 cells. *International Journal of Biological
Macromolecules* 146:353-362.

Hassan, F., S.S. Ni, T.L. Becker, C.M. Kinstedt, J.L. Adul-Samad, L.A. Actis, M.A.
Kennedy 2019. Evaluation of the Antibacterial Activity of 75 Mushrooms
Collected in the Vicinity of Oxford, Ohio (USA). *International Journal of
Medicinal Mushrooms* 21(2):131-141.

Hossain, M.S., A. Barua, M.A.H. Tanim, M.S. Hasan, M.J. Islam et al. 2021.
Ganoderma applanatum mushroom provides new insights into the
management of diabetes mellitus, hyperlipidemia and hepatic degeneration:
A comprehensive analysis. *Food Science and Nutrition* 9(8):4364-4374.

Hossen, S.M.M., M.J. Islam, R. Hossain, A. Barua, G. Uddin, N.U. Emon. 2021. CNS anti-depressant, anxiolytic and analgesic effects of Ganoderma applanatum (mushroom) along with ligand-receptor binding screening provide new insights: Multi-disciplinary approaches. *Biochemistry and Biophysics Reports* 27:101062.

Jiao, Y., T. Xie, L.H. Zou, Q. Wei, L. Qiu, L.X. Chen. 2016. Lanostane triterpenoids from Ganoderma curtisii and their NO production inhibitory activities of LPS-induced microglia. *Bioorganic and Medicinal Chemistry Letters* 26(15):3556-3561.

Kiddane, A.T., M.J. Kang, T.C. Ho, A.T. Getachew, M.P. Patil, B.S. Chun, G.D. Kim. 2022. Anticancer and Apoptotic Activity in Cervical Adenocarcinoma HeLa Using Crude Extract of *Ganoderma applanatum. Current Issues in Molecular Biology* 44(3):1012-1026.

Kumaran, S., A.K. Pandurangan, R. Shenbhagaraman, N.M. Esa. 2017. Isolation and Characterization of Lectin from the Artist's Conk Medicinal Mushoom, Ganoderma applanatum (Agaricomycetes), and Evaluation of Its Antiproliferative Activity in HT-29 Colon Cancer Cells. *International Journal of Medicinal Mushrooms* 19(8):675-684.

Laimuansangi, C., M. Zosangzuali, M. Lairemruati, L. Tochhawng, Z. Siama. 2022. Evaluation of the protective effects of Ganoderma applanatum against doxorubicin-induced toxicity in Dalton's Lymphoma Ascites (DLA) bearing mice. *Drug and Chemical Toxicology* 45(3):1243-1253.

Li, M.Y., L.L. Yu, Q.X. Zhai, B.S. Liu, J.X. Zhao, H. Zhang, W. Chen, F.W. Tian. 2022. *Ganoderma applanatum* polysaccharides and ethanol extracts promote the recovery of colitis through intestinal barrier protection and gut microbiota modulations. *Food and Function* 13(2):688-701.

Luo, D., J.Z. Xie, L.H. Zou, L. Qiu, D.P. Huang, Y.F. Xie, H.J. Xu, X.D. Wu. 2020. Lanostane-type triterpenoids from Ganoderma applanatum and their inhibitory activities on NO production in LPS-induced BV-2 cells. *Phytochemistry* 177:112453.

Mfopa, A., F.K. Mediesse, C. Mvongo, S. Nkoubatchoundjwen, A.A. Lum, E. Sobngwi, R. Kamgang, T. Boudjeko. 2021. Antidyslipidemic Potential of Water-Soluble Polysaccharides of *Ganoderma applanatum* in MACAPOS-2-Induced Obese Rats. *Evidence Based Complementary and Alternative Medicine* 2021:2452057.

Peng, X.R., Q. Wang, H.R. Wang, K. Hu, W.Y. Xiong, M.H. Qiu. 2021. FPR2-based anti-inflammatory and anti-lipogenesis activities of novel meroterpenoid dimers from Ganoderma. *Bioorganic Chemistry* 116:105338.

Raseta, M., M. Popovic, I. Beara, F. Sibul, G. Zengin, S. Krstic, M. Karaman. 2021. Anti-inflammatory, Antioxidant and Enzyme Inhibition Activities in Correlation with Mycochemical Profile of Selected Indigenous Ganoderma spp. from Balkan Region (Serbia). *Chemistry and Biodiversity* 18(2):e20000828.

Rogers, R. 2011. *The Fungal Pharmacy: The Complete Guide to Medicinal Mushrooms and Lichens of North America.* North Atlantic Books, Berkeley, CA.

Rogers, R. & D. Sept. 2020. *Medicinal Mushrooms of Western North America.* Calypso Publishing. Sechelt, B.C.

Su, H.G., Q. Wang, L. Zhou, X.R. Peng, W.Y. Xiong, W.H. Qiu. 2021. Functional triterpenoids from medicinal fungi *Ganoderma applanatum*: A continuous search for antiadipogenic agents. *Bioorganic Chemistry* 112:104977.

Susilo, R.J.K., D. Winarni, S. Hayaza, R.A. Doong, S.PA. Wahyunignsih, W. Darmanto. 2022. Effect of crude *Ganoderma applanatum* polysaccharides as a reno-protective against against carbon tetrachloride-induced early kidney fibrosis in mice. *Veterinary World* 15(4):1022-1030.

Tang, L., Z.F. Zhu, L.P. Cao, M. Shen, Y. Gao, C.J. Tu, Z.H. Zhang, W.G. Shan. 2020. Thermosensitive gel of polysaccharide from Ganoderma applanatum combined with paclitaxel for mice with 4T1 breast cancer. *Zhongguo Zhong Yao Za Zhi* 45(11):2533-2539.

Yong, T.Q., S.D. Chen, Y.Z. Xie, D.L. Chen, J.Y. Su, O. Shuai, C.W. Jiao, C. Zuo. 2018. Hypouricemic Effects of *Ganoderma applanatum* in Hyperuricemia Mice through OAT1 and GLUT9. *Frontiers in Pharmacology* 8:996.

Yong, T.Q., D.L. Liang, C. Xiao, L.H. Huang, S.D. Chen, Y.Z. Xie, X. Gao, Q.P. Wu et al. 2022. Hypouricemic effect of 2,4-dihyroxybenzoic acid methyl ester in hyperuricemic mice through inhibiting XOD and down-regulating URAT1. *Biomedicine and Pharmacotherapy* 153:113303.

Zhou, H., X.R. Peng, T. Hou, N. Zhao, M.H. Qiu, X.L. Zhang, X.M. Liang. 2020. Identification of novel phytocannabinoids from Ganoderma by label-free dynamic mass redistribution assay. *Journal of Ethnopharmacology* 246:112218.

BAROMETER EARTHSTAR References:

Arpha, K., C. Phosri, N. Suwannasai, W. Mongkolthanaruk, S. Sodngam. 2012. Astraodoric acids A-D: new lanostane triterpenes from edible mushroom Astraeus odoratus and their anti-Mycobacterium tuberculosis H37Ra and cytotoxic activity. *Journal of Agricultural and Food Chemistry* 60(39): 9834-9841.

Biswas, G., S. Sarkar, K. Acharya. 2011. Hepatoprotective activity of the ethanolic extract of *Astraeus hygrometricus* (Pers.) Morg. *Digest Journal Nanomaterials and Biostructures* 6(2): 637-641.

Biswas, G., S. Rana, S. Sarker, K. Acharya. Cardioprotective activity of the ethanolic extract of *Astraeus hygrometricus* (Pers) Morg. *Pharmacology Online* 2:808-817.

Biswas, G. K. Acharya. 2013. Hypoglycemic activity of ethanolic extract of *Astraeus hygrometricus* (Pers.) Morg in alloxan-induced diabetic mice. *International Journal of Pharmacy and Pharmaceutical Sci*ences 5(1): 391-394.

Biswas, G., S. Nandi, D. Kuila, K. Acharya. 2017. A Comprehensive Review on Food and Medicinal Prospects of *Astraeus hygrometricus*. *Pharmacognosy Journal* 9(6): 799-806.

Dasgupta, A., D. Dey, D. Ghosh, T.K. Lai, N. Bhuvanesh, S. Dolui, R. Velayuthan, K. Acharya. 2019. Astrakkurkurone, a sesquiterpene from wild edible mushroom, targets liver cancer cells by modulating Bcl-2 family proteins. *International Union of Biochemistry and Molecular Biology Life* 71(7): 992-1002.

Hussain, A., S. Ghosh, K. Roy, S. Nath, B. Sarkar, A. Dutta et al. 2021. A mushroom derived "carbohydrate-fraction" reinstates host-immunity and protects from Leishmania donovani infection. Parasite Immunology 43(3): e12806.

Khan, F. & R. Chandra. 2019. Bioprospecting of Wild Mushrooms from India with Respect to Their Medicinal Aspects. *International Journal of Medicinal Mushrooms* 21(2): 181-192.

Lai, T.K., G. Biswas, S. Chatterjee, A. Dutta, C. Pal, J. Banerji, N. Bhuvanesh, J.H. Reibenspies, K. Acharya. 2012. *Chemistry and Biodiversity* 9(8): 1517-1524.

Mallick, S.K., S. Maiti, S.K. Bhutia, T.K. Maiti. 2010. Immunostimulatory properties of a polysaccharide isolated from Astraeus hygrometricus. Journal of Medicinal Food 13(3): 665-672.

Mallick, S.K. S. Maiti, S.K. Bhutia, T.K. Maiti. 2010a. Antitumor properties of a heteroglucan isolated from Astraeus hygrometricus on Dalton's lymphoma bearing mouse. *Food and Chemical Toxicology* 48(8-9): 2115-2121.

Mallick, S.K., S. Maiti, S.K. Bhutia, T.K. Maiti. 2011. Activation of RAW 264.7 cells by Astraeus hygrometricus-derived heteroglucan through MAP kinase pathway. *Cell Biology International* 35(6): 617-621.

Mallick, S., S. Dey, S. Mandal, A. Dutta, D. Mukkerjee et al. 2015. A novel triterpene from Astraeus hygrometricus induces reactive oxygen species leading to death in Leishmania donovani. *Future Microbiology* 10(5): 763-789.

Mallick, S., A. Dutta, A. Chaudhuri, D. Mukherjee, S. Dey, S. Halder, J. Ghosh, D. Mukherjee, S.S. Sultana et al. 2016. Successful Therapy of Murine Visceral Leishmaniasis with Astrakurkurone, a Triterpene Isolated from the Mushroom Astraeus hygrometricus, Involves the Induction of Protective Cell-Mediated Immunity and TLR9. *Antimicrobial Agents Chemotherapy* 60(5): 2696-2708.

Nandi, S., S. Chandra, R. Sikder, S. Bhattacharya, M. Ahir, D. Biswal, A. Adhikary, N.R. Pramanik, T.K. Lai, M.G.B. Drew, K. Acharya. 2019. *Journal of Agricultural and Food Chemistry*. 67(27): 7660-7673.

Nandi, S., A. Adhikary, K. Acharya. 2022. *Food Biochemistry* 46(1): e14021.

Phadannok, P., A. Naladta, K. Noipha, N. Nualknew. 2020. Enhancing glucose uptake by Astraeus odoratus and Astraeus asiaticus extracts in L6 myotubes. *Pharmacognosy Magazine* 16(67): 33-42.

Stanikunaite, R., M.M. Radwan, J.M. Trappe, F. Fronczek, S.A. Ross. 2008. Lanostane-type triterpenes from the mushroom Astraeus pteridis with antituberculosis activity. *Journal of Natural Products* 71(12): 2077-2079.

Yadav, R.P., S. Chatterjee, A. Chatterjee, D.K. Pal, S. Ghosh, K. Acharya, M. Das. 2022. Identification of novel mycocompounds as inhibitors of PI3K/AKT/mTOR pathway against RCC. *Journal of Receptors and Signal Transduction Research* doi: 10.1080/10799893.2022.2123515.

BIG BROWN CAT References:

Liu, Y.T., J. Sun, Z.Y. Luo, S.Q. Rao, Y.J. Su, R.R. Xu, Y.J. Yang. 2012. Chemical composition of five wild edible mushrooms collected from Southwest China and their anti-hyperglycemic and antioxidant activity. *Food and Chemical Toxicol*ogy 50(5): 1238-1244.

Liu, Y.T., J. Sun, S.G. Rao, Y.J. Su, Y.J. Yang. 2013. Antihyperglycemic, antihyperlipidemic and antioxidant activities of polysaccharides from Catathelasma ventricosum in streptozotocin-induced diabetic mice. *Food and Chemical Toxicology* 57: 39-45.

Liu, Y.T., C.M. Li, Z.H. Luo et al. 2015. Characterization of selenium-enriched mycelia of Catathelasma ventricosum and their anti-hyperglycemic and antioxidant properties. *Journal of Agricultural and Food Chemistry* 63(2): 562-568.

Liu, Y.T., D. Chen, Y.X. You, S.Q. Zeng, Y. Hu, X.Y Duan et al. 2016. Structural characterization and antidiabetic activity of a glycopyranose-rich heteropolysaccharide from Catathelasma ventricosum. *Carbohydrate Polymers* 149: 399-407.

Liu, Y.T., Y.X. You, Y.W. Li, L. Zhang, L.L. Yin et al. 2017. The characterization, selenylation and antidiabetic activity of mycelial polysaccharides from Catathelasma ventricosum. *Carbohydrate Polymers* 174: 72-81.

Liu, Y.T., S.Q. Zeng, Y.X. Liu, W.J. Wu, Y.B. Shen, L. Zhang, C. Li et al. 2018. Synthesis and antidiabetic activity of selenium nanoparticles in the presence of polysaccharides from Catathelasma ventricosum. *International Journal of Biological Macromolecules* 1114: 632-639.

Liu, L., X. Ding, Y.L. Hou. 2019. Structural characterization and immune regulation of a new heteropolysaccharide from *Catathelasma imperiale* (Fr.) Sing. *Pharmacognosy Magazine* 15(65): 621-630.

Trudell, S.A., J.P Xu, I. Saar, A. Justo, J. Cifuentes. 2017. North American matsutake: names clarified and a new species described. *Mycologia* 109(3): 379-390.

Zhang, L., Y. Shen, H.J. Zhu, F. Wang, Y. Leng, J.K Liu. 2009. Pentanol derivatives from basidiomycete Catathelasma imperiale and their 11beta-hydroxysteroid dehydrogenases inhibitory activity. *Journal of Antibiotics* (Tokyo) 62(5): 239-242.

CAULIFLOWER MUSHROOM References:

Bang, S.H., H.S. Chae, C.Y. Lee, H.G. Choi, J.Y. Ryu et al. 2017. New Aromatic Compounds from the Fruiting Body of Sparassis crispa (Wulf.) and Their Inhibitory Activities on Proprotein convertase Subtilisin/Kexin Type 9 mRNA Expression. *Journal of Agricultural and Food Chemistry* 65(3): 6152-6157.

Hu, S., D. Wang, J.R. Zhang, M.Y. Du, Y.K. Cheng, Y. Liu, N. Zhang, D. Wang, Y. Wu. 2016. Mitochondria Related Pathway Is Essential for Polysaccharides Purified from Sparassis crispa Mediated Neuro-Protection against Glutamate-Induced Toxicity in Differentiated PC12 Cells. *International Journal of Molecular Science* 17(2): 133.

Jeong, S.Y., S. Kang, C.S. Hua, Z. Ting, S. Park. 2017. Synbiotic (sic) effects of B-glucans from Cauliflower mushroom and *Lactobacillus fermentum* on metabolic changes and gut microbiome in estrogen-deficient rats. *Genes and Nutrition* 12:31.

Lan, M.J., M.F. Weng, Z.Y. Lin, J. Wang, F. Zhao, B. Qiu. 2021. Metabolomic analysis of antimicrobial mechanism of polysaccharides from Sparassis crispa based on HPLC-Q-TOF/MS. *Carbohydrate Research* 503: 108299.

Kawagishi, H., K. Hayashi, S. Tokuyama, N. Hashimoto, T. Kimura. 2007. Novel bioactive compound from the Sparassis crispa mushroom. *Bioscience Biotechnology and Biochemistry* 71(7): 1804-1806.

Kim, H.S. 2010. Induction of dendritic cells maturation by beta-glucan from *Sparassis crispa*. *International Immunopharmacology* 10(10): 1284-1294.

Kimura, T., M. Hashimoto, M. Yamanda, Y. Nishikawa. 2013. *Sparassis crispa* (*Hanabiratake*) ameliorates skin conditions in rats and humans. *Bioscience Biotechnology Biochemistry* 77(9): 1961-1963.

Niazi, A.R. & H. Ijaz. 2021. Proximate Analysis and In Vitro Biological Activities of Caulilfower Mushroom, Sparassis crispa (Agaricomycetes), from Pakistan. *International Journal of Medicinal Mushrooms* 23(2): 79-84.

Ngoc, L.T.N., Y.K. Oh, Y.J. Lee, Y.C. Lee. 2018. Effects of *Sparassis crispa* in medical therapeutics: A systematic review and meta-analysis of randomized controlled trials. *International Journal of Molecular Science* 19(5): 1487.

Nishioka, J.J., K. Hiramoto, K. Suzuki. 2020. Mushroom Sparassis crispa (Hanabiratake) Fermented with Lactic Acid Bacteria Significantly Enhances Innate Immunity of Mice. *Biological and Pharmaceutical Bulletin* 43(4): 629-638.

Nowacka-Jechalke, N., R. Nowak, M.K. Lemieszek, W. Rzeski, U. Gawlik-Dziki, N. Szpakowska, Z. Kaczynski. 2021. Promising Potential of Crude Polysaccharides from *Sparassis crispa* against Colon Cancer: An In Vitro Study. *Nutrients* 13(1): 161.

Ohno, N., T. Harada, N.M. Miura, Y. Adachi et al. 2003. Immunomodulating activity of a b-glucan preparation SCG, extracted from a culinary-medicinal mushroom *Sparassis crispa* and application to cancer patients. *International Journal of Medicinal Mushrooms* 5(4): 359-368.

Uchida, M., N. Horii, N. Hasegawa, E. Oyanagi, H. Yano, Mo. Iemitsu. 2019. *Sparassis crispa* Intake Improves the Reduced Lipopolysaccharide-Induced TNF-a Production That Occurs upon Exhaustive Exercise in Mice. *Nutrients* 11(9): 2049.

Wang, J., H.X. Wang, T.B. Ng. 2007. A peptide with HIV-1 reverse transcriptase inhibitory activity from the medicinal mushroom *Russula paladosa*. *Peptides* 28(3): 560-565.

Wang, Z.X., J.Y. Liu, X.J. Zhong, J.J. Li, X. Wang, L.L. Ji, X.Y. Shang. 2019. Rapid Characterization of Chemical Compoenents in Edible Mushroom Sparassis crispa by UPLC-Orbitrap MS Analysis and Potential Inhibitory Effects on Allergic Rhinitis. *Molecules* 24(16): 3014.

Yamamoto, K., T. Kimura. 2014. Orally and topically administered *Sparassis crispa* (Hanabiratake) improved healing of skin wounds in mice with streptozotocin-induced diabetes. *Bioscience Biotechnology Biochemstry* 77: 1303-1305.

Yoskikawa, K., M. Kokudo, T. Hashimoto, K. Yamamoto, T. Inose, T. Kimura. 2010. Novel phthalide compounds from Sparassis crispa (Hanabiratake), Hanabiratakelide A-C, exhibiting anti-cancer related activity. *Biological and Pharmaceutical Bulletin* 33(8): 1355-1359.

Zhang, W.Y., B. Hu, M. Han, Y.H. Guo, Y.L. Cheng, H. Qian. 2022. Purification, structural characterization and neuroprotective effect of a neutral polysaccharide from Sparassis crispa. *International Journal of Biological Macromolecules* 201: 389-399.

Zhang, W.Y, B. Hu, C. Liu, H. Hua, Y. Guo, Y.L. Cheng et al. 2022a. Comprehensive analysis of Sparassis crispa polysaccharide characteristics during the in vitro digestion and fermentation model. *Food Research International* 154:111005.

CHICKEN OF THE WOODS References:

Appleton RE. 1988. *Laetiporus sulphureus* causing visual hallucination and ataxia in a child. *Canadian Medical Association Journal* 139(1):48-49.

Ershova E, Tikhonova OV, Lur'e LM, Efremenkova OV, Kamzolkina OV & Dudnik IuV. 2003. Antimicrobial activity of *Laetiporus sulphureus* strains grown in submerged culture. *Antibiotic Khimioter* 48(1):18-22.

Fan QY, Yin X, Li ZH, Li Y, Liu JK, Feng T, Zhao BH. 2014. Mycophenolic acid derivatives from cultures of the mushroom *Laetiporus sulphureus*. 2014. *Chinese Journal Natural Medicine.* 12(9):685-8.

Francisco L, Jose Q, Augusto R, Francisco E, Jaime B. 2004. Lanostanoid triterpenes from *Laetiporus sulphureus* and apoptosis induction on HL-60 human myeloid leukemia cells. *Journal of Natural Products* 67:2008-11.

Garcia-Corzo L, Luna-Sanchez M, Doerrier C, Garcia JA et al. 2013. Dysfunctional CoQ9 protein causes predominant encephalomyopathy associated with CoQ deficiency. *Human Molecular Genetics.* 22(6)1233-48.

He JB, Tao J, Miao XS, Bu VV, Zhang S et al. 2015. Seven new drimane-type sesquiterponoids from cultures of fungus *Laetiporus sulphureus. Fitoterapia* 102:1-6.

Hwang HS, Lee SH, Baek YM, Kim SW, Jeong YK, Yun JW. 2008. Production of extracellular polysaccharides by submerged mycelial culture of *Laetiporus sulphureus* var. *miniatus* and their insulinotrophic properties. *Applied Microbiology Biotechnology* 78:419-29.

Jayasooriya RG, Kang CH, Seo MJ, Choi YH, Jeong YK & Kim GY. 2011. Exopolysaccharide *of Laetiporus sulphureus* var. *miniatus* down-regulates LPS-induced production of NO, PGE$_2$, and TNF-alpha in BV2 microglia cells via suppression of the NF-$_k$B pathway. *Food Chem Toxicology* 49(11):2758-64.

Jiang-Bo He, Jian Tao, Xi-Song Miao, Wei Bu et al. 2015. Seven new drimane-type sesquiterpenoids from cultures of fungus *Laetiporus sulphureus. Fitoterapia* 102:1-6.

Jonathan, G., J. Chikwem, A. Hull, A. Daniel, M.D. Asemoloye. 2021. Antimicrobial Activities of Laetiporus conifericola (Agaricomycetes) from the United States. *International Journal of Medicinal Mushrooms* 23(6): 69-77.

Kang CY, Lee CO, Chung KS, Choi EC, Kim BK. 1982. An antitumor component of *Laetiporus sulphureus* and its immunostimulating activity. *Archives Pharmaceutical Research.* 5(2):39-43.

Lear MJ, Simon O, Foley TL, Burkart MD et al. 2009. Laetirobin from the parasitic growth of *Laetiporus sulphureus* on Robinia pseudoacacia. *Journal Natural Products* 72(11):1980-7.

Lee JW, Lee SM, Gwak KS, Lee JY, Choi IG. 2006. Screening of edible mushrooms for the production of lovastatin and its HMG-CoA reductase inhibitory activity. *Korean Journal of Microbiology*. 42(2):83.

León F, Quintana J, Rivera A, Estévez F & Bermejo J. 2004. Lanostanoid triterpenes from *Laetiporus sulphureus* and apoptosis induction on HL-60 human myeloid leukemia cells. *Journal Natural Products* 67(12):2008-11.

Lindner DL, Banik MT. 2008. Molecular phylogeny of Laetiporus and other brown rot polypore genera in North America. *Mycologia* 100(3):417-30.

Lu D, Yang L, Li Q, Gao X, Wang F, Zhang G. 2012. Egonol gentiobioside and egonol gentiotrioside from Styrax perkinsiae promote the biosynthesis of estrogen by aromatase. *European Journal of Pharmacology*. 691(1-3):275-82.

Menshova RV, Ermakova SP, Anastyuk SD, Isakov VV et al. 2014. Structure, enzymatic transformation and anticancer activity of branched high molecular weight laminaran from brown alga *Eisenia bicyclis*. *Carbohydrate Polymers* 99:101-9.

Mlinaric A, Kac J, Pohleven F. 2005. Screening of selected wood-damaging fungi for the HIV-1 reverse transcriptase inhibitors. *Acta Pharmaceutica* 55(1):69-79.

Okamura T, Takeno T, Dohi M, Yasumasa I et al. 2000. Development of mushrooms for thrombosis prevention by protoplast fusion. *Journal of Bioscience and Bioengineering* 89(5):474-8.

Park HK, Kim IH, Kim J, Nam TJ. 2013. Induction of apoptosis and the regulation of ErbB signaling by lamarin in HT-29 human colon cancer cells. *International Journal of Molecular Medicine* 32(2):291-5.

Pavic, A., T. Ilic-Tomic, J. Glamoclija. 2021. Unravelling Anti-Melanogenic Potency of Edible Mushrooms *Laetiporus sulphureus* and *Agaricus silvaticus* In Vivo Using the Zebrafish Model. *Journal of Fungi* (Basel) 7(10):834.

Petrovic J, Stojkovic D, Reis FS, Barros L et al. 2014. Study on chemical, bioactive and food preserving properties of *Laetiporus sulphureus* (Bull.: Fr.) Murr. *Food Function* 5(7):1441-51.

Pleszczynska M, Wiater A, Siwulski M & Szczodrak J. 2013. Successful large-scale production of fruiting bodies of *Laetiporus sulphureus* (Bull.:Fr.) Murrill on an artificial substrate. *World Journal Microbiology Biotechnology* 29(4):753-8.

Popoff EH, Kapich, AN. 2010 The effect of ionizing radiation on testosterone binding globulin characteristics: correction of the protein parameters by lipid polyene complexes of fungus *Laetiporus sulfureus*. *International Journal Radiation Biology*. 86(3):238-51.

Ríos JL, Andújar I, Recio MC, Giner RM. 2012. Lanostanoids from fungi: a group of potential anticancer compounds. *Journal of Natural Products*. 75:2016-44.

Sato M, Tai T, Nunoura Y, Kawashima S, Tanaka K. 2002. Dehydrotrametenolic acid induces preadipocyte differentiation and sensitizes animal models of noninsulin-dependent diabetes mellitus to insulin. *Biological and Pharmaceutical Bulletin* 25(1):81-86.

Skarlovnik A, Janic M, Lunder M, Turk M, Sabovic M. 2014. Coenzyme Q10 supplementation decreases statin-related mild-to-moderate muscle symptoms: a randomized clinical study. Medical Science Monitor 20:2183-8.

Slanc P, Doljak B, Mlinaric A, Strukeji B. 2004. Screening of wood damaging fungi and macrofungi for inhibitors of pancreatic lipase. *Phytotherapy Research*. 18:758-62.

Turkoglu A, Duru ME, Mercan N, Kivrak I, Gezer K. 2007. Antioxidant and antimicrobial activity of *Laetiporus sulphureus* (Bull.) Murrill. *Food Chemistry* 101:267-73.

Vasaitis R, Menkis A, Lim YW, Seok S, Tomsovsky M et al. 2009. Genetic variation and relationships in *Laetiporus sulphureus* s. lat., as determined by ITS rDNA sequences and in vitro growth rate. *Mycological Research* 113(Pt 3):326-36.

Wang LW, Jabbour A, Hayward CS, Furlong TJ, Girgis L, Macdonald PS, Keogh AM. 2015 Potential role of coenzyme Q10 in facilitating recovery from statin-induced rhabdomyolysis. *Internal Medicine Journal*. 45(4):451-3.

Wiater A, Szczodrak J, Pleszczynska M. 2008. Mutanase induction in *Trichoderma harzianum* by cell wall of *Laetiporus sulphureus* and its application for mutan removal from oral biofilms. *Journal Microbiology Biotechnology* 18(7):1335-41.

Yoshikawa K, Bando S, Arihara S, Matsumura E, Katayama S. 2001.A benzofuran glycoside and an acetylenic acid from the fungus *Laetiporus sulphureus* var. *miniatus*. *Chemical Pharmaceutical Bulletin* 49(3):327-9.

CLOUDED FUNNEL References:

Avanzo, P., J. Sabotic, S. Anzlovar, T. Popovic, A. Leonardi, R.H. Pain, J. Kos, J. Brzin. 2009. Trypsin-specific inhibitors from the basidiomycete Clitocybe nebularis with regulatory and defensive functions. *Microbiology* 155 (Pt 12): 3971-3981.

Chen, M.H., W.S. Li, Y.S. Lue, C.L. Chu, I.H. Pan, C.H. Ko et al. 2013. Clitocybe nuda Activates Dendritic Cells and Acts as a DNA Vaccine Adjuvant. *Evidence Based Complementary and Alternative Medicine* 2013: 761454.

Chen, M.H., C.H. Lin, C.C. Shih. 2014. Antidiabetic and Antihyperlipidemic Effects of Clitocybe nuda on Glucose Transporter 4 and AMP-Activated Protein Kinase Phosphorylation in High-Fat-Fed Mice. *Evidence Based Complementary and Alternative Medicine* 2014: 981046.

Dizeci, N. O. Onar, B. Karaca, N. Demirtas, A.C. Cihan, O. Yildrim. 2021. Comparison of the chemical composition and biological effects of *Clitocybe nebularis* and *Infundibylicybe geotropa*. *Mycologia* 113(6): 1156-1168.

Doljak, B., M. Stegnar, U. Urleb, S. Kreft, A. Umek, M. Ciglaric, B. Strukelj, T. Popovic. 2001. Screening for selective thrombin inhibitors in mushrooms. *Blood Coagulation and Fibrinolysis* 12(2): 123-128.

Emsen, B., B. Guven, Y. Uzun, A. Kaya. 2020. Antioxidant and Genotoxic Effects of Aqueous and Methanol Extracts from Two Edible Mushrooms from Turkey in Human Peripheral Lymphocytes. *International Journal of Medicinal Mushrooms* 22(2): 161-170.

Fortin, H., S. Tomasi, J.G. Delcros, J.Y. Bansard, J. Boustie. 2006. In vivo antitumor activity of clitocine, an exocyclic amino nucleoside isolated from Lepista inversa. *ChemMedChem* 1(2): 189-196.

Friesen, W.J., C.R. Trotta, Y. Tomizawa, J. Zhuo, B. Johnson et al. 2017. The nucleoside analog clitocine is a potent and efficacious readthrough agent. *RNA* 23(4): 567-577.

Guo, D.D., J.Y. Lei, L.J. Xu, Y.F. Cheng, C.P. Feng et al. 2022. Two Novel Polysaccharides from *Clitocybe squamulosa*: Their Isolation, Structures, and Bioactivities. *Frontiers in Nutrition* 9:934769.

Guo, D.D., J.Y. Lei, C. He, Z.J. Peng, R.Z. Liu, X. Pan et al. 2022a. In vitro digestion and fermentation by human fecal microbiota of polysaccharides from Clitocybe squamulosa. *International Journal of Biological Macromolecules* 208: 343-355.

Huo, Y., Q.L. Li, M.Y. Chen, H.F. Wu, J. Yang, Z.C. Sun, X.D. Xu, G.X. Ma. 2022. Novel geranylhydroquinone derived meroterpenoids from the fungus Clitocybe clavipes and their cytotoxic activity. *Fitoterapia* 161: 105251.

Hu, S.H., P.C.K. Cheung, R.P. Hung, Y.K. Chen, J.C. Wang, S.J. Chang. 2015. Antitumor and Immunomodulating Activities of Exopolysaccharide Produced by Big Cup Culinary Medicinal Mushroom Clitocybe maxima (Higher Basidiomycetes) in Liquid Submerged Culture. *International Journal of Medicinal Mushrooms* 17(9): 891-901.

Lee, J.E., I.S. Lee, K.C. Kim, I.D. Yoo, H.M. Yang. 2017. ROS Scavenging and Anti-Wrinkle Effects of Clitocybin A Isolated from the Mycelium of the Mushroom *Clitocybe aurantiaca*. *Journal of Microbiology and Biotechnology* 27(5): 933-938.

Nanut, M.P., S. Zurga, S. Konjar, M. Prunk, J. Kos, J. Sabotic. 2022. The fungal Clitocybe nebularis lectin binds distinct cell surface glycoprotein receptors to induce cell death selectively in Jurkat cells. *Federation of American Society for Experimental Biology Journal* 36(4): e22215.

Pišlar, A., J. Sabotic, J. Šlenc, J. Brzin, J. Kos. 2016. Cytotoxic L-amino-acid oxidases from Amanita phalloides and Clitocybe geotropa induce caspase-dependent apoptosis. *Cell Death Discovery* 2: 16021.

Sabotic, J., J. Kos. 2019. CNL- *Clitocybe nebularis* Lectin- The Fungal GaINAcbeta!-4GlcNAc-binding Lectin. *Molecules* 24(23): 4204.

Schrey, H., T. Scheele, C. Ulonska, D.L. Nedder, T. Neudecker, P. Spiteller, M. Stadler. 2022. Allicane-Type Secondary Metabolites from Submerged Cultures of the Basidiomycete *Clitocybe nebularis*. *Journal of Natural Products* doi: 10.1021/acs.jnatprod.2c00554.

Shih, C.C., 2014. Validation of the Antidiabetic and Hypolipidemic Effects of Clitocybe nuda by Assessment of Glucose Transporter 4 and Gluconeogenesis and AMPK Phosphorylation in Streptozotocin-Induced Mice. *Evidence Based Complementary and Alternative Medicine* doi: 10.1155/2014/705636.

Sugaya, K., M. Ino, N. Matsuo, J.I. Onose, N. Abe. 2020. Variegatic acid from the edible mushroom *Tylopilus ballouii* inhibits TNF-a production and PKCbeta1 activity in leukemia cells. *Bioorganic & Medicinal Chemistry Letters* 30(4).

Sun, J.G., H. Li, X. Li, X.L. Zeng, P. Wu, K.P. Fung, F.Y. Liu. 2014. Clitocine targets Mcl-1 to induce drug-resistant human cancer cell apoptosis in vitro and tumor growth inhibition in vivo. *Apoptosis* 19(5): 871-882.

Sun, J.G., F. Ruan, X.L. Zeng, J. Xiang, X. Li, P. Wu, K.P. Fung, F.Y. Liu. 2016. Clitocine potentiates TRAIL-mediated apoptosis in human colon cancer cells by promoting Mcl-1 degradation. *Apoptosis* 21(10): 1144-1157.

Sun, Z.C., X.D. Xu, H.Q. Liang, X.Y. Xia, G.X. Ma, L.L. Shi. 2019. Five New Meroterpenoids from the Fruiting Bodies of the Basidiomycete *Clitocybe clavipes* with Cytotoxic Activity. *Molecules* 24(22): 4015.

Sun, Z.C., D. Chen, L.Y. Li, Y. Hou, M.Y. Chen, G.D. Huang, G.X. Ma, Z.Y. Li. 2021. Clavipyrrine A, a unique polycylic nitrogenous meroterpenoid with promising anti-glioma effects isolated from the fungus Clitocybe clavipes. *Bioorganic Chemistry* doi: 10.1016/j.bioorg.2021.105468.

Vaz, J.A., G.M. Almeida, I.C.F.R. Ferreira, A. Martins, M.H. Vasconcelos. 2012. Clitocybe alexandri extract induces cell cycle arrest and apoptosis in a lung cancer cell line: Identification of phenolic acids with cytotoxic potential. *Food Chemistry* 132(1): 482-486.

Yoo, K.D., E.S. Park, Y. Lim, S.I. Kang et al. 2012. Clitocybin A, a novel isoindolinone, from the mushroom Clitocybe aurantiaca, inhibits cell proliferation through G1 phase arrest by regulating the PI3K/Akt cascade in vascular smooth muscle cells. *Journal of Pharmacological Sciences* 118(2): 171-177.

Yoo, K.D., E.S. Park, Y. Lim, S.I. Kang, S.H. Yoo, H.H. Won et al. 2012a. Clitocybin B inhibits rat aortic smooth muscle cell proliferation through suppressing PDGF-Rbeta phosphoration. *Vascular Pharmacology* 56(1-2): 91-97.

COLLYBIA References:

Engler, M., T. Anke, O. Sterner. 1998. Production of antibiotics by Collybia nivalis, Omphalotus olearis, a Favolaschia and a Pterula species on natural substrates. *Zeitschrift fur Naturforschung Section C, Journal of Bioscience* 53(5-6): 318-324.

Gao, Z., J. Li, X.L. Song, J.J. Zhang, X.X. Wang, H.J. Jing, Z.Z. Ren, S.S. Li, C. Zhang, L. Jia. 2017. Antioxidative, anti-inflammation and lung-protective effects of mycelia selenium polysaccharides from Oudemansiella radicata. *International Journal of Biological Macromolecules* 104(Pt A): 1158-1164.

Gao, Z., C. Zhang, C.Y. Tian, Z.Z. Ren, X.L. Song, X.X. Wang et al. 2018. Characterization, antioxidation, anti-inflammation and renoprotection effects of selenized mycelia polysaccharides from Oudemansiella radiata. *Carbohydrate Polymers* 181: 1224-1234.

Gupta, A., I. Gomes, E.N. Bobeck, A.K. Fakira, N.P. Massaro, I. Sharma, A. Cavé, H.E. Hamm, J. Parello, LA. Devi. 2016. Collybolide is a novel biased agonist of k-opioid receptors with potent antipruritic activity. *Proceedings of the National Academy of Science USA*. 113(21): 6041-6046.

Lee, S.W., J.G. Song, B.S. Hwang, D.W. Kim, Y.J. Lee, E.E. Woo, J.Y. Kim, I.K. Lee, B.S. Yun 2014. Lipoxygenase Inhibitory Activity of Korean Indigenous Mushroom Extracts and Isolation of an Active Compound from Phellinus baumii. *Mycobiology* 42(2): 185-188.

Leonhardt, K., T. Anke, E. Hillen-Maske, W. Steglich. 1987. 6-Methylpurine, 6-methyl-9-beta-D-ribofuranosylpurine, and 6-hydroxymethyl-9-beta-D-ribofuranosylpurine as antiviral metabolites of Collybia maculata (Basidiomycetes). *Zeitschrift fur Naturforschung Section C, Journal of Bioscience* 42(4): 420-424.

Liu, Q., M.J. Zhu, Z.R. Geng, H.X. Wang, T.B. Ng. 2017. Characterization of Polysaccharides with Antioxidant and Hepatoprotective Activities from the Edible Mushroom Oudemansiella radicata. *Molecules* 22(2): 234.

Liu, Y.T., Y.W. Li, Y. Ke, C. Li, Z.Q. Zhang, Y.L. Wu, B. Hu, A.P. Liu, Q.Y. Luo, W.J. Wu. 2021. In vitro saliva-gastrointestinal digestion and fecal fermentation of Oudemansiella radicata polysaccharides reveal its digestion prolife and effect on the modulation of the gut microbiota. *Carbohydrate Polymers* 251: 117041.

Liu, Q., X. Cui, Z.B. Song, W.W. Kong, Y.C. Kang, W.L. Kong, T.B. Ng. 2021. Coating shiitake mushrooms (Lentinus edodes) with a polysaccharide from Oudemansiella radicata improves product quality and flavor during postharvest storage. *Food Chemistry* 352: 129357.

Mujic, I., Z. Zekovic, S. Vidovic, M. Radojkovic, J. Zivkovic, D. Godevac. 2011. Fatty acid profiles of four wild mushrooms and their potential benefits for hypertension treatment. *Journal of Medicine and Food* 14(11): 1330-1337.

Pacheco-Sánchez, M., Y. Boutin, P. Angers, A. Gosselin, R.J. Tweddell. 2007. Inhibitory effect of CDP, a polysaccharide extracted from the mushroom Collybia dryophila, on nitric oxide synthase expression and nitric oxide production in macrophages. *European Journal of Pharmacology* 555(1): 61-66.

Simon, B., T. Anke, U. Anders, M. Neuhaus, F. Hansske. 1995. Collybial, a new antibiotic sesquiterpenoid from Collybia confluens (Basidiomycetes). *Zeitschrift fur Naturforschung Section C, Journal of Bioscience* 50(3-4): 173-180.

Wang, L., & Y.H. Hou. 2011. Determination of trace minerals in anti-influenza virus mushrooms. *Biological Trace Element Research* 143(3): 1799-1807.

Wang, Z, S.F. Zhang, L.Y. Zhao, F.C. Zhao, Z.Y. Yang. 2015 Effect of Collybia radiata (sic) on intestinal flora and secretory immunoglobulin A in mice. *Science and Technology of Food Industry* 13: 376-379.

Wang, Y.F., Y.Q. Tian, J.G. Shao, Z. Shu, J.X. Jia, X.J. Ren, Y. Guan. 2018. Macrophage Immunomodulatory activity of the polysaccharide isolated from Collybia radicata mushroom. *International Journal of Biological Macromolecules* 108: 300-306.

Wang, X.X., M. Liu, C. Zhang, S.S. Li, Q.H. Yang et al. 2018a. Antioxidant Activity and Protective Effects of Enzyme-extracted Oudemansiella radiata (sic) Polysaccharides on Alcohol-Induced Liver Injury. *Molecules* 23(2): 481.

Yang, K., S.C. Jeong, H.J. Lee, D.H. Sohn, C.H. Song. 2006. Antidiabetic and hypolipidemic effects of Collybia confluens mycelia produced by submerged culture in streptozotocin-diabetic rats. *Archives of Pharmacal Research* 29(1): 73-79.

Yang, B.K., Y.S. Jung, C.H. Song. 2007. Hypoglycemic effects of Ganoderma applanatum and Collybia confluens exo-polymers in streptozotocin-induced diabetic rats. *Phytotherapy Research* 21(11): 1066-1069.

DIAMOND WILLOW & CONCEALED POLYPORE References:

Bao, Z.S. 2004. www.globethesis.com/?t= 2144360092990645.

Blanchette, Robert A. 1997. *Haploporus odorus*: A sacred fungus in traditional native American culture of the Northern Plains. *Mycologia* 89(2): 233-240.

Carlezon, W. A. Jr., S. D. Maque, A. M. Parow, A. L. Stoll, B. M. Cohen and P. F. Renshaw. 2005. Antidepressant-like effects of uridine and omega-3 fatty acids are potentiated by combined treatment in rats. *Biological Psychiatry* 57(4): 343-350.

Cavdar, H., M. Senturk, M. Guney, S. Durdagi, G. Kayik, C.T. Supuran, D. Ekinci. 2019. Inhibition of acetylcholinesterase and butyrycholinesterase with uracil derivatives: kinetic and computational studies. *Journal of Enzyme Inhibition and Medicinal Chemistry* 34(1): 429-437.

Chen, L. 2009. www.globalthesis.com/?t= 2144360272476705.

Duan, C., X. Ge, J.C. Wang, Z.Y. Wei, W.H. Feng, J.F. Wang. 2021. Ergosterol peroxide exhibits antiviral and immunomodulatory abilities against porcine deltacoronavisus (PDCoV) via suppression of NF-$_\kappa$B and p38/MAPK signaling pathways in vitro. *International Immunopharmacology* 93:107317.

Gao, L., Y. Sun, J.Si, J. Lui, G. Sun, X. Sun et al. 2014. *Cryptoporus volvatus* Extract Inhibits Influenza Virus Replication *In Vitro* and *In Vivo*. *PLoS One* 9(12): e113604.

Gao, L., J. Han, J. Si, J. Wang, H. Wang, Y. Sun et al. 2017. Cryptoporic acid E from *Cryptoporus volvatus* inhibits influenza virus replication in vitro. *Antiviral Research* 143: 106-112.

Ling-Yun., Zhou, Xiao-Hong., Yu, Bin.,Lu, Yan., Hua. 2016. Bioassay-Guided Isolation of Cytotoxic Isocryptoporic Acids from *Cryptoporus volvatus*. *Molecules* 21(12): 1692.

Liu, Y., X. Wang, J. Wang, J. Zhang, C. Duan, J.F. Wang. 2022. Ergosterol Peroxide Inhibits Porcine Epidemic Diarrhea Virus Infection in Vero Cells by Suppressing ROS Generation and p53 Activation. *Viruses* 14(2): 402.

Narisawa, T., Y. Fukaura, H. Kotanagi, Y. Asakawa. 1992. Inhibitory Effect of Cryptoporic Acid E, a Product from Fungus *Cryptoporus volvatus*, on Colon Carcinogenesis Induced with N-Methyl-N-Nitrosourea in Rats and with 1,2 Dimethylhydrazine in Mice. *Japanese Journal of Cancer Research* 83(8): 830-834.

Palasz, A., & D. Ciez. 2015. In search of uracil derivatives as bioactive agents. Uracils and fused uracils: Synthesis, biological activity and applications. *European Journal of Medicinal Chemistry*. 97: 582-611.

Pham, H.T., K.H. Lee, E. Jeong, S.M. Woo, J.S. Yu, W.Y. Kim, Y.W. Lim, K.H. Kim, K.B. Kang. 2021. Species Priorization Based on Spectral Dissimilarity: A Case Study of Polyporoid Fungal Species. *Journal of Natural Products* 84(2): 298-309.

Rogers, Robert. 2016. *Mushroom Essences: Vibrational Healing from the Kingdom Fungi*. North Atlantic Books. Berkeley CA. page 90.

Svanberg, I. 2018. Ethnomycological notes on *Haploporus odorus* and other polypores in Northern Fennoscandia. *Journal of Northern Studies*. 8(6): 73-91.

Zhang, H. & W.Q. Liang. 2004. Studies on the extraction process of Cryptoporus volvatus oil by orthogonal design method. *Zhong Yao Cai* 27(5): 373-374.

Zhou, L., Z. Zhao, F. Xiong, Y. Chen, Y. Sun. 2022. Anti-tumor mechanism of sesquiterpenoids from *Cryptoporus volvatus* based on molecular docking. *Nan Fang Yi Ke Da Xue Xue Bao* 42(1): 71-77.

Zmirovich, I.V., S.P. Arefyev, M.A. Bondartseva, N.V. Belova, Y.R. Khimich et al. 2019. Profiles of Little-Known Medicinal Polypores: *Haploporus odorus* (Agaricomycetes). *International Journal of Medicinal Mushrooms* 21(8): 783-791.

Wang, J.C., G. Z. Li, L. Gao, L. Cao et al. 2015. Two new cryptoporic acid derivatives from the fruiting bodies of *Cryptoporus volvatus*. *Phytochemistry Letters* 14: 63-66.

FAIRY RING MUSHROOM References:

Abraham, Wolf Rainier. 2001. Bioactive sesquiterpenes produced by fungi: Are they useful for humans as well? *Current Medical Chemistry* 8(6): 583-606.

Juillot, S., C. Cott, J. Madi, J. Claudionon et al. 2016. Uptake of *Marasmius oreades* agglutinin disrupts integrin-dependent cell adhesion. *Biochemica et Biophysica Acta* 392-401.

Kayode, R.M.O., S.A. Laba, B.I. Kayode, T.H. Aliyu et al. 2016. Chemical composition of *Marasmius oreades*: A wild edible mushroom among Kabba-Bunu inhabitants of Nigeria. *FUTA Journal of Research in Sciences* 1:1-8.

Liao, Y.F., Y.K. Rao, Y.M. Tzeng. 2017. Anti-cancer activities of extracts from *Marasmius oreades. Journal of Cancer Science and Therapy* 9(4): 53.

Ngai, P.H., Z. Zhao, T.B. Ng. 2005. Agrocybin, an anti-fungal peptide from the edible mushroom *Agrocybe cylindracea. Peptides* 26(2): 191-6.

Petrova, R.D., J. Mahajna, A.Z. Reznick, S.P. Wasser et al. 2007. Fungal substances as modulators of NF-kappaB activation pathway. *Molecular Biology Reports* 34(3): 145-154.

Rogers, Robert. 2016. *Mushroom Essences: Vibrational Healing from the Kingdom Fungi*. North Atlantic Books, Berkeley CA. pages 140-143.

Rosa, L.H., E.M. Souza-Fagundes, Katia M.G. Machado et al. 2006. Cytotoxic, immunosuppressive and trypanocidal activities of agrocybin, a polyacetylene produced by *Agrocybe perfecta* (Basidiomycota). *World Journal of Microbiology and Biotechnology* 22(6): 539-545.

Ruimi, N., R.D. Petrova, R. Agabria, S. Sussan, S. Wasser et al. Inhibition of TNFalpha-induced iNOS expression in HSV-tk transduced 9L glioblastoma cell lines by *Marasmius oreades* substances through NFkappa-B and MAPK-dependent mechanisms. *Molecular Biology Reports* 37(8): 3801-3812.

Song, J., X. Wang, Y. Huang, Y. Qu, G. Zhang & D. Wang. 2018. Analgesic effects of *Marasmius androsaceus* mycelia ethanol extract and possible mechanisms in mice. *Brazilian Journal Med Biol Research* 51(4): e7124.

Song, J., X. Wang, Y. Huang, Y. Qu, L. Teng et al. 2017. Antidepressant-like effects of *Marasmius androsaceus* metabolic exopolysaccharides on chronic unpredictable mild stress-induced rat model. *Molecular Medicine Reports* 16(4): 5043-5049.

Song, J., X.Q. Geng, Y. Su, X.Y. Zhang, L. Tu, Y. Zheng, M. Wang. 2020. Structure feature and antidepressant-like activity of a novel exopolysaccharide isolated from Marasmius androsaceus fermentation broth. *International Journal of Biological Macromolecules* 165(pt B):1646-1655.

Steinbrecht, S., J. Kiebist, R. Konig, M. Thiessen et al. 2020. Synthesis of cyclophosphamide metabolites by a peroxygenase from Marasmius rotula for toxicological studies on human cancer cells. *AMB Express* 10(1): 128.

Vieira, V., A. Marques, L. Barros, J.C.M. Barreira, & C.F.R. Ferreira. 2012. Insights in the antioxidant synergistic effects of combined edible mushrooms: phenolic and polysaccharidic extracts of *Boletus edulis* and *Marasmius oreades. Journal of Food and Nutrition Research* 51(2): 109-116.

Wang, X., Q.M. Liang, T.T. Li, R. Zhi, N. Zhang, & J.H. Lu. 2006. Study on extraction and anti-oxidation of *Marasmius androsaceus* mycelium polysaccharides. *Food Science and Technology* 12.

Wang, H.G., Y. Zhao, X.H. Li. 2007. Experimental research on immunocompetence of *Marasmius androsaceus* polysaccharide in mice. *Traditional Chinese Drug Research and Clinical Pharmacology* 2007:05.

Zhang, L et al. 2009. Antihypertensive effect of 3,3,5,5-tetramethyl-4-piperiodone, a new compound extracted from *Marasmius androsaceus. Journal of Ethnopharmacology* 123(1): 34-39.

FALSE TURKEY TAIL References:

Aqueveque, P., C.L. Céspedes, J. Becerra, M. Dávila, O. Sterner. 2015. Bioactive compounds isolated from submerged fermentations of the Chilean fungus Stereum rameale. *Zeitschrift fur Naturforschung C Journal of Biosciences* 70(3-4): 97-102.

Cateni, F., B. Doljak, M. Zacchigna, M. Anderluh, A. Piltaver, G. Scialino, E. Banfi. 2007. *Bioorganic & Medicinal Chemistry Letters* 17(22): 6330-6334.

Cayan, F., G. Tel-Cayan, E. Deveci, M. Öztürk, M.E. Duru. 2019. Chemical Profile, In Vitro Enzyme Inhibitory, and Antioxidant Properties of Stereum Species (Agaricomycetes) from Turkey. *International Journal of Medicinal Mushrooms* 21(11): 1075-1087.

Doljak, B., F. Cateni, M. Anderluh, G. Procida, J. Zilic, M. Zacchigna. 2006. Glycerolipids as selective thrombin inhibitors from the fungus Stereum hirsutum. *Drug Development and Industrial Pharmacy* 32(5): 635-643.

Hybelbauerova, S., J. Sejbal, M. Dracinsky, A. Hahnova, B. Koutek. 2008. Chemical Constituents of Stereum subtomentosum and Two Other Birch-Associated Basidiomycetes: An Interspecies Comparative Study. *Chemistry and Biodiversity* 5: 743-540.

Imtiaj, A., C. Jayasinghe, G.W. Lee, T.S. Lee. 2007. Antibacterial and Antifungal Activities of Stereum ostrea, an inedible Wild Mushroom. *Mycobiology* 35(4): 210-214.

Isaka, M., U. Srisanoh, W. Choowong, T. Boonpratuang. 2011. Ssterostreins A-E, new terpenoids from cultures of the Basidiomycete Stereum ostrea BCC 22955. *Organic Letters* 13(18): 4886-4889.

Kang, H.S. & J.P. Kim. 2016. Ostalactones A-C, B- and e-Lactones with Lipase Inhibitory Activity from the Cultured Basidiomycete Stereum ostrea. *Journal of Natural Products* 79(12): 3148-3151.

Kim, S.E., I.K. Lee, Y.A. Jung, J.H. Yeom, D.W. Ki et al. 2012. Mushrooms collected from deogyu mountain, muju, Korea and their antioxidant activity. *Mycobiology* 40(2): 134-137.

Kim, Y.H., B.S. Yun, I.J. Ryoo, J.P. Kim, H. Koshino, I.D. Yoo. 2006. Methyloxylaricinolic acid, a new sesquiterpene from the fruiting bodies of Stereum ostrea. *Journal of Antibiotics* (Tokyo) 59(7): 432-434.

Kleinwächter, P., H.M. Dahse, U. Luhmann, B. Schiegel, K. Dornberger. 2001. Epicorazine C, an antimicrobial metabolite from Stereum hirsutum HKI 0195. *Journal of Antibiotics* (Tokyo) 54(6): 521-525.

Ma, K., L. Bao, J.J. Han, T. Jin, X.L. Yang, F. Zhao et al. 2014. New benzoate derivatives and hirsutane type sesquiterpenoids with antimicrobial activity and cytotoxicity from the sold-state fermented rice by the medicinal mushroom Stereum hirsutum. *Food Chemistry* 143: 239-245.

Miskovic, J., M. Raseta, E. Capelja, N. Krsmanovic, A. Novakovic, M. Karaman. 2021. Mushroom Species Stereum hirsutum as Natural Source of Phenolics and Fatty Acids as Antioxidants and Acetylcholinesterase Inhibitors. *Chemistry and Biodiversity* 18(11): e2100409.

Pu, K.J., Q.Y. Hu, S.S. Li, G.H. Li, P.J. Zhao. 2021. Sesquiterpenoids and their quaternary ammonium hybrids from the mycelium of mushroom Stereum hirsutum by medium optimization. *Phytochemistry* 189:112852.

Qi, Q.Y., J.W. Ren, L.W. Sun, L.W. He, L. Bao, W. Yue et al. 2015. Structurally Diverse Sesquiterpenes Produced by a Chinese Tibet Fungus Stereum hirsutum and Their Cytotoxic and Immunosuppressant Activities. *Organic Letters* 17(12): 3098-3101.

Sevindik, M., B. Ozdemir, C. Bal, Z. Selamoglu. 2021. Bioactivity of EtOH and MeOH Extracts of Basidiomycetes Mushroom (Stereum hirsutum) on Atherosclerosis. *Archives of Razi Institute* 76(1): 87-94.

Tian, M.Q., P.J. Zhao, G.H. Li, K.Q. Zhang. 2020. In Depth Natural Discovery from the Basidiomycetes Stereum Species. *Microorganisms* 8(7): 1049.

Wang, B.T., Q.Y. Qi, K. Ma, Y.F. Pei, J.J. Han, W. Xu, E.W. Li, H.W. Liu. 2004. Depside a-glucosidase inhibitors from a culture of the mushroom Stereum hirsutum. *Planta Medica* 80(11): 918-924.

Yao, J.N., L. Chen, H.P. Chen, Z.Z. Zhao, S.B. Zhang, Y. Huang, Y. Tang et al. 2018. Miscellaneous lanostane triterpenoids with cytotoxicities from fruiting bodies of the basidiomycete Stereum sp. *Fitoterapia* 125: 227-234.

Yoo, N.H., J.P. Kim, B.S. Yun, I.J. Ryoo, I.K. Lee, E.S. Yoon et al. 2006. Hirsutenols D, E and F, new sesquiterpenes from the culture broth of Stereum hirsutum. *Journal of Antibiotics* 59(2): 110-113.

FRIED CHICKEN MUSHROOM References:

Ike, K., N. Kameyama, A. Ito, S. Imai. 2012. Induction of a T-Helper 1 (Th1) immune response in mice by an extract from the Pleurotus eryngii (Eringi) mushroom. *Journal of Medicinal Food* 15(12): 1124-1128.

Ishihara, A., N. Sugai, T. Bito, N. Ube, K. Ueno, Y. Okuda, E. Fusushima-Sakuno. 2019. Isolation of 6-hydroxy-L-tryptophan from the fruiting body of *Lyophyllum decastes* for use as a tyrosinase inhibitor. *Bioscience Biotechnology and Biochemistry* 83(10): 1800-1806.

Kimura, C.K., M. Nukina, K. Igarashi, Y. Sugawara. 2005. Beta-hydroxy ergothioneine, a new ergothioneine derivative from the mushroom Lyophyllum connatum, and its protective activity against carbon tetrachloride-induced injury in primary culture hepatocytes. *Bioscience Biotechnology and Biochemistry* 69(2): 357-363.

Krupodorova, T., S. Rybalko, V. Barshteyn. 2014. Antiviral activity of Basidiomycete mycelia against influenza type A (serotype H1N1) and herpes simplex virus type 2 in cell culture. *Virologica Sinica* 29(5): 284-290.

Miura, T., M. Kubo, Y. Itoh, N. Iwamoto, M. Kato, S.R. Park, Y. Ukawa, Y. Kita, I. Suzuki. 2002. Antidiabetic activity of Lyophyllum decastes in genetically type 2 diabetic mice. *Biological and Pharmaceutical Bulletin* 25(9): 1234-1237.

Moon, S.M., J.S. Kim, H.J. Kim, M.S. Choi, B.R. Park, S.G. Kim et al. 2014. Purification and characterization of a novel fibrinolytic alpha chymotrypsin like serine metalloprotease from the edible mushroom, Lyophyllum shimeji. *Journal of Bioscience and Bioengineering* 117(5): 544-550.

Nakamura, T., Y. Itokawa, M. Tajima, Y. Ukawa, K.H. Cho, J.S. Choi, T. Ishid, Y. Gu. 2007. Radioprotective effect of Lyophyllum decastes and the effect on immunological functions in irradiated mice. *Journal of Traditional Chinese Medicine* 27(1): 70-75.

Suzuki, I. et al. 2001. Antihypertensive effect of *Lyophyllum decastes* Sing. In spontaneously hypertensive rats. *International Journal of Medicinal Mushrooms* 3(2-3): 231.

Takaki, K., K. Yoshida, T. Saito, T. Kusaka, R. Yamaguchi, K. Takahashi, Y. Sakamoto. 2014. Effect of Electrical Stimulation on Fruit Body Formation in Cultivating Mushrooms. *Microorganisms* 2(1): 58-72.

Ukawa, Y., H. Ito, M. Hisamatsu. 2000. Antitumor effects of $(1{\rightarrow}3)$-beta-D-glucan and $(1 \rightarrow 6)$-beta-D-glucan purified from newly cultivated mushroom, Hatakeshimeji (Lyophyllum decastes Sing.) *Journal of Bioscience and Bioengineering* 90(1): 98-104.

Ukawa, Y., Y. Furuichi, Y. Kokean, T. Nishii, M. Hisamatsu. 2002. Effect of Hatakeshimeji (Lyophyllum decastes Sing.) Mushroom on serum lipid levels in rats. *Journal of Nutritional Science Vitaminology* (Tokyo) 48(1): 73-76.

Ukawa, Y., Y. Izuma, T. Ohbuchi, T. Takahashi, S. Ikemizu, Y. Kojima. 2007. Oral administration of the extract from Hatakeshimeji (Lyophyllum decastes sing.) mushroom inhibits the development of atopic dermatitis-like skin lesions in NC/Nga mice. *Journal of Nutritional Science Vitaminology* (Tokyo) 53(3): 293-296.

Wang, T., J.J. Han, H.Q. Dai, J.Z. Sun, J.W. Ren, W.Z. Wang et al. 2022. Polysaccharides from Lyophyllum decastes reduce obesity by altering gut microbiota and increasing energy expenditure. *Carbohydrate Polymers* 295:119862.

Zhang, F.P., H. Xu, Y. Yuan, H.C. Huang, X.P. Wu, J.L. Zhang, J.S. Fu. 2022. Lyophyllum decastes fruiting body polysaccharide alleviates acute liver injury by activating the Nrf2 signaling pathway. *Food and Function* 13(4): 2057-2067.

GOLDEN CHANTERELLE References:

Fogarasi, M., M.I. Soccaciu, C.D. Salagean, F. Ranga et al. 2021. Comparison of Different Extraction Solvents for Characterization of Antioxidant Potential and Polyphenolic Composition in *Boletus edulis* and *Cantharellus cibarius* Mushrooms from Romania. *Molecules* 26(24): 7508.

Kolundzic, M., T. Stanojkovic, J. Radovic, A. Tacic, M. Dodevska, M. Milenkovic, F. Sisto, C. Masia, G. Farronato, V. Nikolic, T. Kundakovic. 2017. Cytotoxic and Antimicrobial Activities of Cantharellus cibarius Fr. (Cantarellacea). *Journal of Medicinal Food* 20(8): 790-796.

Kozarski, M., A. Klaus, J. Vunduk, Z. Zizak, M. Niksic, D. Jakovljevic, M.M. Vrvic, L.J.L.D. Van Griensven. 2015. Nutraceutical properties of the methanolic extract of edible mushroom Cantharellus cibarius (Fries): primary mechanisms. *Food and Function* 6(6): 1875-1886.

Lemieszek, M.K., F.M. Nunes, C. Cardoso, G. Marques, W. Rzeski. 2018. Neuroprotective properties of Cantharellus cibarius polysaccharide fractions in different in vitro models of neurodegeneration. *Carbohydrate Polymers* 197: 598-607.

Lemieszek, M.K., P.S. Marques, M. Ribeiro, D. Ferreira, G. Marques, R. Chaves, P. Pozarowski, F.M. Nunes, W. Rzeski. 2019. Mushroom small RNAs as potential anticancer agents: a closer look at Cantharellus cibarius proapoptotic and antiproliferative effects in colon cancer cells. *Food and Function* 10(5): 2739-2751.

Lemieszek, M.K., F.M. Nunes, W. Rzeski. 2019a. Branched mannans from the mushroom Cantharellus cibarius enhance the anticancer activity of natural killer cells against human cancers of lung and colon. *Food and Function* 10(9): 5816-5826.

Lemieszek, M.K., F.M. Nunes, G. Marques, W. Rzeski. 2019b. Cantharellus cibarius branched mannans inhibit colon cancer cells growth by interfering with signal transduction in NF-kappaB pathway. *International Journal of Biological Macromolecules* 134: 770-780.

Marathe, S.J., W. Hamzi, A.M. Bashein, J. Deska, T. Seppänen-Laakso, R.S. Singhal, S. Shamekh. 2022. Anti-angiogenic Effect of *Cantharellus cibarius* Extracts, its Correlation with Lipoxygenase Inhibition, and Role in the Bioactives Therein. *Nutrition and Cancer* 74(2): 724-734.

Meng, Y., Y.H. Qu, W.J. Wu, L. Chen, L. Sun, G.H. Tai, Y.F. Zhou, H.R. Cheng. 2019. Galactan isolated from Cantharellus cibarius modulates antitumor immune response by converting tumor-associated macrophages toward M1-like phenotype. *Carbohydrate Polymers* 226: 115295.

Muszynska, B., K. Sulkowska-Ziaja, H. Ekiert. 2013. Analysis of indole compounds in methanolic extracts from the fruiting bodies of Cantharellus cibarius (the Chanterelle) and from the mycelium of this species cultured in vitro. *Journal of Food Science and Technology* 50(6): 1233-1237.

Nasiry, D., A.R. Khalatbary, M.A. Ebrahimzadeh. 2017. Anti-Inflammatory and Wound-Healing Potential of Golden Chanterelle Mushroom, Cantharellus cibarius (Agaricomycetes). *International Journal of Medicinal Mushrooms* 19(10): 893-903.

Qu, Y.H., X.L. Zhao, H.J. Guo, Y. Meng, Y.M. Wang, Y. Zhou, L. Sun. 2021. Structural analysis and macrophage activation of a novel B-glucan isolated from *Cantharellus cibarius. International Journal of Molecular Medicine* 47(4): 50.

Uthan, E.T., H. Senturk, M. Uyanoglu, M. Yamac. 2021. First Report on the In Vivo Prebiotic, Biochemical, and Histological Effects of Crude Polysaccharide Fraction of Golden Chanterelle Mushroom, Cantharellus cibarius (Agaricomycetes). *International Journal of Medicinal Mushrooms* 23(5): 67-77.

Watanabe, F., J. Schwarz, S. Takenaka, E. Miyamoto, N. Ohishi, E. Nelle, R. Hochstrasser, Y. Yabuta. 2012. Characterization of vitamin B_{12} compounds in the wild edible mushrooms black trumpet (Craterellus cornucopioides) and golden chanterelle (Cantharellus cibarius). *Journal of Nutritional Science & Vitaminology* (Tokyo) 58(6): 438-441.

Zhao, D.Q., X. Ding. Y.L. Hou, W.R. Hou, L. Liu, T. Xu, D. Yang 2018. Structural characterization, immune regulation and antioxidant activity of a new heteropolysaccharide from Cantharellus cibarius Fr. *International Journal of Molecular Medicine* 41(5): 2744-2754.

HAWK WING References:

Alves, M.J., I. Ferreira, I. Lourenco, E. Costa, A. Martins, M. Pintado. 2014. Wild mushroom extracts as inhibitors of bacterial biofilm formation. *Pathogens* 3(3): 667-679.

Cao, C.Y., Y.X. Yang, Z. Xie, X. Chen, X.W. Shi, X. Yin. 2022. Derivatives of sarcodonin A isolated from Sarcodon scabrosus reversed LPS-induced M1 polarization in microglia through MAPK/NF-$_K$B pathway. *Bioorganic Chemistry* 125: 105854.

Chen, Y., M. Hu, C. Wang, Y.L. Yang, J.H. Chen, J.N. Ding, W.Q. Guo. 2013. Characterization and in vitro antitumor activity of polysaccharides from the mycelium of *Sarcodon aspratus*. *International Journal of Biological Macromolecules* 52: 52-58.

Chen, J., J.J. Liu, C.C. Yan, C. Zhang, W.J. Pan, W. Zhang, Y.M. Lu, L. Chen, Y. Chen. 2020. Sarcodon aspratus polysaccharides ameliorated obesity-induced metabolic disorders and modulated gut microbiota dysbiosis in mice fed a high-fat diet. *Food and Function* 11(3): 2588-2602.

Dong, M., S.P. Chen, K. Kita, Y. Ichimura, W.Z. Guo et al. 2009. Anti-proliferative and apoptosis-inducible activity of sarcodonin G from *Sarcodon scabrosus* in HeLa cells. *International Journal of Oncology* 34(1): 201-207.

Dong, H.B., J.L. Yang, Y. Wang, Y. Jiang, J. Chen, W. Zhang, Y.M. Lu, L. Chen, Y. Chen. 2020. Polysaccharide SAFP from Sarcodon aspratus attenuates oxidative stress-induced cell damage and bleomycin-induced pulmonary fibrosis. *International Journal of Biological Macromolecules* 164: 1215-1236.

Hirota, H., K. Morimura, H. Shibata. 2002. Anti-inflammatory compounds from the bitter mushroom, *Sarcodon scabrosus*. *Bioscience Biotechnology and Biochemistry* 66(1): 179-184.

Jantunen, H., N.S. Wasenius, M.A. Guzzardi, P. Iozzo, E. Kajantie et al. 2020. Physical activity and telomeres in old age: A longitudinal 10-year follow-up study. *Gerontology* 66(4): 315-322.

Kaygusuz, O., M. Secme, M. Kaygusuz. 2021. Nutritional composition and antioxidant, antimicrobial and cytotoxic activities of the Scaly Tooth wild mushroom, *Sarcodon squamosus* (Agaricomycetes), from Turkey. *International Journal of Medicinal Mushrooms* 23(6): 57-68.

Kita, T., Y. Takaya, Y. Oshima, T. Ohta, K. Aizawa, T. Hirano, T. Inakuma. 1998. Scabronines B, C, D, E and F, novel diterpenoids showing stimulating activity of nerve growth factor-synthesis, from the mushroom *Sarcodon scabrosus*. *Tetrahedron* 54(39): 11877-11886.

Larsson, K.H., S. Svantesson, D. Miscevic, U. Koljalg, E. Larsson. 2019. Reassessment of the generic limits for *Hydnellum* and *Sarcodon* (Thelephorales, Badisiomycota). *Mycokeys* 54: 31-47.

Liu, J.J., J. Chen, Y. Wang, C.C. Yan, C. Zhang, S. Mehmood, W.J. Pan et al. 2020. Reduction of 5-fluorouracil-induced toxicity by Sarcodon aspratus polysaccharides in Lewis tumor-bearing mice. *International Journal of Biological Macromolecules* 163: 232-239.

Lubart, E., R. Segal, E. Haimov, M. Dan, Y. Baumoehl, A. Leibovitz. 2011. Bacteremia in a multilevel geriatric hospital. *Journal of the American Medical Directors Association* 12(3): 204-207.

Luo, Y., Y. Huang, X.H. Yuan, L. Zhang, X.Y. Zhang, P. Gao. 2017. Evaluation of fatty acid composition and antioxidant activity of wild-growing mushrooms from southwest China. *International Journal of Medicinal Mushrooms* 19(10): 937-947.

Johannesson, H., S. Ryman, H. Lundmark, E. Danell. 1999. *Sarcodon imbricatus* and *S. squamosus* – two confused species. *Mycological Research* 103(11): 1447-1452.

Shi, X.W., L. Liu, J.M. Gao, A.L. Zhang. 2011. Cyathane diterpenes from Chinese mushroom *Sarcodon scabrosus* and their neurite outgrowth-promoting activity. *European Journal of Medicinal Chemistry* 46(7): 3112-3117.

Shomali, N., O. Onar, T. Alkan, N. Demirtas, I. Akata, O. Yildirim. 2019. *Turkish Journal of Pharmaceutical Sciences* 16(2): 155-160.

Tan, X.P., W. Chen, C.W. Jiao, H.J. Liang, H. Yun, C.Y. He, J.M. Chen, X.W. Ma, Y.Z. Xie. 2020. Anti-tumor and immunomodulatory activity of the aqueous extract of *Sarcodon imbricatus in vitro* and *in vivo*. *Food & Function* 11(1): 1110-1121.

Wang, D.D., Q.X. Wu, W.J. Pan, S. Hussain, S. Mehmood, Y. Chen. 2018. A novel polysaccharide from the Sarcodon aspratus triggers apoptosis in HeLa cells via induction of mitochondrial dysfunction. *Food and Nutrition Research* doi: 10.29219/fnr.v62.1285.

Wang, D.D., W.J. Pan, S. Mehmood, X.D. Cheng, Y. Chen. 2018a. Polysaccharide isolated from Sarcodon aspratus induces RAW264.7 activity via TLR4-mediated $NF_{\kappa}B$ and MAPK signaling pathways. *International Journal of Biological Macromolecules* 120(pt A): 1039-1047.

Wang, X., Y. Qu, Y.F. Zhang, S.P. Li, Y.Y. Sun, Z.P. Chen, L.R. Teng, D. Wang. 2018a. Antifatigue potential activity of *Sarcodon imbricatus* in acute excise (sic)-treated and chronic fatigue syndrome in mice via regulation of Nrf2-mediated oxidative stress. *Oxidative Medicine and Cellular Longevity* 2018:9140896.

Wang, X., Z.Q. Wang, H.H. Wu, W. Jia, L.S. Teng, J. Song, X.G. Yang, D. Wang 2018b. *Sarcodon imbricatus* polysaccharides protect against cyclophosphamide-induced immunosuppression via regulating Nrf2-medicated oxidative stress. *International Journal of Biological Macromolecules* 120 (Pt A): 736-744.

Wang, X., Q.B. Chu, X. Jiang, Y. Yu, L.B. Wang, Y.Q. Cui, J.H. Lu, L.R. Teng, D. Wang. 2018. *Sarcodon imbricatus* polysaccharides improve mouse hematopoietic function after cyclophosphamide-induced damage via G-CSF mediated JAK2/STAT3 pathway. *Cell Death and Disease* 9(6): 578.

Zhang, F.M., Y.H. Wang, P. Zhao, F.Q. Yu. 2019. A new *p*-terphenyl derivative from the fruiting bodies of *Sarcodon imbricatus* (L.) P. Karst. *Natural Product Research* doi: 10.1080.14786419.2019.1680664.

Zhang, D.L., M. Xiang, Y. Jiang, F. Wu, H.Q. Wu, H.Q Chen, M. Sun, L.Z. Zhang, X.F. Du, L. Chen. 2022. The Protective Effect of Polysaccharide SAFP from Sarcodon aspratus on Water Immersion and Restraint Stress-Induced Gastric Ulcer and Modulatory Effects on Gut Microbiota Dysbiosis. *Foods* 11(11): 1567.

Xu, B.J., C. Li, C.K. Sung. 2014. Telomerase inhibitory effects of medicinal mushrooms and lichens, and their anticancer activity. *International Journal of Medicinal Mushrooms* 16(1): 17-28.

HEMLOCK VARNISH CONK References:

Chen, M.L., C.C. Hsieh, B.L. Chiang, B.F. Lin. 2015. Triterpenoids and Polysaccharide Fractions of Ganoderma tsugae Exert Different Effects on Antiallergic Activities. *Evidence Based Complementary and Alternative Medicine* 2015:754836.

Chien, R.C., S.Y. Tsai, E.Y.C. Lai, J.L. Mau. 2015. Antiproliferative Activities of Hot Water Extracts from Culinary-Medicinal Mushrooms, Ganoderma tsugae and Agrocybe cylindracea (Higher Basidiomycetes) on Cancer Cells. *International Journal of Medicinal Mushrooms* 17(5):453-62.

Fryssouli, V., G. Zervakis, E. Polemis, M.A. Typas. 2020. A global meta-analysis of ITS rDNA sequences from material belonging to the genus Ganoderma (Basidiomycota, Polyporales) including new data from selected taxa. *MycoKeys* 75:71-143.

Hseu, Y.C., Y.C. Shen, M.C. Kao, D.C. Mathew, P. Karuppaiya, M.L. Li, H.L. Yang. 2019. Ganoderma tsugae induced ROS-independent apoptosis and cytoprotective autophagy in human chronic myeloid leukemia cells. *Food and Chemical Toxicology* 124:30-44.

Huang, S.Y., G.J. Huang, H.C. Wu, M.C. Kao, W.C. Huang. 2018. *Ganoderma tsugae* inhibits the SREBP-1/AR Axis Leading to Suppression of Cell Growth and Activation of Apoptosis in Prostate Cancer Cells. *Molecules* 23(10):2539.

Huang, W.C., M.S. Chang, S.Y. Huang, C.J. Tsai et al. 2019. Chinese Herbal Medicine *Ganoderma tsugae* Displays Potential Anti-Cancer Efficacy on Metastatic Prostate Cancer Cells. *International Journal of Molecular Sciences* 20(18): 4418.

Jiang, N., S. Hu, B. Peng, Z.H. Li, X.C. Yuan, S.J. Xiao, Y.P. Fu. 2021. Genome of *Ganoderma* Species Provides Insights Into the Evolution, Conifers Substrate Utilization, and Terpene Synthesis for *Ganoderma tsugae*. *Frontiers in Microbiology* 12:724451.

Kuo, H.P., S.C. Hsu, C.C. Ou, J.W. Li, H.H. Tseng, T.C. Chuang et al. 2013. Ganoderma tsugae Extract Inhibits Growth of HER-2 Overexpressing Cancer Cells via Modulation of HER2/PI3K/Akt Signaling Pathway. *Evidence Based Complementary and Alternative Medicine* 2013:219472.

Kuo, H.C., S.Y. Tong, M.W. Chao, C.Y. Tseng. 2022. Ganoderma tsugae prevents cognitive impairment and attenuates oxidative damage in d-galactose-induced aging in the rat brain. *PLoS One* 17(4):e0266331.

Kuok, Q.Y., C.Y. Yeh, B.C. Su, P.L. Hsu, H. Ni, M.Y. Liu, F.E. Mo. The triterpenoids of Ganoderma tsugae prevent stress-induced myocardial injury in mice. *Molecular Nutrition and Food Research* 57(10):1892-1896.

Lin, K.W., D. Maitraie, A.M. Huang, J.P. Wang, C.N. Lin. 2016. Triterpenoids and an alkamide from Ganoderma tsugae. *Fitoterapia* 108:73-80.

Loyd, A.L., B.S. Richter, M.A. Jusino, C. Truong, M.E. Smith, R.A. Blanchette, J.A. Smith. 2018. Identifying the "Mushroom of Immortality": Assessing the *Ganoderma* Species Composition in Commercial Reishi Products. *Frontiers in Microbiology* 9:1557.

Tsai, Y.T., P.H. Kuo, H.P. Kuo, C.Y. Hsu, Y.J. Lee, C.L. Kuo et al. 2021. Ganoderma tsugae suppresses the proliferation or endometrial carcinoma cells via Akt signaling pathway. *Environmental Toxicology* 36(3):320-327.

Tseng, C.Y., M.C. Chung, J.S. Wang, Y.J. Chang, J.F. Chang, C.H. Lin, R.S. Hseu, M.W. Chao. 2016. Potent In Vitro Protection Against $PM_{2.5}$-Caused ROS Generation and Vascular Permeability by Long-Term Pretreatment with Ganoderma tsugae. *American Journal of Chinese Medicine* 44(2):355-76.

Yao, Y.J., Y. Li, Z. Du, K. Wang, X.C. Wang, P.M. Kirk, B.M. Spooner. 2020. On the typification of Ganoderma sichuanense (Agaricomycetes)-the Widely Cultivated Lingzhi Medicinal Mushroom. *International Journal of Medicinal Mushrooms* 22(1):45-54.

KING BOLETE References:

Bovi, M., L. Cenci, M. Perduca, S. Capaldi, M.E. Carrizo et al. 2013. BEL beta-trefoil: a novel lectin with antineoplastic properties in king bolete (*Boletus edulis*) mushrooms. *Glycobiology* 23(5): 578-592.

Byerrum, R.U., D.A. Clarke, E.H. Lucas et al. 1957. Tumor inhibitors in *Boletus edulis* and other Holobasidiomycetes. *Antibiotics & Chemotherapy* (Northfield) 7(1): 1-4.

Garcia, J., F. Rodrigues, F. Castro, A. Aires, G. Marques, M.J. Saavedra. 2022. Antimicrobial, Antibiofilm, and Antioxidant Properties of *Boletus edulis* and *Neoboletus luridiformis* Against Multidrug-Resistant ESKAPE Pathogens. *Frontiers in Nutrition* 8:773346.

Helbling, A., N. Bonadies, K.A. Brander, W.J. Pichler. 2002. Boletus edulis: a digestion-resistance allergen may be relevant for food allergy. *Clinical and Experimental Allergy* 32(5): 771-775.

Kosanic, M., B. Rankovic, M. Dasic. 2012. Mushrooms as possible antioxidant and antimicrobial agents. *Iranian Journal of Pharmaceutical Research* 11(4): 1095-1102.

Landi, N., S. Ragucci, R. Culurciello, R. Russo, M. Valletta, P.V. Pedone, E. Pizzo, A.D. Maro. 2021. Ribotoxin-like proteins from Boletus edulis: structural properties, cytotoxicity and in vitro digestibility. *Food Chemistry* 259: 129931.

Lemieszek, M.K., M. Ribeiro, H.G. Alves, G. Marques, F.M. Nunes, W. Rzeski. 2016. *Boletus edulis* ribonucleic acid—a potent apoptosis inducer in human colon adenocarcinoma cells. *Food and Function* 7(7): 3163-3175.

Lemieszek, M.K., M. Ribeiro, G. Margues, F.M. Nunes, P. Pozarowski, W. Rzeski. 2017. New insights into the molecular mechanism of *Boletus edulis* ribonucleic acid fraction (BE3) concerning proliferation activity on human colon cancer cells. *Food and Function* 8(5): 1830-1839.

Lemieszek, M.K., F.M. Nunes, K. Sawa-Wejksza, W. Rzeski. 2017a. A King Bolete, *Boletus edulis* (Agaricomycetes), RNA fraction stimulates proliferation and cytotoxicity of natural killer cells against myelogenous leukemia cells. *International Journal of Medicinal Mushrooms* 19(4): 347-353.

Meng, T., S.S. Yu, H.Y. Ji, X.M. Xu, A.J. Liu. 2021. A novel polysaccharide from Boletus edulis: extraction, characteristics and antitumor activities in vitro. *Glycoconjugate Journal* 38(1): 13-24.

Muszynska, B., K. Sutkowska-Ziaja, H. Ekiert. 2011. Indole compounds in some culinary-medicinal higher basidiomycetes from Poland. *International Journal of Medicinal Mushrooms* 13(5): 449-454.

Novakovic, A., M. Karaman, S. Kaisarevic, T. Radusin, N. Llic. 2017. Antioxidant and antiproliferative potential of fruiting bodies of the wild-growing King Bolete mushroom, *Boletus edulis* (Agaricomycetes), from western Serbia. *International Journal of Medicinal Mushrooms* 19(1): 27-34.

Rogers, R. 2020. *Medicinal Mushrooms: The Human Clinical Trials*. Prairie Deva Press, Edmonton Alberta. Page 14.

Rosa, G.B., W.G. Sganzeria, A.L.A. Ferreira, L.O. Xavier, N.C. Veloso et al. 2020. Investigation of nutritional composition, antioxidant compounds, and antimicrobial activity of wild culinary-medicinal mushrooms *Boletus edulis* and *Lactarius deliciosus* (Agaricomycetes) from Brazil. *International Journal of Medicinal Mushrooms* 22(10): 931-942.

Valenti, M.T., G. Marchetto, M. Perduca, N. Tiso, M. Mottes, L.D. Carbonare. 2020. BEL beta-trefoil reduces the migration ability of RUNX2 expressing melanoma cells in xenotransplanted zebrafish. *Molecules* 25(6): 1270.

Vamanu, E., & S. Nita. 2013. Antioxidant capacity and the correlation with major phenolic compounds, anthocyanin, and tocopherol content in various extracts from the wild edible *Boletus edulis* mushroom. *BioMed Research International* 2013: 313905.

Wang, D., S.Q. Sun, W.Z. Wu, S.L. Yang, J.M. Tan. 2014. Characterization of a water-soluble polysaccharide from *Boletus edulis* and its antitumor and immunomodulatory activities on renal cancer in mice. *Carbohydrate Polymers* 105: 127-134.

Witkowska, A.M., M. E. Zujiko, I. Mironczuk-Chodakowska. 2011. Comparative study of wild edible mushrooms as sources of antioxidants. *International Journal of Medicinal Mushrooms* 13(4): 335-341.

Wu, S.Q., G.L. Wang, R.H. Yang, Y.B. Cui. 2016. Anti-inflammatory effects of *Boletus edulis* polysaccharide on asthma pathology. *American Journal of Translational Research* 8(10): 4478-4489.

Youonis, A.M., M.M. Abdel-Aziz, M. Yosri. 2019. Evaluation of some biological applications of *Pleurotus citronpileatus* and *Boletus edulis* fruiting bodies. *Current Pharmaceutical Biotechnology* 20(15): 1309-1320.

Zhang, H.Y., D. Pu, B.G. Sun, F.Z. Ren, Y.Y. Zhang, H.T. Chen. 2018. Characterization and comparison of key aroma compounds in raw and dry porcini mushroom (*Boletus edulis*) by aroma extract dilution analysis, quantitation and aroma recombination experiments. *Food Chemistry* 258: 260-268.

Zhang, W.W., G.T. Tian, S.S. Feng, J.H. Wong, Y.C. Zhao, X. Chen et al. 2015. *Boletus edulis* nitrite reductase reduces nitrite content of pickles and mitigates intoxication in nitrite-intoxicated mice. *Scientific Reports* 5: 14907.

Zhang, L.P., B. Meng, L.Z. Li, Y.Z. Wang, Y.Z. Zhang, X.X. Fang, D. Wang. 2020. *Boletus aereus* protects against acute alcohol-induced liver damage in the C57BL/6 mouse via regulating the oxidative stress-mediated NF-$_\kappa$B pathway. *Pharmaceutical Biology* 58(1):905-914.

Zhang, Y., R. Zhou, F. Liu, T.B. Ng. 2021. Purification and characterization of a novel protein with activity against non-small-cell lung cancer in vitro and in vivo from the edible mushroom Boletus edulis. *International Journal of Biological Macromolecules* 174: 77-88.

Zhang, M.H., R. Zhou, F. Liu, T.B. Ng. 2021a. Purification of a novel protein with cytotoxicity against non-small-cell lung cancer cells from Boletus bicolor. *Archive of Pharmacy* (Weinheim) 254(9):e2100135.

Zheng, J.L., T.T. Zhang, J. Fan, Y.L. Zhuang, L.P. Sun. 2021. Protective effects of a polysaccharide from Boletus aereus on S180 tumor-bearing mice and its structural characteristics. *International Journal of Biological Macromolecules* 188:1-10.

Zhu, H.Q., X. Ding, Y.L. Hou, Y.M. Li, M. Wang. 2019. Structure elucidation and bioactivities of a new polysaccharide from Xiaojin Boletus speciosus Frost. *International Journal of Biological Macromolecules* 126:697-716.

LESSER-KNOWN MEDICINAL POLYPORES OF THE PACIFIC NORTHWEST References:

Ayed, A.B., I. Akrout, Q. Albert, S. Greff, C. Simmier, J. Armengaud et al. 2022. Biotransformation of the Fluoroquinolone, Levofloxacin, by the White-Rot *Coriolopsis gallica*. *Journal of Fungi* (Basel) 8(9): 965.

Barad, A., S. Javed, S., C.H. Lee. 2016. *Trichaptum abietinum* from British Columbia exhibited anti-proliferative and immune-modulatory activities. *Planta Medica* 82(S 01): S1-S381; doi: 10.1055/s-0036-1596674.

Bertinetti, B., M. Scandiani, G. Cabrera. 2011. Analogs of Antifungal Indoles Isolated from *Aporpium Caryae* with Activity against Sudden-Death Syndrome of Soybean. *American Journal of Plant Sciences* (2): 245-254.

Buzina, W., C. Lass-Florl. G. Kropshofer, M. C. Freund, E. Marth. 2005. The Polypore Mushroom *Irpex lacteus*, a New Causative Agent of Fungal Infections. *Journal of Clinical Microbiology* 43(4): 2009-2011.

Cateni, F., V. Lucchini, M. Anderluh, P. Martinuzzi et al. 2010. Triterpenes from *Gloeophyllum odoratum* as potential leads towards potent thrombin inhibitors. *Letters in Drug Design & Discovery* 7(7):521-527.

Chand, S., A. Nazir, R. Chaw, R. Arora, B. Ahmed et al. 2006. The endophytic fungus *Trametes hirsuta* as a novel alternative source of podophyllotoxin and related aryl-tetralin lignans. *Journal of Biotechnology* 122(4): 494-510.

Chen, S. C., M. K. Lu, J. J. Cheng, D. L. Wang. 2005. Antiangiogenic activities of polysaccharides isolated from medicinal fungi. *FEMS Microbiology Letters* 249(2): 247-254.

Deng, Z. S., J. X. Li, P. Teng, P. Li, X. R. Sun. 2008. Biocatalyzed Cross-Coupling of Sinomenine and Guaiacol by *Antrodiella semisupina*. *Organic Letters* 10(6): 1119-1122.

Deng, Z., A. Deng, D. Luo, D. Gong, K. Zuo, Y. Peng, Z. Guo. 2015. Biotransformation of (-)-(10E,15S)-10,11-dehydrocurvularin. *Natural Product Communications* 10(7): 1277-1278.

Deo, G.S., J. Khatra, S. Buttar et al. 2019. Antiproliferative, Immunostimulatory, and Anti-inflammatory Activities of Extracts derived from Mushroom Collected in Haida Gwaii, British Columbia (Canada). *International Journal of Medicinal Mushrooms* 21(7): 629-643.

Dizeci, N., B. Karaca, O. Onar, A.C. Cihan, I. Akata, O. Yildirim. 2021. The Remarkable Antibiofilm Activity of the Sweet Tooth Mushroom, Hydnum repandum (Agaricomycetes), Displaying Synergistic Interactions with Antibiotics. *International Journal of Medicine Mushrooms* 23(10):45-60.

Dogan, H.H., S. Karagoz, R. Duman. 2018. *In vitro* evaluation of the antiviral activity of some mushrooms from Turkey. *International Journal of Medicinal Mushrooms* 20(3): 201-212.

Doskocil, I., J. Havlik, R. Verlotta, J. Tauchen, L. Vesela et al. 2016. In vitro immunomodulatory activity, cytotoxicity and chemistry of some central European polypores. *Pharmaceutical Biology* 54)11): 2369-2376.

Fakoya, S., S. Oloketuyl. 2012. Antimicrobial efficacy and phytochemical screening of mushrooms, *Lenzites betulinus* and *Coriolopsis gallica* extracts. *TAF Preventive Medicine Bulletin* 11(6):1.

Gao, L., Y. P. Sun, J. Y. Si, J. Hl Liu, G. B. Sun, X. O. Sun, L. Cao. 2014. *Cryptoporus volvatus* Extract Inhibits Influenza Virus Replication *In Vitro* and *In Vivo*. *PLoS One* 9(2).

Gao, L., J. Han, J. Si, J Wang, Y. Sun, Y. Bi, J. Liu, L. Cao. 2017. Crytoporic acid E from *Cryptoporus volvatus* inhibits influenza virus replication in vitro. *Antiviral Research* 143: 106-112.

Grienke, U., J. Zwirchmayr, U. Peintner, E. Urban, M. Zehl et al. 2019. Lanostane Triterpenes from *Gloeophyllum odoratum* and Their Anti-Influenza Effects. *Planta Medica* 85(3): 195-202.

Hossen, S.M.M., M.S. Hossain, S. Akbar, U. Tahmida, J. Mawa, N.U. Emon. 2021. Wild mushrooms showed analgesic and cytotoxic properties along with phytoconstituent's binding affinity to COX-1, COX-2 and cytochrome P450 2C9. *Heliyon* 7(9):e07997.

Im, K.H., T.K. Nguyen, J.K. Kim, J.H. Choi, T.S. Lee. 2016. Evaluation of Anticholinesterase and Inflammation Inhibitory Activity of Medicinal Mushroom *Phellinus pini* (Basidiomycetes) Fruiting Bodies. *International Journal of Medicinal Mushrooms* 18(11):1011-1022.

Im, K.H., J. Choi, S.A. Baek, T.S. Lee. 2018. Hyperlipidemic Inhibitory Effects of *Phellinus pini* in Rats Fed with a High Fat and Cholesterol Diet. *Mycobiology* 46(2).

Javid, S., W.M. Li, M. Zeb, A. Yaqoob, L.E. Tackaberry, H.B. Massicotte, K.N. Egger, P.C.K. Cheung, G.W. Payne, C.H. Lee. 2019. Anti-inflammatory Activity of the Wild Mushroom, *Echinodontium tinctorium*, in RAW264.7 Macrophage Cells and Mouse Microcirculation. *Molecules* 24(9):3509.

Kaur, N., N. Kaushai, N., Singh, M., Singh, A.P., Dhingra, G.S. 2019. Investigations on Antioxidative Potential of Poroid Medicinal Mushroom Porodaedalea pini (Agaricomycetes). *International Journal of Medicinal Mushrooms* 21(6): 549-559.

Knezevic, A., M. Stajic, L. Zivkovic, I. Milovanovic, B. Spremo-Potparevic, J. Vukojevic. 2017. Antifungal, Antioxidative, and Genoprotective Properties of Extracts from the Blushing Bracket Mushroom, *Daelaleopsis confragosa* (Agaricomycetes). *International Journal of Medicinal Mushrooms* 19(6):509-520.

Knezevic, A., M. Stajic, I. Sofrenic, T. Stanojikovic et al. 2010. Antioxidative, antifungal, cytotoxic and antineurodegenerative activity of selected *Trametes* species from Serbia. *PLoS One* 13(8).

Krupodorova, T., S. Rybalko, V. Barshteyn. 2014. Antiviral activity of Basidiomycete mycelia against influenza type A (serotype HINI) and herpes virus type 2 in cell culture. *Virologica Sinica* 29(5): 284-290.

Krupodorova, T., V. Barshteyn, I. Scharakov, M. M. Marchenko. 2016. Anticancer potential of *Trametes versicolor* (L.) Lloyd and *Auriporia aurea* (Peck) Ryvarden mycelia in rat Guerin's carcinoma. *Advances in Biomedicine and Pharmacy* 3(1): 1-8.

Kwon, J., H. Lee, Y. D. Yoon, B. Y. Kwang, Y. Guo et al. 2016 Lanostane Triterpenes Isolated from *Antrodia heteromorpha* and Their Inhibitory Effects on RANKL-Induced Osteoclastogenesis. *Journal of Natural Products* 79(6): 1689-1693.

Lee, S.M., S.M. Kim, Y.H. Lee, W.J. Kim et al. 2010. Macromolecules isolated from *Phellinus pini* fruiting body: Chemical characterization and antiviral activity. *Macromolecular Research* 18(6):602-609.

Levy, L. M., G. M. Cabrera, J. E. Wright, A. M. Seldes. 2003. 5*H*-Furan-2-ones from fungal cultures of *Aporpium caryae*. *Phytochemistry* 62(2): 239-243.

Li, S.Y., Z. H. Jiang, F. J. Xin. 2017. Characterization of a New Fungal Immunomodulatory Protein, FIP-dsq2 from *Dichomitus squalens*. *Journal of Biotechnology* 02.006.

Li, X, J. Gao, M.M. Li, H. Cui, W. Jiang, Z.C. Tu, T. Yuan. 2021. Aromatic Cadinane Sesquiterpenoids from the Fruiting Bodies of *Phellinus pini* Block SARS-CoV-2 Spike-ACE2 Interaction. *Journal of Natural Products* 84(8):2385-2389.

Li, Z.Y., G.H. Leng, J.B. Wen, G.Q. Deng, J.Y. Jiang. 2022. Cordycepin production by a novel endophytic fungus Irpex lacteus CHG05 isolated from Cordyceps hawkesii Gray. *Folia Microbiologia* (Praha) doi: 10/1007/s12223-022-00981-6

Liu, F., Y. Wang, K. Zhang et al. 2017. A novel polysaccharide with antioxidant, HIV protease inhibiting and HIV integrase inhibiting activities from *Fomitiporia punctata* (P. karst.) Murrill (Basidiomycota, hymenochaetales). *International Journal of Biological Macromolecules* 97: 339-347.

Ma, Z. Q., W. W. Zhang, L. Wang, M. G. Zhu et al. 2013. A Novel Compound from the Mushroom *Cryptoporus volvatus* inhibits Porcine Reproductive and Respiratory Syndrome Virus (PRRSV) *in Vitro*. *PLoS One* 8(11).

Manna, D., S. Pust, M. L. Torgensen, G. Cordara, M. Künzler, U. Krengel, K. Sandvig. 2017. *Polyporus squamosus* Lectin 1a (PSL1a) Exhibits Cytotoxicity in Mammalian Cells by Disruption of Focal Adhesions, Inhibition of Protein Synthesis and Induction of Apoptosis. *PLoS One* 12(1): e0170716.

Matuszewska, A., M. Karp, M. Jaszek, G. Janusz et al. 2016. Laccase purified from *Cerrena unicolor* exerts antitumor activity against leukemic cells. *Oncology Letters* 11(3): 2009-2018.

Matuszewska, A., M. Jaszek, D. Stefaniuk, T. Ciszewski, L. Matuszewski. 2018. Anticancer, antioxidant, and antibacterial activities of low molecular weight bioactive subfractions isolated from cultures of wood degrading fungus *Cerrena unicolor*. *PLoS One* 13(6): e0197044.

Matuszewska, A., D. Stefaniuk, M. Jaszek et al. 2019. Antitumor potential of new low moleculular weight antioxidative preparations from the white rot fungus *Cerrena unicolor* against human colon cancer cells. *Scientific Reports* 9(1): 1975.

Mizerska-Dudka, M., M. Jaszek, A. Blachowicz, T. P. Rejczak et al. 2015. Fungus *Cerrena unicolor* as an effective source of new antiviral, immunomodulatory, and anticancer compounds. *International Journal of Biological Macromolecules* 79:459-468.

Mocan, A., A. Fernandes, L. Barros, G. Crisan, M. Smiljkovic, M. Sokovic, I.C. Ferreria. 2018. Chemical composition and bioactive properties of the wild mushroom *Polyporus squamosus* (Huds.) Fr: a study with samples from Romania. *Food Function* 9(1):160-170.

Na, M. W., E.J. Lee, D.M. Kang, S.Y. Jeong et al. 2022. Identification of Antibacterial Sterols from Korean Wild Mushroom *Daedaleopsis confragosa* via Bioactivity—and LC-MS/MS Profile-Guided Fractionation. *Molecules* 27(6):1865.

Newman, D.J., G.M. Cragg. 2016. Natural products as sources of new drugs from 1981 to 2014. *Journal Natural Products*. 79(3): 629-61.

Pop, R.M., Puia, I.C., Puia, A., Chedea, V.S., Leopold, N., Bocsan, I.C., Buzoianu, A.D. 2018. Characterization of *Trametes versicolor*: Medicinal Mushroom with Important Health Benefits. *Notulae Botanicae Horti Abrobotanica Cluj-Napoca* 46(2): 343-349.

Popova, M., B. Trusheva, M. Gyosheva, I. Tsvetkova, V. Bankova. 2009. Antibacterial triterpenes from the threatened wood-decay fungus *Fomitopsis rosea*. 80(5):263-266. *Fitoterapia* 80(5): 263-266.

Rogers, Robert D. 2011. *The Fungal Pharmacy: The Complete Guide to Medicinal Mushrooms and Lichens of North America*. North Atlantic Books, Berkeley, CA.

Rogers, Robert D. 2019. *Rejuvenate Your Brain Naturally*. Prairie Deva Press. Edmonton Alberta Canada. Page 36.

Rogers, Robert D. 2020. *Medicine Mushrooms: The Human Clinical Trials*. Prairie Deva Press. Edmonton Alberta. Pages 20-23.

Ryang, J., F. Liu, T.B. Ng. 2021. Purified antioxidant from the medicinal mushroom Phellinus pini protects rat H9c2 cell against H_2O_2-induced oxidative stress. *Journal of Food Biochemistry* 45(7):e13818.

Sitkof, A. O. Froehlich, C. Wenner. 2017. Cytotoxic Effects of Hot Ethanol and Hot Aqueous Extract of *Fomitopsis cajanderi* on Jurkat Cell Line. https://reishiandrosesbotanicals.com/2017/03/20/fomitopsis-cajanderi-rhodofomes-cajanderi-healing-inquiries/

Smith, A., J. Sumreen, B. Ankush, V. Myhre, W. M. Li, K. Reimer et al. 2017. Growth-inhibitory and Immuno-modulatory Activities of Wild Mushrooms from North-Central British Columbia (Canada). *International Journal of Medicinal Mushrooms*. 19(6): 485-497.

Smith, A. W. T. 2017a. Investigating British Columbia Wild Mushrooms for Growth Inhibitory Activity. Master Thesis UNBC. (2012).

Stefaniuk, D., T. Misztal, M. Piet, A. Zajac et al. 2021. Thromboelastometric analysis of Anticancer Cerrena unicolor Subfractions Reveal Their Potential as Fibrin Glue Drug Carrier Enhancers. *Biomolecules* 11(9): 1263.

Tang, Y., Z. Z. Zhao, J. N. Yao, T. Feng et al. 2018. Irpeksins A-E, 1, 10-seco-Eburicane-Type Triterpenoids from the Medicinal Fungus *Irpex lacteus* and their anti-NO Activity. *Journal of Natural Products* October 8.

Tang, Y., Z. Z. Zhao, Z. H. Li, T. Feng, H. P. Chen, J. K. Liu. 2018a. Irpexoates A-D, Four Triterpenoids with Malonyl Modifications from the Fruiting Bodies of the Medicinal Fungus *Irpex lacteus*. *Natural Products and Bioprospecting* 8(3):171-176.

Tel-Cayan, Gulsen. 2019. Phenolic profiles, antioxidant and anticholinesterase activities of three Gloeophyllum species with chemometric approach. *Journal of Food Biochemistry* 43(4).

Teplyakova, T. V., N.V. Psurtseva, T. A. Kosogova, N. A. Mazurkova et al. 2012. Antiviral activity of polyporoid mushrooms (higher Basidiomycetes) from Altai Mountains (Russia). *International Journal of Medicinal Mushrooms* 14(1):37-45.

Wang, J., J. Song, D. Wang, N. Zhang, J. Lu et al. 2016. The anti-membranous glomerulonephritic activity of purified polysaccharides from *Irpex lacteus* Fr. *International Journal of Biological Macromolecules* 84:87-93.

Yang, K., Y.H. Jin, M. Cai, P.F. He, B.M. Tian, R. Guan, G.R. Yu, P.L. Sun. 2021. Separation, characterization and hypoglycemic activity *in vitro* evaluation of a low molecular weight heteropolysaccharide from the fruiting body of *Phellinus pini*. *Food and Function* 12(8):3493-3503.

Yuan, B., F. Chen, Y. Q. Huang, T. Z. Ju et al. 2011. Chemical constituents, biological activities and fluorescence quenching of *Fomitoporia punctata* fruiting body extract. *Mycostema* (Journal of Fungal Sciences) 30(3):464-471.

Zeb, M., L.E. Tackaberry, H.B. Massicotte, K.N. Egger, K. Reimer, G. Lu, C. Heiss, P. Azadi, C.H. Lee. 2021. Structural elucidation and immune-stimulatory activity of a novel polysaccharide containing glucuronic acid from the fungus Echinodontium tinctorium. *Carbohydrate Polymers* 25j8:117700.

Zeb, M., W.M. Li, C. Heiss, I. Black, L.E. Tackaberry, H.B. Massicotte, K.N. Egger, K. Reimer, P. Azadi, C.H. Lee. 2022. Isolation and characterization of an anti-proliferative polysaccharide from the North American fungus Echinodontium tinctorium. *Scientific Reports* 12(1):17298.

Zhang, N., Y. Liu, J. H. Lu, J. Wang et al. 2012. Isolation, Purification and Bioactivities of Polysaccharides from *Irpex lacteus*. *Chemistry Research Chinese Universities* 28(2): 249-254.

Zheng, W., Y. Zhao, X. Zheng, Y. Liu, S. Pan, Y. Dai, F. Liu. 2011. Production of anti-oxidant and antitumor metabolites by submerged cultures of *Inonotus obliquus* cocultured with *Phellinus punctatus*. *Applied Microbiology and Biotechnology* 89(1): 157-167.

LEUCOPAXILLUS References:

Alves, M.J., I.C.F.R. Ferreira, J. Dias, V. Teixeira, A. Martins, M. Pintado. 2012. A review on antimicrobial activity of mushroom (Basidiomycetes) extracts and isolated compounds. *Planta Medica* 78(16): 1707-1718.

Alves, M.J. I.C.F.R. Ferreira, A. Martins, M. Pintado. 2012a. Antimicrobial activity of wild mushroom extracts against clinical isolates resistant to different antibiotics. *Journal of Applied Microbiology* 113(2): 466-475.

Alves, M.J., I.C.F.R. Ferreira, I. Lourenco, A. Castro, L. Pereira, A. Martins, M. Pintado. 2014. Wild mushroom extracts potentiate the action of standard antibiotics against multiresistant bacteria. *Journal of Applied Microbiology* 116(1): 32-38.

Alves, M.J., I.C.F.R. Ferreira, I. Lourenco, E. Costa, A. Martins, M. Pintado. 2014a. Wild mushroom extracts as inhibitors of bacterial biofilm formation. *Pathogens* 3(3): 667-679.

Clericuzio, M. et al. Cucurbitane triterpenes from Leucopaxillus gentianeus. *Journal of Natural Products* 67(11): 1823-1828.

Clericuzio, M., S. Tabasso, M.A. Bianco, G. Pratesi, G. Beretta, S. Tinelli, F. Zunino, G. Vidari. 2006. Cucurbitane triterpenes from the fruiting bodies and cultivated mycelia of Leucopaxillus gentianeus. *Journal of Natural Products* 69(12): 1796-1799.

Eberl, L., P. Vandamme. 2016. Members of the genus *Burkholderia*: good and bad guys. *F1000Research* 1007 doi: 10.12688/f1000research8221.1.

Friesen, W.J., C.R. Trotta, Y. Tomizawa, J. Zhuo, B. Johnson, J. Sierra, B. Roy, M. Weetall, J. Hendrick, J. Sheedy et al. 2017. The nucleoside analog clitocine is a potent and efficacious readthrough agent. *RNA* 23(4): 567-577.

Geng, X.R., G.T. Tian, W.W. Zhang, Y.C. Zhao, L.Y. Zhao, et al. 2015. Isolation of an Angiotensin 1-Converting Enzyme Inhibitory Protein with Antihypertensive Effect in Spontaneously Hypertensive Rats from the Edible Wild Mushroom Leucopaxillus tricolor. *Molecules* 20(6): 10141-10153.

Geng, X.R., J. Fan, L.J. Xu, H.X. Wang, T.B. Ng. 2018. Hydrolysis of oligosaccharides by a fungal a-galactoside from the fruiting bodies of a wild mushroom Leucopaxillus tricolor. *Journal of Basic Microbiology* 58(12): 1043-1052.

Howard, A., M. O'Donoghue, A. Feeney, R.D. Sleator. 2012. Acinetobacter baumannii: An emerging opportunistic pathogen. *Virulence* 3(3): 243-250.

Liu, H.G., J. Zhang, T. Li, Y.D. Shi, Y.Z. Wang. 2012. Mineral element levels in wild edible mushrooms from Yunnan, China. *Biological Trace Element Research* 147(1-3): 341-345.

Mayla, I.Y., J. Wu, E. Harada, M. Toda, C.N. D'Alessandro-Gabazza, T. Yasuma et al. 2020. Plant growth regulators and Axl and immune checkpoint inhibitors from the edible mushroom *Leucopaxillus giganteus*. *Bioscience Biotechnology & Biochemistry* 84(7): 1332-1338.

Niu, L.L., Y.Wu, H.P. Liu, Q. Wang, M.Y. Li, Q. Jia. 2021. The Structural Characterization of a Novel Water-Soluble Polysaccharide from Edible Mushroom Leucopaxillus giganteus and Its Antitumor Activity on H22 Tumor-Bearing Mice. *Chemistry and Biodiversity* 18(6): 2001010.

Pfister, J.R. 1988. Isolation and Bioactivity of 2-Aminoquinolone from Leucopaxillus albissimus. *Journal of Natural Products* 51(5): 969-70.

Schwan, W.R., C. Dunek, M. Gebhardt, K. Engelbrecht, T. Klett et al. 2010. Screening a mushroom extract library for activity against Acinebacter baumanii and Burkholderia cepacian and the identification of a compound with anti-Burkholderia activity. *Annals of Clinical Microbiology and Antimicrobials* 9:4 doi: 10.1186/1476-0711-9-4.

Sun, J.G., C.A. Yeung, N.N. Co, T.Y. Tsang, E. Yau, K.W. Luo, P. Wu, J.C.Y. Wa, K.P. Fung, T.T. Kwok. F.Y. Liu. 2012. Clitocine reversal of P-glycoprotein associated multi-drug resistance through down-regulation of transcription factor NF-$_k$B in R-HepG2 cell line. *PLoS One* 7(8): e40720.

MILK CAPS References:

Abbas, H.A., R.M. Goda. 2021. Sotolon is a natural virulence mitigating agent in Serratia marcescens. *Archives of Microbiology* 203(2): 533-541.

Aldawsari, M.F., E.S. Khafagy, A.A. Saqr, A. Alalaiew, H.A. Abbas, M.S. Shaldam, W.A.H. Hegazy, R.M. Goda. 2021. Tackling virulence of *Pseudomonas aeruginosa* by the Natural Furanone Sotolon. *Antibiotics* (Basel) 10(7): 871.

Bakun, P., B. Czarczynska-Goslinska, T. Goslinski, S. Lijewski. 2021. In vitro and in vivo biological activities of azulene derivatives with potential applications in medicine. *Medicinal Chemical Research* 30(4):834-846.

Barros, L., P. Baptista, L.M. Estevinho, I.C.F.R. Ferreira. 2007. Effect of fruiting body maturity stage on chemical composition and antimicrobial activity of Lactarius sp. mushrooms. *Journal of Agricultural and Food Chemistry* 55(21): 8766-8771.

Cheng, X.D., Q.X. Wu, J. Zhao, T. Su, Y.M. Lu, W.N. Zhang, Y. Wang, Y. Chen. 2019. Immunomodulatory effect of a polysaccharide fraction on RAW 264.7 macrophages extracts from the wild Lactarius deliciosus. *International Journal of Biological Macromolecules* 128: 732-739.

Dogan, H.H., S. Aydin. 2013. Some biological activities of Lactarius vellereus (Fr.) Fr. in Turkey. *Pakistan Journal of Biological Sciences* 16(21): 1279-1286.

Dogan, A., A. Ulyar, S. Hasar, O.F. Keles. 2022. The protective effects of the *Lactarius deliciosus* and *Agrocybe cylindracea* mushrooms on histopathology of carbon tetrachloride induced oxidative stress in rats. *Biotechnic & Histochemistry* 97(2): 143-151.

Esseddik, T.M., R. Redouane, K.F. Farouk, M. Fateh, B. Khaled, B. Laid, P. Massimiliano, N. Youcef. 2020. In Vivo Immunomodulatory Potential of Partial Purified Lectin from the Saffron Milk Cap Mushroom, Lactarius deliciosus (Agaricomycetes), against Colloidal Carbon Particles. *International Journal of Medicinal Mushrooms* 22(11): 1043-1055.

Guerin-Laguette, A., N. Cummings, R.C. Butler, A. Willows, N. Hesom-Williams, S.H. Li, Y. Wang. 2014. Lactarius deliciosus and Pinus radiata in New Zealand: towards the development of innovative gourmet mushroom orchards. *Mycorrhiza* 24(7): 511-523.

Hou, Y.L., M. Wang, D.Q. Zhao, L. Liu, X. Ding, W.R. Hou. 2019. Effect on macrophage proliferation of a novel polysaccharide from *Lactarius deliciosus* (L. ex Fr.) Gray. 2019. *Oncology Letters* 17(2): 2507-2515.

Karahan, S., A. Erden, A. Cetinkaya, D. Avci, A.I. Ortakoyluoglu, H. Karagoz, K. Bulut, M. Basak. 2016. Acute Pancreatitis Caused By Mushroom Poisoning: A Report of Two Cases. *Journal of Investigative Medicine High Impact Case Reports* 4(1): 2324709615627474.

Kim, K.H., H.J. Noh, S.U. Choi, K.M. Park, S.J. Seok, K.R. Lee. 2010. Lactarane sesquiterpenoids from Lactarius subvellereus and their cytotoxicity. *Bioorganic & Medicinal Chemistry Letters* 20(18): 5385-5388.

Kosanic, M., B. Rankovic, A. Rancic, T. Stanojkovic. 2016. Evaluation of metal concentration and antioxidant, antimicrobial, and anticancer potentials of two edible mushrooms Lactarius deliciosus and Macrolepiota procera. *Journal of Food and Drug Analysis* 24(3): 477-484.

Kosanic, M., N. Petrovic, O. Milosevic-Djordjevic, D. Grujicic, J. Tubic, A. Markovic, T.P. Stanojkovic. 2020. The Health Promoting Effects of the Fruiting Bodies Extract of the Peppery Milk Cap Mushroom Lactarius piperatus (Agaricomycetes) from Serbia. *International Journal of Medicinal Mushrooms* 22(4): 347-357.

Krawczyk, E., M. Kniotek, M. Nowaczyk, T. Dzieciatkowski, M. Przybylski, A. Majewska, M. Luczak. 2006. N-acetylphenylisoserinates of Lactarius sesquiterpenoid alcohols—cytotoxic, antiviral, antiproliferative and immunotropic activities in vitro. *Planta Medica* 72(7): 615-620.

Król, K., M. Pudelek, G. Krzysiek-Maczka, M. Wierdak, B. Muszynska, K. Sulkowska-Ziaja, A. Krakowska, D. Ryszawy, J. Czyz. 2021. Bioactive compounds from Lactarius deterrimus interfere with the invasive potential of gastric cancer cells. *Acta Biochimica Polonica* 68(4): 505-513.

Mihailovic, M., J.A. Jovanovic, A. Uskokovic, N. Grdovic, S. Dinic, S. Vidovic, G. Poznanovic, I. Mujic, M. Vidakovic. 2015. Protective Effects of the Mushroom Lactarius deterrimus Extract on Systemic Oxidative Stress and Pancreatic Islets in Streptozotocin-Induced Diabetic Rats. *Journal of Diabetes Research* 2015: 576726.

Nowakowski, P., R. Markiewicz-Zukowska, K. Gromkowska-Kepka, S. K. Naliwajko, J. Moskwa, J. Bielecka, M. Grabia, M. Borawska, K. Socha. 2021. Mushrooms as potential therapeutic agents in the treatment of cancer: Evaluation of anti-glioma effects of Coprinus comatus, Cantharellus cibarius, Lycoperdon perlatum and Lactarius deliciosus extracts. *Biomedicine & Pharmacotherapy* 133: 111090.

Ruthes, A.C., E.R. Carbonero, M.M. Cordova, C.H. Baggio, A.R.S. Santos, G.L. Sassaki, T.R. Cipriani, P.A. James Gorin, M. Iacomini. 2013. Lactarius rufus (1>3), (1>6)-B-D-glucans: structure, antinociceptive and anti-inflammatory effects. *Carbohydrate Polymers* 94(1): 129-136.

Xu, Z., L. Fu, S.L. Feng, M. Yuan, Y. Huang, J.Q. Liao, L.J. Zhou, H.Y. Yang, C.B. Ding. 2019. Chemical composition, antioxidant and antihyperglycemic activities of the wild *Lactarius deliciosus* from China. *Molecules* 24(7): 1357.

Zhong, R.F., J.J. Yang, J.H. Geng, J. Chen. 2021. Structural characteristics, anti-proliferative and immunomodulatory activities of a purified polysaccharide from Lactarius volemus Fr. *International Journal of Biological Macromolecules* 192: 967-977.

MILKY WHITE MUSHROOM Reference:

Amin, R, A. Khair, N.A. Alam, T.S. Lee. 2010a. Effect of Different Substrates and Casing Materials on the Growth and Yield of *Calocybe indica*. *Mycobiology* 38(2): 97-101.

________2010. Influence of different supplements on the commercial cultivation of milky white mushrooms. *Mycobiology* 38(3): 184-188.

Datta, S., J. Dubey, S. Gupta, A. Paul, P. Gupta, A.K. Mitra. 2020. Tropical Milky White Mushroom, *Calocybe indica* (Agaricomycetes): An Effective Antimicrobial Agent Working in Synergism with Standard Antibiotics. *International Journal of Medicinal Mushrooms* 22(4): 335-346.

Ghosh, S.K., T. Sanyai. 2020. Antiproliferative and apoptotic effect of ethanolic extract of Calocybe indica on PANC-1 and MIAPaCa2 cell lines of pancreatic cancer. *Experimental Oncology* 42(3): 178-182.

Maiti, S., S.K. Bhutia, S.K. Mallick, A. Kumar, N. Khadgi, T.K. Maiti. 2008. Antiproliferative and immunostimulatory protein fraction from edible mushrooms. *Environmental Toxicology and Pharmacology* 26(2): 187-191.

Mandal, E.K., K. Maity, S. Maity, S.K. Gantait, S. Maiti, T.K. Maiti, S.R. Sikdar, S.S. Islam. Structural characterization of an immunoenhancing cytotoxic heteroglycan isolated from an edible mushroom *Calocybe indica* var. APK2. *Carbohydrate Research* 346(14): 2237-2243.

Mishra, K.K., R.S. Pal, R. Arunkumer. 2014. Antioxidant activities and bioactive compound determination from caps and stipes of specialty medicinal mushrooms Calocybe indica and Pleurotus sajor-caju (higher Basidiomycetes) from India. *International Journal of Medicinal Mushrooms* 16(6): 555-567.

Nataraj, A., S. Govindan, P. Ramani, K.A. Subbaiah, S. Sathianarayanan et al. 2022. Antioxidant, Anti-Tumour, and Anticoagulant Activities of Polysaccharide from *Calocybe indica* (APK2). *Antioxidants* (Basel) 11(9): 1694.

Rathore, H., A. Sharma, S. Prasad, S. Sharma. 2018. Selenium bioaccumulation and associated nutraceutical properties in *Calocybe indica* mushroom cultivated on Se-enriched wheat straw. *Journal of Bioscience and Bioengineering* 126(4): 482-487.

Rathore, H, S. Prasad, S. Sehwag, S. Sharma. 2020. Vitamin D_2 fortification of *Calocybe indica* mushroom by natural and artificial UVB radiations and their potential effects on nutraceutical properties. *3 Biotech* 10(2): 41.

Shashikant, M., A. Bains, P. Chawla, M. Sharma, R. Kaushik, S. Kandi, R.C. Kuhad. 2022. In-vitro antimicrobial and anti-inflammatory activity of modified solvent evaporated ethanolic extract of Calocybe indica: GCMS and HPLC characterization. *International Journal of Food Microbiology* 376: 109741.

Singh, V., G.K. Bedi, R. Shri. 2017. In Vitro and In Vivo Antidiabetic Evaluation of Selected Culinary-Medicinal Mushrooms (Agaricomycetes). *International Journal of Medicinal Mushrooms*. 19(1): 17-25.

MUSHROOMS AND BEES References:

Bunyard, B.A. 2021. World Mushroom Production: *An Overview. Fungi* 14(1): 8-13.

Cicero, A.F.G., F. Fogacci, M. Banach. 2019. Red Yeast Rice for Hypercholesterolemia. *Methodist Debakey Cardiovascular Journal*. 15(3): 192-199.

Cicero, A.F.G., F. Fogacci, A. Zambon. 2021. Red Yeast Rice for Hypercholesterolemia: JACC Focus Seminar. *Journal of the American College of Cardiology* 77(5): 620-628.

Gage, S.L., F. Ahumada, A. Rivera, H. Graham, G. DeGrandi-Hoffman. 2018. Smoke Conditions Affect the Release of the Venom Droplet Accompanying Sting Extension in Honey Bees (Hymenoptera: Apidae). *Journal of Insect Science* 18(4): 7; 1-7.

Galvinic, U., J. Stavanovic, M. Ristanic, M. Rajkovic, D. Davitkov, N. Lakic, Z. Stanimirovic. 2021. Potential of fumagillin and *Agaricus blazei* Mushroom Extract to Reduce *Nosema ceranae* in Honey Bees. *Insects* 12(4): 282.

Glavinic, U., M. Rajkovic, J. Vunduk, B. Vejnovic. J. Stevanovic, I. Milenkovic, Z. Stanimirovic. 2021a. Effects of *Agaricus bisporus* Mushroom Extract on Honey Bees Infected with *Nosema ceranae*. *Insects* 12(10): 915.

Gimenez-Martinez, P., C. Ramirez, G. Mitton, F.M. Arcerito, F. Ramos, H. Cooley, S. Fuselli, M. Maggi. 2022. Lethal concentrations of Cymbopogon nardus essential oils and their main component citronellal on Varroa destructor and Apis mellifera. *Experimental Parasitology* 108279.

Han, J.O., N.L. Naeger, B.K. Hopkins, D. Sumerlin, P.E. Stamets, L.M. Carris, W.S. Sheppard. 2021. Directed evolution of *Metarhizium* fungus improves its biocontrol against *Varroa* mites in honey bee colonies. *Scientific Reports* 11: 10582.

Harris, J.W. & J. Woodring. 2002. Effects of dietary precursors to biogenic amines on the behavioral response from groups of caged worker honey bees (Apis mellifera) to the alarm pheromone component isopentyl acetate. *Physiological Entomology* 24(3): 285-291.

Minamizuka, T., M. Koshizaka, M. Shoji, M. Yamaga, A. Hayashi et al. 2021. Low dose red yeast rice with monacolin K lowers LDL cholesterol and blood pressure in Japanese with mild dyslipidemia: a multicenter, randomized trial. *Asian Pacific Journal of Clinical Nutrition* 30(3): 424-435.

Paludo, C.R., G. Pishchany, A. Andrade-Dominguez, E. A. Silva-Junior, C. Menezes, F.S. Nasccimento, C.R. Currie, R. Kolter, J. Clardy, M.T. Pupo. 2019. Microbial community modulates growth of symbiotic fungus required for stingless bee metamorphosis. *PLoS ONE* 14(7) e0219696.

Parish, J.B., E.S. Scott, K. Hogendoorn. 2020. Nutritional benefit of fungal spores for honey bee workers. *Scientific Reports* 10:15671.

Raymann, K., Z. Shaffer, N.A. Moran. 2017. Antibiotic exposure perturbs the gut microbiota and elevates mortality in honeybees. *PLoS ONE* 15(3): e20011861.

Stamets, P.E., N.L. Naeger, J.D. Evans, J.O. Han, B.K. Hopkins, D. Lopez, H.M. Moershel, R. Nally et al. 2018. Extracts of Polpore Mushroom Mycelia Reduce Viruses in Honey Bees. *Science Reports* 8(1): 13936.

Stevanovic, J., Z. Stanimirovic, P. Simeunovic, N. Lakic, I. Radovic, M. Sokovic, L.J.L.D. Van Griensven. 2018. The effect of *Agaricus brasiliensis* extract supplementation on honey bee colonies. *Agrarian Sciences* 90(1).

NAMEKO References:

Abreu, H., F.F. Simas, F.R. Smiderie, V. Sovrani, J.L. Dallazen et al. 2019. Gelling functional property, anti-inflammatory and antinociceptive bioactivities of B-D-glucan form the edible mushroom Pholiota nameko. *International Journal of Biological Macromolecules* 22: 1128-1135.

Bratt H., P. Rottiers, D. W. Hommes, N. Huyghebaert et al. 2006. A phase 1 trail with transgenic bacteria expressing interleukin-10 in Crohn's disease. *Clinical Gastroenterology and Hepatology* 4(6): 754-759.

Brennan F. M., P. Green, P. Amjadi, H. J. Robertshaw et al. 2008. Interleukin-10 regulates TNF-alpha converting enzyme (TACE/ADAM-17) involving a TIMP-3 dependent and independent mechanism. *European Journal of Immunology* 38(4): 1106-1117.

Chang S., W. Hayes. 1978. *The Biology and Cultivation of Edible Mushrooms.* Academic Press. New York. Pages 475-496.

Cotter,Tradd. 2014. Organic Mushroom Farming and Mycoremediation. Chelsea Green Pub. White River Junction Vermont. https://www.youtube.com/watch?v=H_ZmlscaYx4.

Diyabalange T., V. Mulabagal, G. Mills, D. DeWitt, M. G. Nair. 2009. Liperoxidation and Cyclooxygenase Enzyme Inhibitory Compounds from the Lipophilic Extracts of Some Culinary-Medicinal Higher Basidiomycetes Mushrooms. *International Journal of Medicinal Mushrooms.* 11(4): 375-382.

Ikekawa, Tetsuro. 2005. Cancer Reduction by intake of Mushrooms and Clinical Studies on EEM. *International Journal of Medicinal Mushrooms* 7(3): 347.

Inage, M., H. Takahasi, H. Nakamura, I. Masakane, H. Tomoike. 1996. Hypersensitivity pneumonitis induced by spores of *Pholiota nameko.* *Internal Medicine* 35(4): 301-304.

Li, H., M Zhang, G. Ma. 2010. Hypolipidemic effect of the polysaccharide from *Pholiota nameko. Nutrition* 26(5): 556-562.

Li, H., L. Liu, Y. Tao, P. Zhao, F. Wang et al. 2014. Effects of polysaccharides from Pholiota nameko on maturation of murine bone marrow-derived dendritic cells. *International Journal of Biological Macromolecules* 63: 188-197.

Li, H., P. Zhao, F. Wang, L. Huai, R. Zhu, Y. Xu. 2018. A Polysaccharide from the Culinary-Medicinal Mushroom Pholiota nameko (Agaricomycetes) Inhibits the NF-kB Pathway in Dendritic Cells Through the TLR2 Receptor. *International Journal of Medicinal Mushrooms* 18(11): 977-989.

Lin, H., T.Y. Lin, J.A. Lin, K.C. Cheng, S.P. Santoso, C.H. Chou, C.W. Hsieh. 2021. Effect of *Pholiota nameko* Polysaccharides Inhibiting Methylglyoxal-Induced Glycation Damage In Vitro. *Antioxidants* (Basel) 10(10): 1589.

Lin, H., K.C. Cheng, J.A. Lin, L.P. Hsieh, C.H. Chou et al. 2022. *Pholiota nameko* Polysaccharides Protect against Ultraviolet A-Induced Photoaging by Regulating Matrix Metalloproteinases in Human Dermal Fibroblasts. *Antioxidants* (Basel) 11(4): 739.

McCoy, Peter. 2016 *Radical Mycology: A Treatise On Seeing & Working With Fungi.* Chthaeus Press. Portland Oregon. Page 481.

Qian, L., Y. Zhang, F. Liu. 2016. Purification and characterization of a ~43 kDa antioxidant protein with antitumor activity from *Pholiota nameko. Journal of Science Food and Agriculture.* 96(3): 1044-1052.

Ray, Sarah C., B. Baban, M. A. Tucker, A. J. Seaton, K. C. Chang, E. C. Mannon, J. P. Sun et al. 2018. Oral $NaHCO_3$ Activates a Splenic Anti-Inflammatory Pathway: Evidence That Cholinergic Signals Are Transmitted via Mesothelial Cells. *The Journal of Immunology* 4(14).

Rodriques, D., A. C. Freitas, S. Sousa, M. Amorim et al. 2017. Chemical and structural characterization of *Pholiota nameko* extracts with biological properties. *Food Chemistry* 216: 176-185.

Rogers, Robert. 2011. *The Fungal Pharmacy: The Complete Guide to Medicinal Mushrooms and Lichens of North America.* North Atlantic Books. Berkeley CA.

Sano, M., K. Yoshino, T. Matsuzawa, T. Ikekawa. 2002. Inhibitory Effects of Edible Higher Basidiomycetes Mushroom Extracts on Mouse Type IV Allergy. *International Journal of Medicinal Mushrooms.* Vol 4: 37-41.

Sung, T.J., Y.Y. Wang, K.L. Liu, C.H. Chou, P.S. Lai, C.W. Hseih. 2020. *Pholiota nameko* Polysaccharides Promotes Cell Proliferation and Migration and Reduces ROS Content in H_2O_2- Induced L929 Cells. *Antioxidants* (Basel) 9(1):65.

Takaki, K., N. Yamazaki, S. Mukaigawa, T. Fujiwara et al. 2009. Effect of Pulsed High-Voltage Stimulation on Pholiota Nameko Mushroom Yield. *Acta Physica Polonica A* 115(6):1062-1065.

Zhang, Y., Z. Liu, T. B. Ng, Z. Chen, W. Qiao, F. Liu. 2014. Purification and characterization of a novel antitumor protein with antioxidant and deoxyribonuclease activity from edible mushroom *Pholiota nameko.* *Biochimie* 99: 28-37.

Zhang, J., N. Xu, G. Wang, H. Zhao, L. Lin, M. Jia, L. Jia. 2015. In Vitro and In Vivo Antioxidant Effects of Polysaccharides from Nameko Medicinal Mushroom, *Pholiota nameko* SW-01 (Higher Basidiomycetes). *International Journal of Medicinal Mushrooms* 17(7): 671-680.

Zhang, Y., Y.N. Zhang, W.H. Gao, R. Zhou, F. Liu, T.B. Ng. 2020. A novel antitumor protein from the mushroom Pholiota nameko induces apoptosis of human breast adenocarcinoma MCF-7 cells in vivo and modulates cytokine secretion in mice bearing MCF-7 xenografts. *International Journal of Biological Macromolecules* 164: 3171-3178.

Zhang, S., B. Liu, G.Y. Yan, H. Wu, Y.C. Han, H.X. Cui. 2022. Chemical properties and anti-fatigue effect of polysaccharide from Pholiota nameko. *Journal of Food Biochemistry* 46(1):e14015.

Zheng L., G. Zhai, J. Zhang, L. Wang, Z. Ma, M. Jia, L. Jia. 2014. Antihyperlipidemic and hepatoprotective activities of mycelia zinc polysaccharides from *Pholiota nameko* SW-02. *International Journal of Biological Macromolecules* 70: 523-529.

Zheng, L., M. Liu, G. Y. Zhai, Z. Ma, L. Q. Wang, L. Jia. 2015. Antioxidant and anti-ageing activities of mycelia zinc polysaccharide from *Pholiota nameko* SW-O3. *Journal of the Science of Food and Agriculture* 95(15): 3117-3126.

PARASOL References:

Arora, S., S. Goyal, J. Balani, S. Tandon. 2013. Enhanced antiproliferative effects of aqueous extracts of some medicinal mushrooms on colon cancer cells. *International Journal of Medicinal Mushrooms* 15(3): 301-314.

Arora, S., C. Tandon, S. Tandon. 2014. Evaluation of the cytotoxic effects of CAM therapies: an in vitro study in normal kidney cell lines. *Scientific World Journal* 2014:452892.

Chen, H.P., Z.Z. Zhao, Z.H. Li, Y. Huang, S.B. Zhang, Y. Tang et al. 2018. Anti-Prolferative and Anti-Inflammatory Lanostane Triterpenoids from the Polish Edible Mushroom Macrolepiota procera. *Journal of Agriculture & Food Chemistry* 66(12): 3146-3154.

Georgiev, Y.N., O. Vasicek, B. Dzhambazov, T.G. Batsalova, P.N. Denev et al. 2022. Structural Features and Immunomodulatory Effects of Water-Extractable Polysaccharides from *Macrolepiota procera* (Scop.) Singer. *Journal of Fungi* (Basel) 8(8):848.

Kosanic, M., B. Rankovic, A. Rancic, T. Stanojkovic. 2016. Evaluation of metal concentration and antioxidant, antimicrobial, and anticancer potential of two edible mushrooms Lactarius deliciosus and Macrolepiota procera. *Journal of Food and Drug Analysis* 24(3): 477-484.

Lukanc, T., J. Brzin, J. Kos, J. Sabotic. 2017. Trypsin-specific Inhibitors from the Macrolepiota procera, Armillaria mellea and Amanita phalloides wild mushrooms. *Acta Biochim Pol* 64(1): 21-24.

Mujic, I., Z. Zekovic, S. Vidovic, M. Radojkovic, J. Zivkovic, D. Godevac. 2011. Fatty acid profiles of four wild mushrooms and their potential benefits for hypertension treatment. *Journal of Medicinal Food* 14(11): 1330-1337.

Secme, M., O. Kaygusuz, C. Eroglu, Y. Dodurga, O.F. Colak, P. Atmaca. 2018. Potential Anticancer Activity of the Parasol Mushroom, Macrolepiota procera (Agaricomycetes), against the A549 Human Lung Cancer Cell Line. *International Journal of Medicinal Mushrooms* 20(11): 1075-1086.

Urga, S.Å, M.P. Nanut, J. Kos, J. Sabotic. 2017. Fungal lectin MpL enables entry of protein drugs into cancer cells and their subcellular targeting. *Oncotarget* 8(16): 26896-26910.

Wang, W.S., X.X. Li, Y.H. Zhang, J.J. Zhang, L. Jia. 2022. Mycelium polysaccharides of *Macrolepiota procera* alleviate reproductive impairments induced by nonylphenol. *Food and Function* 13(10):5794-5806.

Zara, R., A. Rasul, T. Sultana, F. Jabeen, Z. Selamoglu. 2022. Identification of *Macrolepiota procera* extract as a novel G6PD inhibitor for the treatment of lung cancer. *Saudi Journal of Biological Sciences* 29(5): 3372-3379.

PHELLINUS IGNIARIUS References:

Doğan, H. H., S. Haragöz, R. Duman. 2018. In Vitro Evaluation of the Antiviral Activity of Some Mushrooms from Turkey. *International Journal of Medicinal Mushrooms* 20(3): 201-212.

Dong Y., Y. He, Z.M. Yu, Y. Zhang, N. Wang, D. Shou, C.Y. Li. 2016. Metabolic investigation of rat serum following oral administration of the willow bracket medicinal mushroom, *Phellinus Igniarius* (Agaricomycetes), by UPLC-HDMS. *International Journal of Medicinal Mushrooms* 18(8): 699-711.

Hsiao P.C., Y. H. Hsieh, J. M. Chow, S. F. Yang, M. Hsiao, K. T. Hua, C.H. Lin, H. Y. Chen, M. H. Chien. 2013. Hispolon induces apoptosis through JNK1/2-mediated activation of a caspase-8, -9, and -3-dependent pathway in acute myeloid leukemia (AML) cells and inhibits AML xenograft tumor growth *in vivo*. *Journal of Agricultural and Food Chemistry* 61(42): 10063-10073.

Jiang Z., M. Jin, W. Zhou, R. Li et al. 2018. Anti-inflammatory Activity of Chemical Constituents Isolated from the Willow Bracket Medicinal Mushroom *Phellinus igniarius* (Agaricomycetes). *International Journal of Medicinal Mushrooms* 20(2): 119-128.

Kim J. H., B. Y. Choi, J. K. Kim, I. Y. Kim, B. E. Lee, et al. 2015. A water-ethanol extract from the willow bracket mushroom, *Phellinus igniarius*, reduces transient cerebral ischemia-induced neuronal death. *International Journal of Medicinal Mushrooms* 17(9): 879-89.

Kim J. Y., D. W. Kim, B. S. Hwang, E. E. Woo, Y. J. Lee, K. W. Jeong, I. K. Lee, B. S. Yun. 2016. Neuraminidase inhibitors from the fruiting body of *Phellinus igniarius*. *Mycobiology* 44(2):117-20.

Lee I. K., B. S. Yun. 2011. Styrylpyrone-class compounds from medicinal fungi *Phellinus* and *Inonotus* spp., and their medicinal importance. *The Journal of Antibiotics* (Tokyo) 64(5): 349-359.

Lee S., J. I. Kim, J. Heo, I. Lee, S. Park, M. W. Hwang, et al. 2013. The anti-influenza virus effect of *Phellinus igniarius* extract. *Journal of Microbiology* 51(5): 676-681.

Lee S. W., J. G. Song, B. S. Hwang, D. W. Kim, Y. J. Lee, et al. 2014. Lipoxygenase inhibitory activity of Korean indigenous mushroom extracts and isolation of an active compound from *Phellinus baumii*. *Mycobiology* 42(2): 185-88.

Lee Y. S., Y. H. Kang, J. Y. Jung, I. J. Kang, S. N. Han, J. S. Chung, H. K. Shin, S. S. Lim. 2008. Inhibitory constituents of aldose reductase in the fruiting body of *Phellinus linteus*. *Biology and Pharmaceutical Bulletin* 31(4): 765-8.

Li L., G. Wu, B. Y. Choi, et al. 2014. A mushroom extract Piwep from *Phellinus igniarius* ameliorates experimental autoimmune encephalomyelitis by inhibiting immune cell infiltration in the spinal cord. *BioMed Research International* 2014;2014: 218274.

Li S. C., X. M. Yang, H. L. Ma, J. K. Yan, D. Z. Guo. 2015. Purification, characterization and antitumor activity of polysaccharides extracted from *Phellinus igniarius* mycelia. *Carbohydrate Polymers* 133: 24-30.

Pleninger, D. B. 2009. Iqmik: Troubled Child of *Phellinus* and *Nicotiana*. *Fungi: Special Issue Ethnomycology* 2(2):5-8.

Rogers R. 2016. *Mushroom Essences: Vibrational Healing from the Kingdom Fungi*. North Atlantic Books, Berkeley CA. page 69.

Rouhana-Toubi A., S. P. Wasser, F. Fares. 2009. Ethyl acetate extracts of submerged cultured mycelium of high basidiomycetes mushroom inhibit human ovarian cancer cell growth. *International Journal of Medicinal Mushrooms* 11(1): 29-37.

Smith A., Javed S., Barad A. et al. 2017. Growth-Inhibitory and Immunomodulatory Activities of Wild Mushrooms from North-Central British Columbia (Canada). *International Journal of Medicinal Mushrooms* 19(6): 485-497.

Song T. Y., H. C. Lin, N. C. Yang, M. L. Hu. 2008. Antiproliferative and antimetastatic effects of the ethanolic extract of *Phellinus igniarius* (Linnearus:Fries) Quelet. *Journal of Ethnopharmacology* 112: 50-56.

Suabjakyong P., K. Nishimura, T. Toida, L. J. Van Griensven. 2015a. Structural characterization and immunomodulatory effects of polysaccharides from *Phellinus linteus* and *Phellinus igniarius* on the IL-6/IL-10 cytokine balance of the mouse macrophage cell lines (RAW264.7). *Food and Function* 6(8): 2834-44.

Suabjakyong P., R. Saiki, L. J. Van Griensven, K. Higashi, K. Nishimura, K. Igarashi, T. Toida. 2015b. Polyphenol extract from *Phellinus igniarius* protects against acrolein toxicity *in vitro* and provides protection in a mouse stroke model. *PLoS One* 10(3): e0122733.

Wang F. F., F. Liu, C. Shi, W. Ma, K. J. Wang, N. Li. 2017. Cytotoxic Activities of Fractions of the Willow Bracket Medicinal Mushroom, Phellinus igniarius (Agaricomycetes), and the Induction of Cell Cycle Arrest and Apoptosis in MGC-803 Cells. *International Journal of Medicinal Mushrooms* 19(6): 561-570.

Wang G. J., T. H. Tsai, T. T. Chang, C. J. Chou, L. C. Lin. 2009. Lanostanes from *Phellinus igniarius* and their iNOS inhibitory activities. *Planta Medica* 75(15): 1602-7.

Wu Q., Y. Kang, H. Zhang, H. Wang, Y. Liu, J. Wang. 2014. The anticancer effects of hispolon on lung cancer cells. *Biochemical and Biophysical Research Communications* 453(3): 385-91.

Yin R. H., Z.Z. Zhao, X. Ji, Z. J. Dong, Z. H. Li, T. Feng, J. K. Liu. 2015. Steroids and sesquiterpenes from cultures of the fungus *Phellinus igniarius*. *Natural Products and Bioprospecting* 5(1): 17-22.

Zeng H., W. F. Wang, M. H. Ma, G. H. Xu, M. Ying-Jie, J. F. Sund. 2016. Comparison of the chemical composition and bioactive components of fruiting bodies and submerged cultured mycelia of the willow bracket medicinal mushroom, *Phellinus igniarius* (Agaricomycetes). *International Journal of Medicinal Mushrooms* 18(9): 833-40.

Zheng S., S. Deng, Y. Huang, M. Huang, P. Zhao et al. 2017. Anti-diabetic activity of a polyphenol-rich extract from Phellinus igniarius in KK-Ay mice with spontaneous type 2 diabetes mellitus. *Food & Function* 22 doi: 10.1039/c7fo01460k.

Zhou C., S. S. Jiang, C. Y. Wang, R. Li, H. L. Che. 2014. Different immunology mechanisms of *Phellinus igniarius* in inhibiting growth of liver cancer and melanoma cells. *Asian Pacific Journal of Cancer Prevention* 15(8): 3659-65.

Zhou L. W., J. Vlasak, W. M. Qin, Y. C. Dai. 2016. Global diversity and phylogeny of the *Phellinus igniarius* complex with the description of five new species. *Mycologia* 108(1): 192-204.

Zhu H., W. Liu, S. X. Wang, B. Z. Tian, S. S. Zhang. 2012. Evaluation of anti-quorum sensing activity of fermentation metabolites from different strains of a medicinal mushroom, *Phellinus igniarius. Chemotherapy* 58(3): 195-9.

PIOPINNO References:

Chen, Y.J., S. Jiang, Y.X. Jin, Y.L. Yin, G.J. Yu, X.Q. Lan et al. 2012. Purification and characterization of an antitumor protein with deoxyribonuclease activity from edible mushroom Agrocybe aegerita. *Molecular Nutrition and Food Research* 56(11): 1729-1738.

Citores, L., S. Ragucci, J.M. Ferreras, A. Di Marco, R. Iglesias. 2019. Ageritin, a Ribotoxin from Poplar Mushroom (Agrocybe aegerita) with Defensive and Antiproliferative Activities. *ACS Chemical Biology* 14(6): 1319-1327.

Ji, Y., M.F. Zheng, S.G. Ye, X.B. Wu, J.Y. Chen. 2013. Agrocybe aegerita polysaccharide combined with chemotherapy improves tumor necrosis factor-alpha and interferon-gamma levels in rat esophageal carcinoma. *Diseases of the Esophagus* 26(8): 859-863.

Jing, H.J., Q. Zhang, M. Liu, J.J. Zhang, C. Zhang, S.S. Li et al. 2018. Polysaccharides with Antioxidative and Antiaging Activities from Enzymatic-Extractable Mycelium by *Agrocybe aegerita* (Brig.) Sing. *Evidence Based Complementary and Alternative Medicine* 2018:1584647.

Lampitella, E.A., N. Landi, R. Oliva, R. Gaglione, A. Bosso, F. De Lise, S. Ragucci et al. 2021. Toxicity and membrane perturbation properties of the ribotoxin-like protein Ageritin. *Journal of Biochemistry* 170(4): 473-482.

Landi, N., S. Pacifico, S. Ragucci, R. Iglesias, S. Piccolella, A. Amica, A.M. Di Giuseppe, A. Di Maro. 2017. Purification, characterization and cytotoxicity assessment of Ageritin: The first ribotoxin from the basidiomycete mushroom Agrocybe aegerita. *Biochimica & Biophysica Acta Gen Subj* 1861(5pt A): 1113-1121.

Li, G.L., X.L. Liu, S.Z. Cong, Y.P. Deng, X.Q. Zheng. 2021. A novel serine protease with anticoagulant and fibrinolytic activities from the fruiting bodies of mushroom Agrocybe aegerita. *International Journal of Biological Macromolecules* 168: 631-639.

Li, Y., Y. Li, J. Xia, Q. Yang, Y.J. Chen, H. Sun. 2021. 3'Sulfo-TF Antigen Determined by CAL_3ST_2/ST_3GAL_1 Is Essential for Antitumor Activity of Fungal Galectin AAL/AAGL. *ACS Omega* 6(27): 17379-17390.

Liang, Y., H.H. Liu, Y.J. Chen, H. Sun. 2014. Antitumor activity of the protein and small molecule component fractions from Agrocybe aegerita through enhancement of cytokine production. *Journal of Medicinal Food* 17(4): 439-446.

Liu, W., G.J. Yu, W.H. Yu, X.D. Ye, Y.X. Jin, A. Shrestha, Q. Yang, H. Sun. 2017. Autophagy Inhibits Apoptosis Induced by agrocybe aegerita lectin in Hepatocellular Carcinoma. *Anti-cancer Agents in Medicinal Chemistry* 17(20: 221-229.

Ma, L.B., B.Y. Xu, M. Huang, L.H. Sun, Q. Yang, Y.J. Chen, Y.L. Yin, Q.G. He, H. Sun. 2017. Adjuvant effects mediated by the carbohydrate recognition domain of Agrocybe aegerita lection interacting with avian influenza H9N2 viral surface glycosylated proteins. *Journal of Zhejiang University Science B* 18(8): 653-661.

Ma, L.B., B.Y. Xu, M. Huang, Q.G. He. 2018. Effects of recombinant Agrocybe aegerita lectin as an immunoadjuvant on immune responses. *Immunopharmacology & Immunotoxicology* 40(1): 6-12.

Petrovic, J., J. Glamoclija, D. Stojkovic, M. Nikolic, A. Ciric et al. 2014. Bioactive composition, antimicrobial activities and the influence of Agrocybe aegerita (Brig.) Sing on certain quorum-sensing-regulated functions and biofilm formation by Pseudomonas aeruginosa. *Food & Function* 5(12): 3296-3303.

Surup, F., F. Hennicke, N. Sella, M. Stroot, S. Bernecker, S. Pfutze, M. Stadler, M. Ruhl. 2019. New terpenoids from the fermentation broth of the edible mushroom *Cyclocybe aegerita*. *Beilstein Journal of Organic Chemistry* 15: 1000-1007.

Wu, S.G., H.N. Sun, J.H. Sun, D.K. Liao. 2010. Technical optimization for extracting hypotensive active peptides from Agrocybe aegerita. *Nan Fang Yi Ke Da Xue Xue Bao* (*Journal of Southern Medical University*) 30(6): 1264-1267.

Ye, X.D., X.Q. Wang, W.H. Yu, Q. Yang, Y. Li, Y.X. Jin et al. 2021. Synergistic effects of AAGL and anti-PD-1 on hepatocellular carcinoma through lymphocyte recruitment to the liver. *Cancer Biology and Medicine* 18(4): 1092-1108.

Yong, T.Q., S.D. Chen, Y.Z. Xie, O. Shuai, X.M. Li, D.L. Chen et al. 2018. Hypouricemic Effects of Extracts from *Agrocybe aegerita* on Hyperuricemia Mice and Virtual Prediction of Bioactives by Molecular Docking. *Frontiers in Pharmacology* 9:498 doi: 10.3389/fphar.2018.00498.

Zhao, C.G., H. Sun, X. Tong, Y.P. Qi. 2003. An antitumour lectin from the edible mushroom Agrocybe aegerita. *Biochemical Journal* 374(pt2): 321-327.

PUFFBALL References:

Burk, W.R. 1983. Puffball Usages Among North American Indians. *Journal of Ethnobiology* 3(1): 55-62.

Dulger, B. 2005. Antimicrobial activity of ten Lycoperdaceae. *Fitoterapia* 76(3): 352-354.

Eruglu, C., M. Secme, P. Atmaca, O. Kaygusuz, K. Gezer, G. Bagci, Y. Dodurga. 2016. Extract of Calvatia gigantea inhibits proliferation of A549 human lung cancer cells. *Cytotechnology* 68(5): 2075-2081.

Jameel, G. H., A.I.A. Al-Ezzy, I.H. Mohammed. 2018. Immunomodulatory, Apoptosis Induction and Antitumor Activities of Aqueous and Methanolic Extract of Calvatia Craniiformis in Mice Transfected with Murine Hepatocellular Carcinoma Cells. *Open Access Macedonian Journal of Medical Sciences* 6(7): 1206-1214.

Kivrak, I., S. Kivrak, M. Harmandar. 2016. Bioactive Compounds, Chemical Composition, and Medicinal Value of the Giant Puffball, Calvatia gigantea (Higher Basidomycetes), from Turkey. *International Journal of Medicinal Mushrooms* 18(2): 97-107.

Lam, Y.W., T.B. Ng, H.X. Wang. 2001. Antiproliferative and antimitogenic activities in a peptide from puffball mushroom Calvatia caelata. *Biochemical and Biophysical Research Communications* 289(3): 744-749.

Lee, S., J.Y. Park, D.H. Lee, S. Seok, Y.J. Kwon. T.S. Jang, K.S. Kang, K.H. Kim. 2017. Chemical constituents from the rare mushroom Calvatia nipponica inhibit the promotion of angiogenesis in HUVECs. *Bioorganic and Medicinal Chemistry Letters* 27(17): 4122-4127.

Lee, S., D.H. Lee, R. Ryoo, J.C. Kim, H.B. Park, K.S. Kang, K.H. Kim. 2020. Calvatianone, a Sterol Possessing a 6/5/6/5-Fused Ring System with a Contracted Tetrahydrofuran B-Ring, from the Fruiting Bodies of *Calvatia nipponica. Journal of Natural Products* 83(9): 2737-2742.

Lee, S., M.J. Kim, B.S. Lee, R. Ryoo, H.K. Kim, K.H. Kim. 2020a. Cumulative Effects of Constituents from the mushroom *Calvatia nipponica* on the contractility of Penile Corpus Cavernosum Smooth Muscle. *Mycobiology* 48(2): 153-156.

Lucas, E.H. et al. 1957. Tumor inhibitors in *Boletus edulis* and other Holobasidiomycetes. *Antibiotics & Chemotherapy* 7(1): 1-4.

Ng, T.B., Y.W. Lam, H.X. Wang. 2003. Calcaelin, a new protein with translation-inhibiting, anti-proliferative and antimitogenic activities from the mosaic puffball mushroom Calvatia caelata. *Planta Medica* 69(3): 212-217.

Ogbole, O.O., A. O. Nikumah, A. U. Linus, M.O. Falade. 2019. Molecular identification, *in vivo* and *in vitro* activities of *Calvatia gigantea* (macro-fungus) as an antidiabetic agent. *Mycology* 10(3): 166-173.

Rogers, R. 2016. *Mushroom Essences: Vibrational Healing from the Kingdom Fungi.* North Atlantic Books, Berkeley CA.

Tsay, J.G., K.T. Chung, C.H. Yeh, W.L. Chen, C.H. Chen, M.H-C. Lin, F.J. Lu, J.F. Chiou, C.H. Chen. 2009. Calvatia lilacina protein-extract induces apoptosis through glutathione depletion in human colorectal carcinoma cells. *Journal of Agricultural and Food Chemistry* 57(4): 1579-1588.

Whitmont, E.C. 1969. *The Symbolic Quest: Basic Concepts of Analytical Psychology.* Princeton University Press. Princeton, NJ.

Wu, J.Y., C.H. Chen, W.H. Chang, K.T. Chung, Y.W. Liu, F.J. Lu, C.H. Chen. 2011. Anti-Cancer Effects of Protein Extracts from Calvatia lilacina, Pleurotus ostreatus and Volvariella volvacea. *Evidence Based Complementary and Alternative Medicine* 2011: 982368.

Zeng, Q.H., R. Singh, Y. Ye, S. Cheng, C. Fan, Q.M. Zeng. 2021. Calvatia Lilacina Extracts Exert Anti-Breast-Cancer Bioactivity through the Apoptosis Induction Dependent on Mitochondrial Reactive Oxygen Species and Caspase Activation. *Nutrition and Cancer* doi: 10.1080/01635581.2021.1936576.

RAMARIA References:

Alves, M.J., I.C.F.R. Ferreira, A. Martins, M. Pintado. 2012. Antimicrobial activity of wild mushroom extracts against clinical isolates resistant to different antibiotics. *Journal of Applied Microbiology* 113(2): 466-475.

Aprotosoale, A.C., D.E. Zavastin, C.T. Mihai, G. Voichita, D. Gherghel, M. Silion, A. Trifan, A. Miron. 2017. Antioxidant and antigenotoxic potential of Ramaria largentii Marr & D.E. Stuntz, a wild edible mushroom collected from Northeast Romania. *Food and Chemical Toxicology* 108 (pt B); 429-437.

Centko, R.M., S. Ramón-Garcia, T. Taylor, B.O. Patrick, C.J. Thompson, V.P. Miao, R.J. Andersen. 2012. Ramariolides A-D, antimycobacterial butenolides isolated from the mushroom Ramaria cystidiophora. *Journal of Natural Products* 75(12): 2178-2182.

Chung, K.S. 1979. The effects of mushroom components on the proliferation of HeLa cell line, in vitro. *Archives of Pharmacal Research* 2(1): 25-34.

Deo, G.S., J. Khatra, S. Buttar, W.M. Li, L.E. Tackaberry, H.B. Massicotte, K.N. Egger, K. Reimer, C.H. Lee. 2019. Antiproliferative, immunostimulatory, and Anit-Inflammatory Activities of Extracts Derived from Mushrooms Collected in Haida Gwaii, British Columbia (Canada). *International Journal of Medicinal Mushrooms* 21(7): 629-643.

Dong, M.M., Y.L. Hou, X. Ding. 2020. Structure identification, antitumor activity and mechanisms of a novel polysaccharide from *Ramaria flaccida* (Fr.) Quél. *Oncology Letters* 20(3): 2169-2182.

Kim, K.C., I.S. Lee, I.D. Yoo, B.J. Ha. 2015. Sesquiterpenes from the fruiting bodies of Ramaria formosa and their human neutrophil elastase inhibitory activity. *Chemical and Pharmaceutical Bulletin* 63(7): 554-557.

Li, H. 2017. Extraction, purification, characterization and antioxidant activities of polysaccharides from *Ramaria botrytis* (Pers.) Ricken. *Chemistry Central Journal* doi: 10.1186/s13065-017-0252-x.

Liu, K., J.L. Wang, L. Zhao, Q. Wang. 2013. Anticancer, antioxidant and antibiotic activities of mushroom Ramaria flava. *Food and Chemical Toxicology* 58: 375-380.

Ozen, T., C. Darcan, O. Aktop, I. Turkekul. 2011. Screening of antioxidant, antimicrobial activities and chemical contents of edible mushrooms wildly grown in the black sea region of Turkey. *Combinatorial Chemistry and High Throughput Screening* 14(2): 72-84.

Sadi, G., A. Kaya, H.A. Yalcin, B. Emsen, A. Kocabas, D.I. Kartal, A. Altay. 2016. Wild Edible Mushrooms from Turkey as Possible Anticancer Agents on HepG2 Cells Together with Their Antioxidant and Antimicrobial Properties. *International Journal of Medicinal Mushrooms* 18(1): 83-95.

Sakemi, Y., H. Nakanishi, Y. Araki, K. Shindo. 2022. Antioxidant Activites of Pistillarin n the Clustered Coral Mushroom, *Ramaria Botrytis* (Agaricomycetes) and Discovery of Pisttillarin B. *International Journal of Medicinal Mushrooms* 24(7): 67-75.

Scheid, H.V., E.S.V. Sallis, F. Riet-Correa, A.L. Schild. 2022. Ramaria flavo-brunnescens mushroom poisoning in South America: A comprehensive review. *Toxicon* 205: 91-98.

Zhang, R., G.T. Tian, Y.C. Zhao, L.Y. Zhao, H.X. Wang, Z.Y. Gong, T.B. Ng. 2015. A novel ribonuclease with HIV-1 reverse transcriptase inhibitory activity purified from the fungus Ramaria formosa. *Journal of Basic Microbiology* 55(2): 269-75.

Zhou, R., Y.J. Han, M.H. Zhang, K.R. Zhang, T.B. Ng, F. Liu. 2017. Purification and characterization of a novel ubiquitin-like antitumour protein with hemagglutinating and deoxyribonuclease activities from the edible mushroom Ramaria botrytis. *AMB Express* 7(1): 47.

Zhou, R., Y.T. Wang, C. Li, S.T. Jia, Y.N. Shi, Y.F. Tang, Y.Q. Li. 2022. A preliminary study on preparation, characterization, and prebiotic activity of a polysaccharide from the edible mushroom Ramaria flava. *Journal of Food Biochemistry* 46(9):e14371.

RED-BELTED CONK References:

Angelini, P., B. Tirillini, G. Bistocchi, A. Arcangeli, A. Rubini, et al. 2018. Overview of the biological activities of a methanol extract from wild Red Belt Conk, *Fomitopsis pinicola* (Agaricomycetes), fruiting bodies from central Italy. *International Journal of Medicinal Mushrooms* 20(11): 1047–1063.

Bishop, K.S. 2020. Characterization of extracts and anti-cancer activities of *Fomitopsis pinicola*. *Nutrients* 12(3): 609.

Cheng, Jing-J, Cha-Yui Lin, Huu-Sheng Lui, Hsuan-Pei Chen, and Mei-Kuang Lu. Properties and biological functions of polysaccharides and ethanolic extracts isolated from medicinal fungus, *Fomitopsis pinicola. Process Biochemistry* 43(8): 829–834.

Dresch, P., M.N. D'Aguanno, K. Rosam, U. Grienke, J.M. Rollinger, and U. Peintner. 2015. Fungal strain matters: colony growth and bioactivity of the European medicinal polypores *Fomes fomentarius, Fomitopsis pinicola* and *Piptoporus betulinus. AMB Express* 5: 4. doi: 10.1186/s13568-014-0093-0.

Du, P., T.X. Cao, L.L. Zhang, Y.Q. Huang, and J.Z. Chen. 2020. Cultivation and medicinal value of the Red Belt Conk mushroom *Fomitopsis pinicola* (Agaricomycetes). *International Journal of Medicinal Mushrooms* 22(10): 1021–1031.

Fäldt, J., M. Jonsell, G. Norlander, and A.K. Borg-Karlson. 1999. Volatiles of bracket fungi *Fomitopsis pinicola* and *Fomes fomentarius* and their functions as insect attractants. *Journal of Chemical Ecology* 25(3): 567–590.

Haight, J.E., K.K. Nakasone, G.A. Laursen, S. A. Redhead, D. Lee Taylor, and J.A. Glaeser. 2019. *Fomitopsis mounceae* and *F. schrenkii*—two new species from North America in the *F. pinicola* complex. *Mycologia* 111(2): 339–357. doi: 10.1080/00275514.2018.1564449.

Hobbs, C. 1995. *Medicinal Mushrooms: An Exploration of Tradition, Healing, & Culture.* Second Edition. Botanica Press. Santa Cruz, CA.

Johnston, A. 1987. *Plants and the Blackfoot.* Occasional Paper No. 15, Lethbridge Historical Society, Lethbridge Alberta.

Li, X., T. Bau, and H.Y. Bao. 2018. FPOA induces apoptosis in HeLa human cervical cancer cells through a caspase-mediated pathway. *Oncology Letters* 15(6): 8357–8362.

Macáková, K., L. Opletal, M. Polásek, and V. Samková. 2010. Free-radical scavenging activity of some European Polyporales. *Natural Product Communications* 5(6): 923–926.

Peng, X.R., H.G. Su, J.H. Liu, Y.J. Huang, et al. 2019. C30 and C32 triterpenoids and triterpene sugar esters with cytotoxic activities from edible mushroom *Fomitopsis pinicola* (Sw. ex Fr.) Krast. *Journal of Agricultural and Food Chemistry* 67(37): 10330–10341.

Ren, G., X.Y. Liu, H.K. Zhu, S.Z. Yang and C.X. Fu. 2006. Evaluation of cytotoxic activities of some medicinal polypore fungi from China. *Fitoterapia* 77(5): 408–410.

Rogers, R. 2016. *Mushroom Essences: Vibrational Healing from the Kingdom Fungi.* North Atlantic Books. Berkeley, CA.

Rosecke, J., M. Pietsch, and W.A. Konig. 2000. Volatile constituents of wood-rotting basidiomycetes. *Phytochemistry* 54(8): 747–750.

Lee, S.I, J.-S. Kim, S.-H. Oh, K.-Y. Park, H.-G. Lee and S.-D. Kim. 2008. Anti-hyperlipidemic effect of *Fomitopsis pinicola* extracts in streptozotocin-induced diabetic rats. *Journal of Medicinal Food* 11(3): 518–524.

Shibata, S, Y. Nichikawa, F.M. Cheng, F. Fukuoka, and M. Nakanishi. 1968. Antitumor studies on some extracts of basidiomycetes. *Gann: Japanese Journal of Cancer Research* 59(2): 159–161.

Suay, L., F. Arenal, F.J. Asensio, et al. 2000. Screening of basidiomycetes for antimicrobial activities. *Antoine van Leeuwenhoek* 78(2): 129–140.

Tu, J., J. Zhao, G.H. Liu, C.Y. Tang, Y.H. Han, et al. 2020. Solid state fermentation by *Fomitopsis pinicola* improves physicochemical and functional properties of wheat bran and the brain-containing products. *Food Chemistry* 328: 127046.

Cha, W.-S., J.-L. Ding, H.-J. Shin, et al. 2009. Effects of *Fomitopsis pinicola* extract on blood glucose and lipid metabolism in diabetic rats. *Korean Journal of Chemical Engineering* 26(6): 1696–1699.

Wu, H.T., F. Lu, Y.C. Su, et al. 2014. In vivo and in vitro anti-tumor effects of fungal extracts. *Molecules* 19(2): 2546–2556.

Vermeulen, F. 2007. *Fungi: Kingdom Fungi Spectrum Materia Medica Volume 2.* Emrys Publishers, Haarlem, The Netherlands; 155 pp.

Yoshikawa, K., M. Inoue, Y. Matsumoto, C. Sakabibara, H. Miyataka, H. Matsumoto, and S. Arihara. 2005. Lanostane triterpenoids and triterpene glycosides from the fruit body of *Fomitopsis pinicola* and their inhibitory activity against COX-1 and COX-2. *Journal of Natural Products* 68(1): 69–73.

Zahid, M.T., M. Idrees, I. Abdullah, W. Ying, A.H. Zaki, and H.Y. Bao. 2020. Antidiabetic properties of the Red Belt Conk medicinal mushroom *Fomitopsis pinicola* (Agaricomycetes) extracts on streptozotocin-induced diabetic rats. *International Journal of Medicinal Mushrooms* 22(8): 731–741.

Zhang, J.J., B.S. Chen, J. Liang, J.J. Han, L.W. Zhou, et al. 2020. Lanostane triterpenoids with PTP1B inhibitory and glucose-uptake stimulatory activities from mushroom *Fomitopsis pinicola* collected in North America. *Journal of Agricultural & Food Chemistry* 68(37): 10036–10049.

RED POLYPORE References:

Chen, X.H., M.X. Li, D. Li, T. Luo, Y.Z. Xie, L. Gao, Y.F. Zhang et al. 2020. Ethanol extract of *Pycnoporus sanguineus* relieves the dextran sulfate sodium-induced experimental colitis by suppressing helper T cell-mediated inflammation via apoptosis induction. *Biomedicine and Pharmacotherapy*127: 110212.

Chou, J.M., J. Chae, S.R. Jeong, M.J. Moon, D.Y. Shin, J.H. Lee. 2020. Immune activation of Bio-Geranium in a randomized, double-blind, placebo-controlled clinical trial with 130 human subjects: Therapeutic opportunities from new insights. *PLoS One* 15(10): e0240358.

Doskocil, I., J. Havlik, R. Verlotta, J. Tauchen, L. Vesela, K. Macakova, L. Opletal, L. Kokoska, V. Rada. 2016. In vitro immunomodulatory activity, cytotoxicity and chemistry of some central European polypores. *Pharmaceutical Biology* 54(11): 2369-2376.

Eggert, C. 1997. Laccase-catalyzed formation of cinnabarinic acid is responsible for antibacterial activity of *Pycnoporus cinnabarinus*. *Microbiological Research 152(3): 315-318.*

Gao, N., C.X. Liu, Q.M. Xu, J.S. Cheng, Y.J. Yuan. 2018. Simultaneous removal of ciprofloxacin, norfloxacin, sulfamethoxazole by co-producing oxidative enzymes system of *Phanerochaete chrysosporium* and *Pycnoporus sanguineus*. *Chemosphere* 195: 146-155.

Garcia-Morales, R., M. Rodriguez-Delgado, K. Gomez-Mariscal, C. Orona-Navar, C. Hernandez-Luna, E. Torres, R. Parra et al. 2015. Biotransformation of Endocrine-Disrupting Compounds in Groundwater: Bisphenol A, Nonylphenol, Ethynylestradiol and Triclosan by a Laccase Cocktail from *Pycnoporus sanguineus* CS43. *Water Air Soil Pollution* 226(8):251.

Goodman, S. 1988. Therapeutic effects of organic germanium. *Medical Hypotheses* 26(3): 207-215.

Jaszek, M., M. Osinska-Jaroszuk, J. Sulej, A. Matuszewska, D. Stefaniuk, K. Maciag, J. Polak, L. Matuszewski, K. Grzywnowicz. 2015. Stimulation of the Antioxidative and Antimicrobial Potential of the Blood Red Bracket Mushroom *Pycnoporus sanguineus* (Higher Basidiomycetes). *International Journal of Medicinal Mushrooms* 17(8): 701-712.

Jouda, J.B., E.M. Njoya, C. D. Mbazoa, Z.Y. Zhou. A.M. Lannang, J. Wandji, Y. Shiono, F. Wang. 2018. Lambertellin from *Pycnoporus sanguineus* MUCL 51321 and its anti-inflammatory effect via modulation of MAPK and NF-$_k$B signaling pathways. *Bioorganic Chemistry* 80: 216-222.

Li, M.X., T. Luo, Y. Huang, J.Y. Su, D. Li, X.H. Chen, Y.F. Zhang, L.H. Huang, S.X. Li, C.W. Jiao, W.Z. Li, Y.Z Xie, W.D. Li. 2020. Polysaccharide from *Pycnoporus sanguineus* ameliorates dextran sulfate sodium-induced colitis via helper T cells repertoire modulation and autophagy suppression. *Phytotherapy Research* 34(10): 2649-2664.

Piet, M., A. Zajac, R. Paduch, M. Jaszek, M. Frant, D. Stefaniuk, A. Matuszewska, K. Grzywnowicz. 2021. Chemopreventative activity of bioactive fungal fractions isolated from milk-supplemented cultures of *Cerrena unicolor* and *Pycnoporus sanguineus* on colon cancer cells. *3 Biotech* 11(1):5.

Reddeman, R.A., R. Glávits, J.R. Endres, T.S. Murbach, G. Hirka, A. Vértesi, E. Béres, I.P. Szakonyiné. 2020. A Toxicological Evaluation of Germanium Sesquioxide (Organic Germanium). *Journal of Toxicology* 2020: 6275625.

Ren, G., X.Y. Liu, H.K. Zhu, S.Z. Yang, C.X. Fu. 2006. Evaluation of cytotoxic activities of some medicinal polypore fungi from China. *Fitoterapia* 77(5): 408.410.

Rogers, R. 2011. *The Fungal Pharmacy: The Complete Guide to Medicinal Mushrooms and Lichens of North America*. North Atlantic Books Berkeley, CA.

Smania, A. et al. 2003. Toxicity and antiviral activity of cinnabarin obtained from *Pycnoporus sanguineus* (Fr.) Murr. *Phytotherapy Research* 17(9): 1069-1072.

Wang, J.F., H.M. Li, D.D. Yang. 2015. Effects of Germanium Concentrations on Germanium Accumulation and Biotransformation of Polysaccarified Germanium in Cordyceps militaris. *Journal of Chinese Medicinal Materials* 38(11): 2331-2334.

Yan, M.X., M.T. Zhang, Z.H. Zhu, J.F. Zhang, G.L. Cheng, N.M. Lin, H.J. Zhao, B. Yang. 2022. Structural characterization and tumor microvascular inhibition activity of total polysaccharide from *Trametes sanguinea* Lloyd. *Chemistry and Biodiversity* doi: 10.1002/cbdv.202100765.

RUSSULA References:

Alves, M.J., I.C.F.R. Ferreira, A. Martins, M. Pintado. 2012. Antimicrobial activity of wild mushroom extracts against clinical isolates resistant to different antibiotics. *Journal of Applied Microbiology* 113(2): 466-475.

Alves, M.J., I.C.F.R. Ferreira, I. Lourenco, E. Costa, A. Martins, M. Pintado. 2014. Wild mushroom extracts as inhibitors of bacterial biofilm formation. *Pathogens* 3(3): 667-679.

Kaewnarin, K., N. Suwannarach, J. Kumla, S. Choonpicharn, K. Tanreuan, S. Lumyong. 2020. Characterization of Polysaccharides from Wild Edible Mushrooms from Thailand and Their Antioxidant, Antidiabetic, and Antihypertensive Activities. *International Journal of Medicinal Mushrooms* 22(3): 221-233.

Lajin, B., S. Braeuer, J. Borovicka, W. Goessler. 2021. Is the water disinfection by-product dichloroacetic acid biosynthesized in the edible mushroom Russula nigricans? *Chemosphere* 281:130819.

Laperriere, G., I. Desgagné-Penix, H. Germain. 2018. DNA distribution pattern and metabolite profile of wild edible lobster mushroom (Hypomyces lactifluorum/Russula brevipes). *Genome* 61(5): 329-336.

Li, Y.L., X.J. Li, Q. Chu, R.Y. Jia, W. Chen, Y.X. Wang, X. Yu, X.D. Zheng. 2020. *Russula alutacea* Fr. Polysaccharide ameliorates inflammation in both RAW264.7 and zebrafish (*Danio rerio*) larvae. *International Journal of Biological Macromolecules* 145: 740-749.

Li, Y.M., R.F. Zhong, J. Chen, Z.G. Luo. 2021. Structural characterization, anticancer, hypoglycemia and immune activities of polysaccharides from Russula virescens. *International Journal of Biological Macromolecules* 184: 380-392.

Lovy, A. et al. 1999. Activity of edible mushrooms against the growth of human T4 leukemia cancer cells and *Plasmodium falciparum*. *Journal of Herbs, Spices and Medicinal Plant*s 6(4): 49-57.

Mallick, S., A. Dutta, S. Dey, J. Ghosh, D Mukherjee, S.S. Sultana et al. 2014. Selective inhibition of Leishmania donovani by active extracts of wild mushrooms used by the tribal population of India: An in vitro exploration for new leads against parasitic protozoans. *Experimental Parasitology* 138: 9-17.

Matsuura, M., S. Kato, Y. Saikawa, M. Nakata, K. Hashimoto. 2016. Identification of Cyclopropylacetyl-(R)-carnitine, a Unique Chemical Marker of the Fatally Toxic Mushroom Russula subnigricans. *Chemical and Pharmaceutical Bulletin* 64(6): 602-608.

Nandi, A.K., S. Samanta, I. K. Sen, K.S.P. Devi, T.K. Maiti, K. Acharya, S.S. Islam. 2013. Structural elucidation of an immunoenhancing heteroglycan isolated from Russula albonigra (Krombh.) Fr. *Carbohydrate Polymers* 94(2): 918-926.

Niazi, A.R., M. Shafique, M. Imran, A.N. Khalid. 2021. Evaluation of Mycochemical Analysis and In Vitro Biological Activities of some Russula Species (Agaricomycetes) from Pakistan. *International Journal of Medicinal Mushrooms* 23(10): 35-43.

O'Callaghan, Y.C., N.M. O'Brien, O. Kenny. T. Harrington, N. Bruton, T.J. Smyth. 2015. Anti-inflammatory effects of wild Irish mushroom extracts in RAW264.7 mouse macrophage cells. *Journal of Medicinal Food* 18(2): 202-207.

Rogers, R. 2011. *The Fungal Pharmacy: The Complete Guide to Medicinal Mushrooms and Lichens of North America*. North Atlantic Books. Berekely CA.

Wang, J.B., H.X. Wang, T.B. Ng. 2007. A peptide with HIV-1 transcriptase inhibitory activity from the medicinal mushroom Russula paludosa. *Peptides* 28(3): 560-565.

Xiao, G.L., F.Y. Liu, Z.H. Chen. 2003. Clinical observation on treatment of Russula subnigricans poisoning patients by Ganoderma lucidum decoction. *Chinese Journal of Integrated Traditional and Western Medicine* 23(4): 278-280.

Zhang, H., C.C. Li, P.F.H. Lai, J.S. Chen, F. Xie, Y.J. Xia, L.Z. Ai. 2021. Fractionation, chemical characterization and immunostimulatory activity of B-glucan and galactoglucan from Russula vinosa Lindblad. *Carbohydrate Polymers* 256: 17559.

Zhao, S., Y.C. Zhao, S.H. Li, J.K. Zhao, G.Q. Zhang, H.X. Wang, T.B. Ng. 2010. A novel lectin with highly potent antiproliferative and HIV-I reverse transcriptase inhibitory activities from the edible wild mushroom Russula delica. *Glycoconjugate Journal* 27(2): 259-265.

Zhao, S., Y.C. Zhao, S.H. Li, G.Q. Zhang, H.X. Wang, T.B. Ng. 2010a. An antiproliferative ribonuclease from fruiting bodies of the wild mushroom Russula delica. *Journal of Microbiology Biotechnology* 20(4): 693-696.

SHAGGY MANE References:

Asatiani, M.D., S.P. Wasser, E. Nevo, N. Ruimi, J. Mahajna, A.Z. Reznick. 2011. The Shaggy Inc Cap medicinal mushroom, Coprinus comatus (O.F. Mull.: Fr.) Pers. (Agaricomycetideae) substances interfere with H2O2 induction of the NF-kappaB pathway through inhibition of Ikappaalpha phosphorylation in MCF7 breast cancer cells. *International Journal of Medicinal Mushrooms* 13(1): 19-25.

Cao, H., D.W. Qin, H. Guo, X.W. Cui, S.S. Wang, Y.M. Wu, W.X. Zheng, X.F. Zhong, H.N. Wang, J.Y. Yu, H. Zhang, C.C. Han. 2020. The Shaggy Ink Cap Medicinal Mushroom, Coprinus comatus (Agaricomycetes), a Versatile Functional Species: A Review. *International Journal of Medicinal Mushrooms* 22(3): 245-255.

Cohen, N., J. Cohen, M.D. Asatiani, V.K. Varshney, H.T. Yu, Y.C. Yang, Y.H. Li, J.L. Mau, S.P. Wasser. 2014. Chemical composition and nutritional and medicinal value of fruit bodies and submerged cultured mycelia of culinary-medicinal higher Basidiomycetes mushrooms. *International Journal of Medicinal Mushrooms* 16(3): 273-291.

Dotan, N, S.P. Wasser, J. Mahajna. 2011. The culinary-medicinal mushroom Coprinus comatus as a natural antiandrogenic modulator. *Integrative Cancer Therapies* 10(2): 148-159.

Dubey, S.K., V.K. Chaturvedi, D. Mishra, A. Bajpeyee, A. Tiwari, M.P. Singh. 2019. Role of edible mushroom as a potent therapeutics for the diabetes and obesity. *3 Biotech* 9(12): 450.

Gao, Z., D.Y. Kong, W.X. Cai, J.J. Zhang, L. Jia. 2021. Characterization and anti-diabetic nephropathic ability of mycelium polysaccharides from Coprinus comatus. *Carbohydrate Polymers* 251: 117081.

Karaman, M., K. Tesanovic, A. Novakovic, D. Jakovljevic, L. Janjusevic, F. Sibul, B. Pejin. 2020. *Coprinus comatus* filtrate extract, a novel neuroprotective agent of natural origin. *Natural Products Research* 34(16): 2346-2350.

________K. Tesanovic, S. Gorjanovic, F.T. Pastor, M. Simonovic, M. Glumac, B. Pejin. 2021. Polarography as a technique of choice for the evaluation of total antioxidant activity: The case study of selected *Coprinus Comatus* extracts and quinic acid, their antidiabetic ingredient. *Natural Product Research* 35(10): 1711-1716.

Li, W.D., Y.X. Wang, M. Sun, Y. Liang, X.L. Wang, D.M. Qi, C.C. Han. 2021. The Saggy Ink Cap Medicinal Mushroom, Coprinus comatus (Agaricomycetes), Protein Attenuates Acute Alcoholic Liver Injury in Association with Changes in the Gut Microbiota of Mice. *International Journal of Medicinal Mushrooms* 23(5): 91-100.

Nowakowski, P., S.K. Naliwajko, R. Markiewicz-Zukowska, M.H. Borawska, K. Socha. 2020. The two faces of Coprinus comatus—Functional properties and potential hazards. *Phytotherapy Research* 34(11): 2932-2944.

Peng, Y., T.L. Li, H.M. Jiang, Y.F. Gu, Q. Chen et al. 2020. Postharvest biochemical characteristics and ultrastructure of *Coprinus comatus. Peer J.* 8: e8508.

Ratnaningtyas, N.I., H. Hernayanti, N. Ekowati, F. Hussen. 2022. Ethanol extract of the mushroom *Coprinus comatus* exhibits antidiabetic and antioxidant activities in streptozotocin-induced diabetic rats. *Pharmaceutical Biology* 60(1):1126-1136.

Rogers, R. 2011. *The Fungal Pharmacy: The Complete Guide to Medicinal Mushrooms and Lichens of North America*. North Atlantic Books, Berkeley, CA.

________2019. *Rejuvenate Your Brain Naturally*. Prairie Deva Press, Edmonton, Alberta.

________2021. *Psilocybin Mushrooms: The Mystery, Science and Research*. Prairie Deva Press, Edmonton, Alberta.

Rouhana-Toubi, A, S.P. Wasser, A. Agbarya, F. Fares. 2013. Inhibitory effect of ethyl acetate extract of the shaggy inc cap medicinal mushroom, Coprinus comatus (Higher Basidiomycetes) fruit bodies on cell growth of human ovarian cancer. *International Journal of Medicinal Mushrooms* 15(5): 457-470.

________S.P. Wasser, F. Fares. 2015. The Shaggy Ink Cap Medicinal Mushroom, Coprinus comatus (Higher Basidiomycetes) Extract Induces Apoptosis in Ovarian Cancer Cells via Extrinsic and Intrinsic Apoptotic Pathways. *International Journal of Medicinal Mushrooms* 17(12): 1127-1136.

Zaidman, B.Z., S.P. Wasser, E. Nevo, J. Mahajna. 2008. Coprinus comatus and Ganoderma lucidum interfere with androgen receptor function in LNCaP prostate cancer cells. *Molecular Biology Reports* 35(2): 107-117.

Zhang, P.L., K.H. Li, G. Yang, C.Q. Xia, J.E. Polston, G.N. Li, S.W. Li, Z. Lin, L.J. Yang, S.D. Bruner, Y.S. Ding. 2017. Cytotoxic protein from the mushroom Coprinus comatus possesses a unique mode for glycan binding and specificity. *Proceedings of the National Academy of Science USA* 114(34): 8980-8985.

Zhao, H.J., D. Li, M. Li, L. Liu, B.G. Deng, L. Jia, F. Yang. 2022. *Coprinus comatus* polysaccharides ameliorated carbon-tetrachloride-induced liver fibrosis through modulating inflammation and apoptosis. *Food and Function* doi: 10.1039/d2fo)1349e.

Zhong, X., Q. Li, H.G. Wang, Z.H. Zhao, H.Z. Yu, H.K. Xue, X. Cai et al. 2020. Dichloromethane extract of Fermentation Broth by Co-Culture of Morchella esculenta and Coprinus comatus Induces Apoptosis in U251 Cells via Mitochondrial Intrinsic Pathway. *International Journal of Medicinal Mushrooms* 22(10): 1001-1010.

SUILLUS References:

Andrade, J.M., P. Pachar, L. Trujillo, L. Cartuche. 2022. Suillin: A mixed-type acetylcholinesterase inhibitor from Suillus luteus which is used by Saraguros indigenous, southern Ecuador. *PLoS One* 17(5): e0268292.

Feng, Y., H.R. Xu, Y.M. Fan, F.M. Ma, B. Du, Y.T. Li et al. 2022. Effects of different monochromatic lights on umami and aroma of dried Suillus granulatus. *Food Chemistry* 404(ptA): 134524.

Gao, X., R.H. Zeng, C.T. Ho, B. Li, S.D. Chen, C. Xiao et al. 2022. Preparation, chemical structure, and immunostimulatory activity of a water-soluble heteropolysaccharide from *Suillus granulatus* fruiting bodies. *Food Chemistry:X* 13:100211.

Gordien, A.Y., A. I. Gray, K. Ingleby, S.G. Franzblau, V. Seidel. 2010. Activity of Scottish plant, lichen and fungal endophyte extracts against Mycobacterium aurum and Mycobacterium tuberculosis. *Phytotherapy Research* 24(5): 692-698.

Hou, Z.S., Y.Y. Wei, L.B. Sun, R.R. Xia, et al. 2022. Effects of drying temperature on umami taste and aroma profiles of mushrooms (Suillus granulatus) *Journal of Food Science* 87(5):1983-1998.

Jia, Z.Q., Y. Chen, Y.X. Yan, J.X. Zhao. 2014. Iso-suillin from Suillus luteus, induces G1 phase arrest and apoptosis in human hepatoma SMMC-7721 cells. *Asian Pacific Journal of Cancer Prevention* 15(3): 1423-1428.

León, F., I. Brouard, F. Torres, J. Quintana, A. Rivera, F. Estévez, J. Bermejo. 2008. A new ceramide from Suillus luteus and its cytotoxic activity against human melanoma cells. *Chemistry and Biodiversity* 5(1): 120-125.

Liu, F.Y., K.W. Luo, Z.M. Yu, N.N. Co, S.H. Wu, P. Wu., K.P. Fung, T.T. Kwok. 2009. Suillin from the mushroom Suillus placidus as potent apoptosis inducer in human hepatoma HepG2 cells. *Chemico-Biological Interactions* 181(2): 168-174.

Mironczuk-Chodakowska, I., & A.M. Witkowska. 2020. Evaluation of Polish wild Mushrooms as Beta-Glucan Sources. *International Journal of Environmental Research in Public Health* 17(19): 7299.

Morel, S. S. Arnould, M. Vitou, F. Boudard, Caroline Guzman, P. Poucheret, F. Fons, S. Rapior. 2018. Antiproliferative and Antioxidant Activities of Wild Boletales Mushrooms from France. *International Journal of Medicinal Mushrooms* 20(1): 13-29.

Tomasi, S., F. Lohézic-Le Dévéhat, P. Sauleau, C. Bézivin, J. Boustie. 2004. Cytotoxic activity of methanol extracts from Basidiomycete mushrooms on murine cancer cell lines. *Pharmazie* 59(4): 290-293.

Tringali, C., C. Geraci, G. Nicolosi, J.F. Verbist, C. Roussakis. 1989. An antitumor principle from Suillus granulatus. *Journal of Natural Products* 52(4): 844-845.

Tringali, C., M. Plattelli, C. Geraci, G. Nicolosi. 1989a. Antimicrobial tetraprenyl-phenols from Suillus granulatus. *Journal of Natural Products* 52(5): 941-947.

Ványolós, A., O. Orbán-Gyapai, J. Hohmann. 2014. Xanthine oxidase inhibitory activity of Hungarian wild-growing mushrooms. *Phytotherapy Research* 28(8):1204-1210.

Vaz, J.A., I.C.F.R. Ferreira, C. Tavares, G.M. Almeida, A. Martins, M.H. Vasconcelos. 2012. Suillus collinitus methanolic extract increases p53 expression and causes cell cycle arrest and apoptosis in a breast cancer cell line. *Food Chemistry* 135(2): 596-602.

Wang, Y.H., J.G. Tang, R.R. Wang, L.M. WANG, Z.J. Dong et al. 2007. Flazinamide, a novel beta-carboline compound with anti-HIV actions. *Biochemical and Biophysical Research Communications* 355(4): 1091-1095.

Wang, Y., Q.S. Zhang, J.X. Zhao, X.J. Zhao, J.X. Zhang, L.A. Wang. 2014. Iso-suillin from the mushroom Suillus flavus induces cell cycle arrest and apoptosis in K562 cell line. *Food and Chemical Toxicology* 67:17-25.

Yan, Y.X., S.J. Yao, Z.Q. Jia, J.Z. Zhao, L. Wang. 2021. Iso-suillin-induced DNA damage leading to cell cycle arrest and apoptosis arised from p53 phosphoryation in A549 cells. *European Journal of Pharmacology* 907: 174299.

Yun, B.S., H.C. Kang, H. Koshino, S.H. Yu, I.D. Yoo. 2001. Suillusin, a unique benzofuran from the mushroom Suillus granulatus. *Journal of Natural Products* 64(9): 1230-1231.

Zhang, J.X., Y.J. Lu, L.Q. Zhao, L.A. Wang. 2021. Hypoglycemic Activity of Total Flavonoids from Slippery Jack Mushroom, Suillus luteus (Agaricomycetes), in Vitro and In Vivo. *International Journal of Medicinal Mushrooms* 23(11): 17-26.

Zhao, J.X., Q.S. Zhang, Y. Chen, S.J. Yao, Y.X. Yan, Y. Wang, J.X. Zhang, L.A. Wang. 2016. Iso-suillin from Suillus flavus Induces Apoptosis in Human Small Cell Lung Cancer H446 Cell line. *Chinese Medical Journal* (English) 129(10): 1215-1223.

Zhou, F., S. Yan, S. Chen, L.Y. Gong, T.T. Su, Z.Y. Wang. 2016. Optimization Extraction Process of Polysaccharides from Suillus granulatus and Their Antioxidant and Immunological Activities in vitro. *Pharmacognosy Magazine* 12(Suppl 2): S277-284.

TIGER MILK MUSHROOM References:

Ellan, K., R. Thayan, C.W. Phan, V. Sabaratnam. 2019. Anti-inflammatory effects of mushrooms in dengue-infected human monocytes. *Tropical Biomedicine* 36(4): 1087-1098.

Ellan, K., R. Thayan, J. Raman, K.I.P.J. Hidari, N. Ismail, V. Sabaratnam. 2019a. Anti-viral activity of culinary and medicinal mushroom extracts against dengue virus serotype 2: an in-vitro study. *BMC Complementary & Alternative Medicine* 19(1): 260.

Goh, N.Y., M.F.M. Razif, Y.H.Y. Yap, C.L. Ng, S.Y. Fung 2022. In silico analysis and characterization of medicinal mushroom cystathionine beta-synthase as an angiotensin converting enzyme (ACE) inhibitory protein. *Computational Biology and Chemistry* 96: 107620.

Jamil, N.A.M., C. Gomes, Z. Kadir, A. Gomes. 2020. Impact of electrical stimulation on the growth of mycelium of lignosus rhinocerus (cooke) ryvarden. *Electromagnetic Biology and Medicine* 39(4): 356-363.

Johnathan, M., S.A. Muhanad, S.H. Gan, J. Stanslas, W.E.M. Fuad, F.A. Hussain, W.A.N.W. Ahmad, A.A. Nurul. 2021. Lignosus rhinocerotis Cooke Ryvarden ameliorates airway inflammation, mucus hypersecretion and airway hyperresponsiveness in a murine model of asthma. *PLoS One* 16(3):e0249091.

Lau, B.F., N. Abdullah, N. Aminudin, H.B. Lee, K.C. Yap, V. Sabaratnam. 2014. The potential of mycelium and culture broth of Lignosus rhinocerotis as substitutes for the naturally occurring sclerotium with regard to antioxidant capacity, cytotoxic effect, and low-molecular-weight chemical constituents. *PLoS One* 9(7):e102509.

Lee, M.K., K.H. Lim, P. Millns, S.K. Mohankumar, S.T. Ng, C.S. Tan, S.M. Then, Y. Mbaki, K.N. Ting. 2018. Bronchodilator effects of Lignosus rhinocerotis extract on rat isolated airways is linked to the blockage of calcium entry. *Phytomedicine* 42: 172-179.

Nallathamby, N., C-W. Phan, S. L-S. Seow, A. Baskaran, H. Lakshmanan, S.N.A. Malek, V. Sabaratnam. 2018. A Status Review of the Bioactive Activities of Tiger Milk Mushroom *Lignosus rhinocerotis* (Cooke) Ryvarden. *Frontiers in Pharmacology* 8: 998.

Nyam, K.L., C.Y. Chang, C.S. Tan, S.T. Ng. 2016. Investigation of the Tiger Milk Medicinal Mushroom, Lignosus rhinocerotis (Agaricomycetes), as an Antiulcer Agent. *International Journal of Medicinal Mushrooms* 18(12): 1093-1104.

Nyam, K.L., C.F. Chow, C.S. Tan, S.T. Ng. 2017. Antidiabetic Properties of the Tiger's Milk Medicinal Mushroom, Lignosus rhinocerotis (Agaricomycetes), in Streptozotocin-Induced Diabetic Rats. *International Journal of Medicinal Mushrooms* 19(7): 607-617.

Pushparajah, V., A. Fatima, C.H. Chong, T.Z. Gambule, C.J. Chan, S.T. Ng et al. 2016. Characterisation of a New Fungal Immunomodulatory Protein from Tiger Milk mushroom, Lignosus rhinocerotis. *Scientific Reports* 6: 30010.

Rashid, N.A.A, B.F. Lau, C.S. Kue. 2022. Differential toxicity and teratogenic effects of the hot water and cold water extracts of Lignosus rhinocerus (Cooke) Ryvarden sclerotium on zebrafish (Danio rerio) embryos. *Journal of Ethnopharmacology* 285: 114787.

Samberkar, S., S. Gandhi, M. Naidu, K.H. Wong, J. Raman, V. Sabaratnam. 2015. Lion's Mane, Hericium erinaceus and Tiger Milk, Lignosus rhinocerotis (Higher Basidiomycetes) Medicinal Mushrooms Stimulate Neurite Outgrowth in Dissociated Cells of Brain, Spinal Cord and Retina: An In Vitro Study. *International Journal of Medicinal Mushrooms* 17(11): 1047-1054.

Seow, S.L.S., L.F. Eik, M. Naidu, P. David, K.H. Wong, V. Sabaratnam. 2015. Lignosus rhinocerotis (Cooke) Ryvarden mimics the neuritogenic activity of nerve growth factor via MEK/ERK1/2 signaling pathway in PC-12 cells. *Scientific Reports* 5: 16349.

Tan, E.S.S., T.K. Leo, C.K. Tan. 2021. Effect of tiger milk mushroom (Lignosus rhinocerus) supplementation on respiratory health, immunity and antioxidant status: an open-label prospective study. *Scientific Reports* 11(1): 11781.

Tan, Y.H. C.S.Y. Lim, K.H. Wong, V. Sabaratnam. 2021a. Neuritin Protein Expression is Positively Correlated with Neurite Outgrowth Induced by the Tiger Milk Mushroom, Lignosus rhinocerotis (Agaricomycetes), in PC12 Cells. *International Journal of Medicinal Mushrooms* 23(6): 1-11.

Usuldin, S.R.A., W.A. Wan-Mohtar, Z. Ilham, A.A. Jamaludin, N.R. Abdullah, N. Rowan. 2021. In vivo toxicity of bioreactor-grown biomass and exopolysaccharides from Malaysian tiger milk mushroom mycelium for potential future health applications. *Sci Rep* 11(1): 23079.

Veeraperumal, S., H.M. Qui, C.S. Tan, S.T. Ng, W.C. Zhang, S.J. Tang, K.L. Cheong, Y. Liu. 2021. Restitution of epithelial cells during intestinal mucosal wound healing: The effect of a polysaccharide from the sclerotium of Lignosus rhinocerotis (Cooke) Ryvarden. *Journal of Ethnopharmacology* 274:114024.

Yap, H.Y.Y., S.Y. Fung, S.T. Ng, C.S. Tan, N.H. Tan. 2015. Shotgun proteomic analysis of tiger milk mushroom (Lignosus rhinocerotis) and the isolation of a cytotoxic fungal serine protease from its sclerotium. *Journal of Ethnopharmacology* 174: 437-451.

Yap, H.Y.Y., M.J. Muria-Gonzalez, B.H. Kong, K.A. Stubbs, C.S. Tan et al. 2017. Heterologous expression of cytotoxic sesquiterpenoids from the medicinal mushroom Lignosus rhinocerotis in yeast. *Microbial Cell Factories* 16(1): 103.

Yap, H.Y.Y., N.H. Tan, S.T. Ng, C.S. Tan, S.Y. Fung. 2018. Inhibition of Protein Glycation by Tiger Milk Mushroom [Lignosus rhinocerus (Cooke) Ryvarden] and Search for Potential Anti-diabetic Activity- Related Metabolic Pathways by Genomic and Transcriptomic Data Mining. *Frontiers in Pharmacology* 9: 103.

Yap, H.Y.Y., B H. Kong, C.S.A. Yap, K.C. Ong, R.B. Zain et al. 2022. Immunomodulatory Effect and an Intervention of TNF Signalling Leading to Apoptotic and Cell Cycle Arrest on ORL-204 Oral Cancer Cells by Tiger Milk Mushroom, *Lignosus rhinoocerus. Food Technology and Biotechnology* 60(1): 80-88,

TRICHOLOMA References:

Anand, J.S., P. Chwaluk, and M. Sut. 2009. Acute poisoning with *Tricholoma equestre. Przeglad Lekarski* 66(6): 339-40.

Bergius, N., and E. Danell. 2000. The Swedish matsutake (*Tricholoma nauseosum* syn. *T. matsutake*) distribution, abundance and ecology. *Scandinavian Journal of Forest Research* 15(3): 318-325.

Chapela, I.H. and M. Garbelotto. 2004. Phylogeography and evolution in matsutake and close allies inferred by analyses of ITS sequences and AFLPs. *Mycologia* 96(4): 730-741.

Deng, H., and Y.J. Yao. 2005. *Tricholoma equestre*, the correct name for *T. flavovirens* (Agaricales). *Mycotaxon* 94: 325-329.

Gülsen, T., A. Müjde, E.D. Mehmet, and M. Öztürk. 2012. Antioxidant and cholinesterase inhibition activities of three *Tricholoma* species with yotal phenolic and flavonoid contents: the edible mushrooms from Anatolia. *Food Analytical Methods* 5(3): 495-504.

Hata, K., F. Sugawara, N. Ohisa, S. Takahashi, and K. Hori. Stimulative effects of (22E,24R)-ergosta-7,22-diene-3β, 5α,6 β -triol from fruiting bodies of *Tricholoma auratum. Biological and Pharmaceutical Bulletin* 25(8): 1040-4.

Kim, J.H., and Y.S. Kim. 2001. Characterization of a metalloenzyme from a Wild Mushroom, *Tricholoma saponaceum. Bioscience, Biotechnology, Biochemistry.* 65: 356-362.

Massart, F. 2003. The golden tricholoma (*T. auratum* [Fr.] Gillet) stands accused. *Documents Mycologiques.* 32(126): 17-20.

Nieminen, P., V. Kärjä, and A.M. Mustonen. 2008. Indications of hepatic and cardiac toxicity caused by sub-chronic *Tricholoma flavovirens* consumption. *Food and Chemical Toxicology* 46(2): 781-86.

Ohtsuka, S. et al. 1973. Polysaccharides having an anticarcinogenic effect and a method of producing them from species of *Basidiomycetes*. US Patent 1331513. Issued: September 26, 1973.

Pachón-Peña, G., F.J. Reyes-Zurita, G. Deffieux, A. Azqueta, J.J. de Cerain, E.E. Creppy, and M. Cascante. 2009. Antiproliferative effect of flavomannin-6,6'dimethylether from *Tricholoma equestre* on Caco-2 cells. *Toxicology* 264(3): 192-197.

Sein, A.J. and P. Chwaluk. 2010. Acute intoxication with *Tricholoma equestre*—clinical course. *Przeglad Lekarski* 67(8): 618-619.

Turner, N.J., C. Laurence, M. Thompson, T. Thompson, and A.Z. York. 1990. *Thompson Ethnobotany: Knowledge and Usage of Plants by the Thompson Indians of British Columbia.* Royal British Columbia Museum Memoir No. 3.

Yamac, M., and F. Bilgili. 2006. Antimicrobial activities of fruit bodies and/or mycelial cultures of some mushroom isolates. *Pharmaceutical Biology* 44(9): 660-667.

Yuvali, G., & D. Onbasil. 2022. Cytotoxicity of Sarcosphaera crassa and Tricholoma terreum extracts on colon cancer cell line (HT-29) in conjunction with their antioxidant properties. *International Journal of Environmental Health Research* 32(10): 2286-2297.

Zhang, F.L., H.X. Yang, X. Wu, J.Y. Wang, J. He, Z.H. Li, T. Feng, J.K Liu. 2020. Chemical constituents and their cytotoxicities from mushroom Tricholoma imbricatum. *Phytochemistry* 177: 112431.

TRUFFLES References:

Beara, I.N., M.M. Lesjak, D.D. Cetojevic-Simin, Z.S. Marjanovic, J.D. Ristic, Z. O. Mrkonjic, N.M. Mimica-Dukic. 2014. Phenolic profile, antioxidant, anti-inflammatory and cytotoxic activities of black (*T. aestivum* Vittad.) and white (*T. magnatum* Pico) truffles. *Fungal Biology & Biotechnology* 7:9.

Khojasteh, S.M., L. Amiri, F. Sheikhzadeh. 2013. Effect of the alcoholic extract of Terfezia boudieri on reproductive hormones in male rats. *International Journal of Pharmacy and Biological Science* 3: 517-522.

Mimeault, M. N. Pommery, N. Wattez, C. Bailly, J.P. Henichart. 2003. Anti-proliferative and apoptotic effects of anandamide in human prostatic cancer cell lines: implication of epidermal growth factor receptor down-regulation and ceramide production. *Prostate* 56: 1-2.

Pacioni, G., C. Rapino, O. Zavari, A. Falconi, M. Leonardi, N. Battista et al. 2015. Truffles contain endocannabinoid metabolic enzymes and anandamide. *Phytochemistry* 110: 104-110.

Pattanayak, M., S. Samanta, P. Maity, D.K. Manna, I.K. Sen, A.K. Nandi et al. 2017. Polysaccharides of an edible truffle Tuber rufum: structural studies and effects on human lymphocytes. *International Journal of Biological Macromolecules* 95: 1037-1048.

Picardi, G., E. Ciaglia, M. Proto, S. Pisanti. 2014. Anandamide inhibits breast tumor-induced angiogenesis. *Translational Medicine at UniSa* (Salerno) 10: 8-12.

Rogers, Robert. 2016. *Mushroom Essences: Vibrational Healing from the Kingdom Fungi*. North Atlantic Books, Berkeley CA page 207.

Rosa-Gruszecka, A., D. Hilszczanska, W. Gil, B. Kosel. 2017. Truffle renaissance in Poland—history, present and prospects. *Journal of Ethnobiology and Ethnomedicine* 13(1): 36.

Segelke, T., S. Schelm, C. Ahlers, M. Fischer. 2020. Food authentication: Truffle (Tuber spp.) species differentiation by FT-NIR and chemometrics. *Foods* 9(7): 922.

Sorrentino, E., A. Reale, P. Tremonte, L. Maiuro, M. Succi, L. Tipaldi et al. 2013. Lactobacillus plantarum 29 Inhibits Penicillium spp. Involved in the Spoilage of Black Truffles (Tuber aestivum). *Journal of Food Science* 78(8): M1188-1194.

Wu, Z.Y., M. Jayachandran, W.S. Cheang, B.J. Xu. 2022. Black Truffle Extract Exerts Antidiabetic Effects through Inhibition of Inflammation and Lipid Metabolism Regulation. *Oxidative Medicine and Cellular Longevity* 2022:6099872.

Zhang, T.Z., M. Jayachandran, K. Ganesan, B.J. Xu. 2018. Black truffle aqueous extract attenuates oxidative stress and inflammation in STZ-induced hyperglycemic rats via Nrf2 and NF-$_K$B pathways. *Frontiers in Pharmacol*ogy 9:1257.

__________2020. The Black Truffle, *Tuber melanosporum* (Ascomycetes), ameliorates hyperglycemia and regulates insulin signaling pathway in STZ-induced diabetic rats. *International Journal of Medicinal Mushrooms* 22(11): 1057-1066.

Zhao, W. X.H. Wang, H.M. Li, S.H. Wang, T. Chen et al. 2014. Isolation and characterization of polysaccharides with the antitumor activity from Tuber fruiting bodies and fermentation system. *Applied Microbiology and Biotechnol*ogy 98: 1991-2002.

TYLOPILUS References:

Arbour, C.A. & B. Imperiali. 2020. Uridine natural products: Challenging targets and inspiration for novel small molecule inhibitors. *Bioorganic and Medicinal Chemistry* 28(18): 115661.

Casale, M., L. Bagnasco, M. Zotti, S.D. Piazza, N. Sitta, P. Oliveri. 2016. A NIR spectroscopy-based efficient approach to detect fraudulent additions within mixtures of dried porcini mushrooms. *Talanta* 160: 729-734.

Connolly, G.P. & J.A. Duley. 1999. Uridine and its nucleotides: biological actions, therapeutic potentials. *Trends in Pharmacological Sciences* 20(5): 218-225.

González-Cortázar, M., J.E. Sánchez, M. Hulcochea-Medina, V.M. Hernàndez-Velàzquez, P. Medoza-de-Gives, A. Zamilpa et al. 2021. *In Vitro* and *In Vivo* Nematicide Effect of Extract Fractions of *Pleurotus djamor* against *Haemonchus contortus*. *Journal of Medicinal Food* 24(3): 310-318.

Lee, S.J., B.S. Yun, D.H. Cho, I.D. Yoo. 1999. Tylopeptins A and B, new antibiotic peptides from Tylopilus neofelleus. *Journal of Antibiotics* (Tokyo) 52(11): 998-1006.

Li, L.F., G.G.L. Yue, B.C.L. Chan, Q. Zeng, Q.B. Han, P.C. Leung, K.P. Fung, J.K. Liu, C.B.S. Lau. 2021. Rubinoboletus ballouii polysaccharides exhibited immunostimulatory activities through toll-like receptor-4 via NF-$_k$B pathway. *Phytotherapy Research* 35(4): 2108-2118.

Li, L.F., B.C.L. Chan, G.G.L. Yue, C.B.S. Lau, Q.B. Han, P.C. Leung, J.K. Liu, K.P. Fung. 2021a. Two immunosuppressive compounds from the mushroom Rubinoboletus ballouii using human peripheral blood mononuclear cells by bioactivity-guided fractionation. *Phytomedicine* 20(13): 1196-1202.

Lima, A.T.M., M.N. Santos, L.A.R. de Souza, T.S. Pinheiro, A.A.O. Paiva, C.M.P.G. Dore et al. 2016. Chemical characteristics of a heteropolysaccharide from Tylopilus ballouii mushroom and its antioxidant and anti-inflammatory activities. *Carbohydrate Polymers* 144: 400-409.

Ramesh, D., B.G. Vijayakumar, T. Kannan. 2020. Therapeutic potential of uracil and its derivatives in countering pathogenic and physiological disorders. *European Journal of Medicinal Chemistry* 207: 112801.

Slanc, P., B. Doljak, A. Mlinaric, B. Strukelj. 2004. Screening of wood damaging fungi and macrofungi for inhibitors of pancreatic lipase. *Phytotherapy Research* 18(9): 758-762.

Sugaya, K., M. Ino, N. Matsuo, J.I. Onose, N. Abe. 2020. Variegatic acid from the edible mushroom Tylopilus ballouii inhibits TNF-a production and PKCb1 activity in leukemia cells. *Bioorganic Medicinal and Chemistry Letters* 30(4): 126886.

Susaniková, I., A. Kvasnicová, Z. Brzková, O. Duriska, P. Mucaji. 2018. New biological findings of ethanol and chloroform extracts of fungi Suillelus rubrosanguineus and Tylopilus felleus. *Interdisciplinary Toxicology* 11(3): 204-208.

Yamamoto, T., H. Koyama, M. Kurajoh, T. Shoji, Z. Tsutsumi, Y. Moriwaki. 2011. Biochemistry of uridine in plasma. *Clinica Chimica Acta* 312(19-20): 1712-1724.

UMBRELLA POLYPORE References:

Bian, Z., J. Li. 1997. Short-term curative observation of polyporus polysaccharide with COEP combined treatment in 50 cases of small cell lung cancer. *Chinese Journal of Cancer Biotherapy* 3: 233-234.

Chen, Z., Q. Luo. 2001. Short-term curative observation of polyporus polysaccharide capsules in the treatment of 28 cases with chronic hepatitis B. *Clinical Focus* 7: 313-314.

Dai, H., X.Q. Han, F.Y. Gong, H.L. Dong P.F. Tu, X.M. Gao. 2012. Structure elucidation and immunological function analysis of a novel B-glucan from the fruiting bodies of *Polyporus umbellatus* (Pers.) Fries. *Glycobiology* 22(12): 1673-1683.

Guo, B. 1981. Application of polyporus polysaccharide in the treatment of lung cancer. *J Norman Bethune University Medical Science* 4: 51-54.

Guo, B. 1984. The efficacy of polyporus polysaccharide and its extract (757) in the treatment of lung cancer. *J Norman Bethune University Medicinal Science* 1: 43-45.

Guo, Z.H., Y.J. Zin, L.J. Zhang. 2019. The efficacy of *Polyporus umbellatus* polysaccharide in treating hepatitis B in China. *Progress in Molecular Biology and Translational Science* 163: 329-360.

Han, P.J., T.R. Liu, Y. Zheng, R.Q. Song, T.G. Nan, X.L. Yang, L.Q. Huang, Y. Yuan. 2022. A Mycorrhizal Bacteria Strain Isolated From *Polyporus umbellatus* Exhibits Broad-Spectrum Antifungal Activity. *Frontiers in Plant Science* 13:954160.

He, P.F., A.Q. Zhang, F. Zhang, R.J. Linhardt, P.L. Sun. 2016. Structure and bioactivity of a polysaccharide containing uronic acid from Polyporus umbellatus sclerotia. *Carbohydrate Polymers* 152: 222-230.

Huang, J.W., C.J.S. Lai, Y.Yuan, M. Zhang, J.H. Zhou, L.Q. Huang. 2017. Correlative analysis advance of chemical constituents of *Polyporus umbellatus* and *Armillaria mellea*. *Zhongguo Zhong Yao Za Zhi* 42(15): 2905-2914.

Ishida, H., Y. Inaoka, J. Shibatani, M. Fukushima, K. Tsuji. 1999. Isolation of hair regrowth substances, acetosyringone and polyporusterone A and B, from *Polyporus umbellatus* Fries. *Biology and Pharmacology Bulletin* 22(11): 1189-92.

Jia, W.Y., S.W. Luo, G. Lai, S.Q. Li, S. Huo, M.F. Li, X. Zeng. 2021. Homogeneous polyporus polysaccharide inhibits bladder cancer by polarizing macrophages to M1 subtype in tumor microenvironment. *BMC Complementary Medicine and Therapies* 21(1): 150.

Jiang, J.T., F.Wang, A. Luo, S.Y. Lin, K.O. Feng, W. Yan et al. 2020. Polyporus Polysaccharide Ameliorates Bleomycin-induced Pulmonary Fibrosis by Suppressing Myofibroblast Differentiation via TGF-B/Smad2/3 Pathway. *Frontiers in Pharmacology* 11:767.

Kim, T.H., J.S. Kim, Z.H. Kim, R.B. Huang, Y.L. Chae, R.S. Wang. 2016. Induction of apoptosis in MCF-7 human breast cancer cells by Khz (fusion of *Ganoderma lucidum* and *Polyporus umbellatus* mycelium). *Molecular Medicine Reports* 13(2): 1243-9.

Lee, W.Y., Y.K. Park, J.K. Ahn. 2007. Improvement of Ergone Production from Mycelial Culture of *Polyporus umbellatus. Mycobiology* 35(2): 82-86.

Li, H., Z. Yan, Q.P. Xiong et al. 2019. Renoprotective effect and mechanism of polysaccharide from *Polyporus umbellatus* sclerotia on renal fibrosis. *Carbohydrate Polymers* 212: 1-10.

Li, X.Q., W. Xu, J. Chen. 2010. Polysaccharide purified from *Polyporus umbellatus* (Per) Fr induces the activation and maturation of murine bone-derived dendritic cells via toll-like receptor4. *Cellular Immunology* 265(1): 50-56.

Liu, X, Y. Yuan, H. Wang et al. 1993. Clinical observation of polyporus polysaccharide injection in the treatment for 156 cases with hepatitis B. *Shangdong Medical Journal* 6: 27-28.

Liu, M.M., D.W. Zhang, Y.M. Xing, S.X. Guo. 2017. Cloning and expression of three thaumatin-like protein genes from *Polyporus umbellatus. Acta Pharmaceutica Sinica B* 7(3): 373-380.

Liu, C.P., X. Li, G.N. Lai, J.H. Li et al. 2020. Mechanisms of Macrophage Immunomodulatory Activity Induced by a New Polysaccharide Isolated from *Polyporus umbellatus* (Pers.) Fries. *Frontiers in Chemistry* 8: 581.

Ohsawa, T., M. Yukawa, C. Takao, M. Murayama, H. Bando. 1992. Studies on constituents of fruit body of *Polyporus umbellatus* and their cytotoxic activity. *Chemical and Pharmaceutical Bulletin* (Tokyo) 40(1): 143-147.

Tan, X.L., L. Guo, G.H. Wang. 2016. *Polyporus umbellatus* inhibited tumor cell proliferation and promoted tumor cell apoptosis by down-regulating AKT in breast cancer. *Biomedicine and Pharmacotherapy* 83: 526-535.

Wang, Y.N., X.Q. Wu, D.D. Zhang, H.H. Hu, J.L. Liu, N.D. Vaziri, Y. Guo, Y.Y. Zhao, H. Miao. 2021. *Polyporus umbellatus* Protects Against Renal Fibrosis by Regulating Intrarenal Fatty Acyl Metabolites. *Frontiers in Pharmacology* 12: 633566.

Xing, X., J.X. Men, L.L. Song, S.X. Guo. 2020. Do the Main Components of the Sclerotia of Umbrella Polypore Mushroom, *Polyporus umbellatus* (Agaricomycetes), Correlate with Armillaria Associates? *International Journal of Medicinal Mushrooms* 22(5): 479-488.

Xiong, L.L. 1993. Therapeutic effect of combined therapy of *Salvia miltiorrhizae* and *Polyporus umbellatus* polysaccharide in the treatment of chronic hepatitis B. *Zhongguo Zhong Xi Yi Jie He Za Zhi* 13(9): 516-57.

Yang, D., S. Li, H. Wang et al. 1999. Prevention of postoperative recurrence of bladder cancer: An experimental and clinical study. *Zhonghua Wai Ke Za Zhi* 37(8): 464-465.

Zhang, G.W., G.F. Qin, B. Han, C.X. Li, H.G. Yang, P.H. Nie, X. Zeng. 2015. Efficacy of Zhuling polyporus polysaccharide with BCG to inhibit bladder carcinoma. *Carbohydrate Polymers* 118: 30-35.

Zhao, Y.Y., R.M. Xie, X. Chao, Y.M. Zhang, R.C. Lin, W.J. Sun. 2009. Bioactivity-directed isolation, identification of diuretic compounds from *Polyporus umbellatus*. *Journal of Ethnopharmacology* 126(1): 184-187.

Zhao, Y.Y., X. Chao, Y.M. Zhang, R.C. Lin, W.J. Sun. 2010. Cytotoxic steroids from *Polyporus umbellatus*. *Planta Medica* 76(15): 1755-1758.

WAX GILLS AND WAX CAPS References:

Alkan, S., A. Uysal, G. Kasik, S. Vlaisavljevic, S. Berezni, G. Zengin. 2020. Chemical Characterization, Antioxidant, Enzyme Inhibition and Antimutagenic Properties of Eight Mushroom Species: A Comparative Study. *Journal of Fungi* (Basel) 6(3): 166.

Carey, C.J., S.I. Glassman, T.D. Bruns, E.L. Aronson, S.C. Hart. 2020. Soil microbial communities associated with giant sequoia: How does the world's largest tree affect some of the world's smallest organisms? *Ecology and Evolution* 10(13): 6593-6609.

Gilardoni, G., M. Clericuzio, S. Tosi, G. Zanoni, G. Vidari. 2007. Antifungal acylcyclopentenediones from fruting bodies of Hygrophorus chrysodon. *Journal of Natural Products* 70(1): 137-139.

Kosanic, M.M., D.S. Seklic, M.M. Jovanovic, N.N. Petrovic, S. D. Markovic. 2020. *Hygrophorus eburneus*, edible mushroom, a promising natural bioactive agent. *EXCLI Journal* 19: 442-457.

MacKinnon, A., K. Luther. 2021. *Mushrooms of British Columbia*. Royal BC Museum Handbook, Victoria, BC.

Miller, B.C., D. Nelson, R.E. Moore, J.R. Rao, J.E. Moore. 2019. Antimicrobial properties of basidiomycota macrofungi to *Mycobacterium abscessus* isolated from patients with cystic fibrosis. *International Journal of Mycobacteriology* 8(1): 93-97.

Otto, A., A. Porzel, J. Schmidt, W. Brandt, L. Wessjohann, N. Arnold. 2016. *Journal of Natural Products* 79(1): 74-80.

Slanc, P., B. Doljak, A. Mlinaric, B. Strukelj. 2004. Screening of wood damaging
fungi and macrofungi for inhibitors of pancreatic lipase. *Phytotherapy
Research* 18(9): 758-762.

Suzucki, T., K. Sugiyama, H. Hirai, H. Ito, T. Morita, H. Dohra et al. 2012. Mannose-
specific lectin from the mushroom Hygrophorus russula. *Glycobiology*
22(5): 616-629.

Teichert, A., T. Lübken, J. Schmidt, C. Kuhnt et al. 2008. Determination of
B-carboline alkaloids in fruiting bodies of *Hygrophorus* spp. by liquid
chromatography/electrospray ionisation tandem mass spectrometry.
Phytochemical Analysis 19(4): 335-341.

Zhu, M.J., L.J. Xu, X. Chen, Z.Q. Ma, H.X. Wang, T.B. Ng. 2013. A novel
ribonuclease with HIV-1 reverse transcriptase inhibitory activity from
the edible mushroom Hygrophorus russula. *Applied Biochemistry and
Biotechnology* 170(1): 219-230.

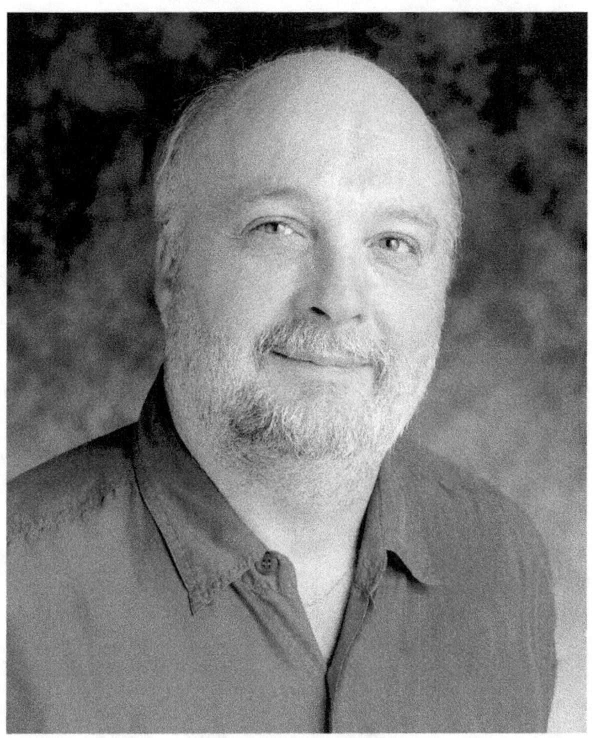

Robert Dale Rogers is a professional member of the American Herbalist Guild, Herbal Elder of Canada, and Fellow of the International College of Nutrition.

He conducted a clinical practice for 20 years and taught herbal medicine at the Northern Star College and Grant McEwan University for 26 years. He previously served on the editorial board of the International Journal of Medicinal Mushrooms, and writes occasional columns for Fungi magazine.

Robert is the author of 59 books on plant and mushroom medicine, including The Fungal Pharmacy: The Complete Guide to Medicinal Mushrooms and Lichens of North America.

He presently continues to research and writes and enjoys leading plant and mushroom walks and talks throughout North America.

www.selfhealdistributing.com

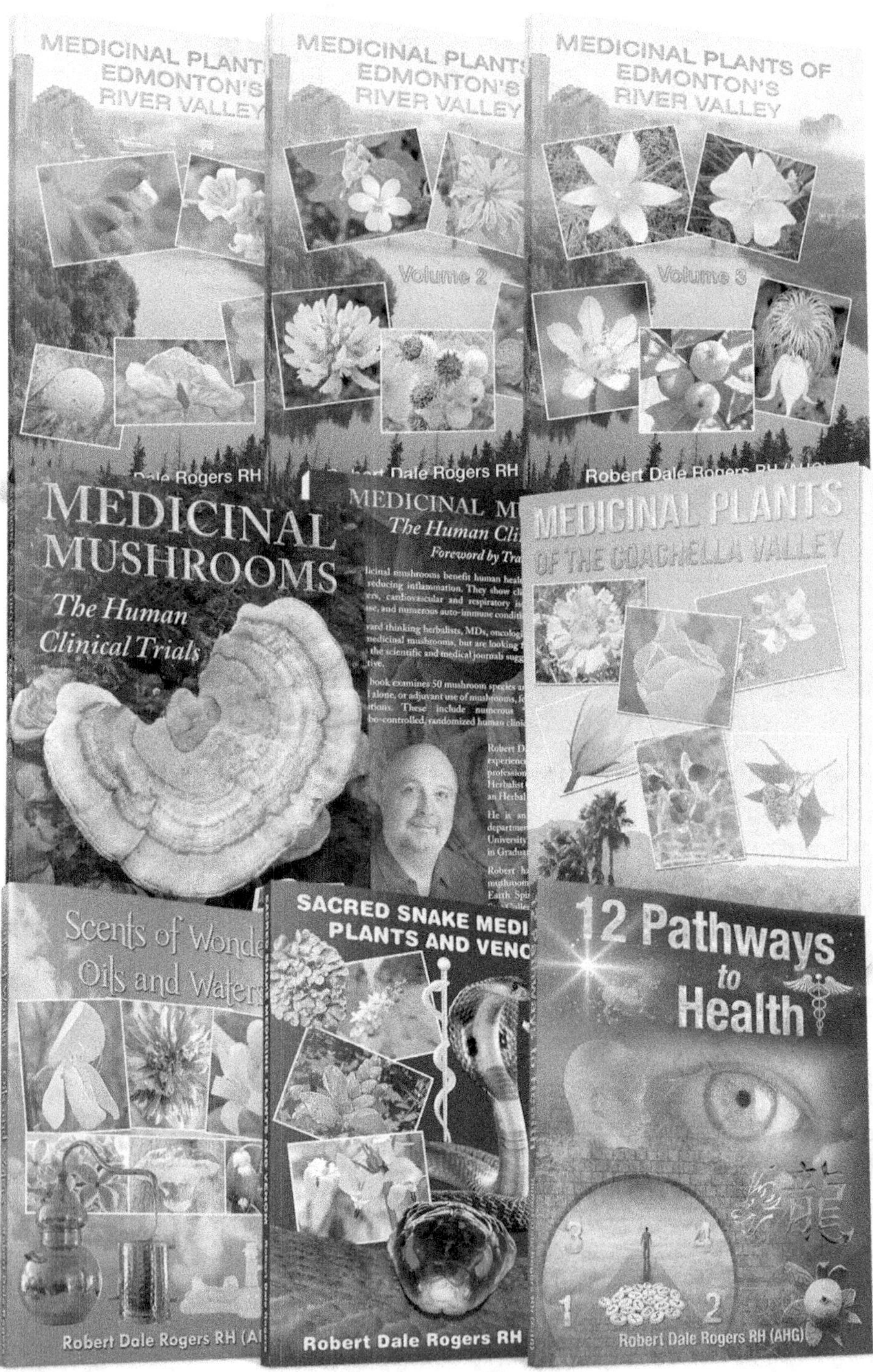

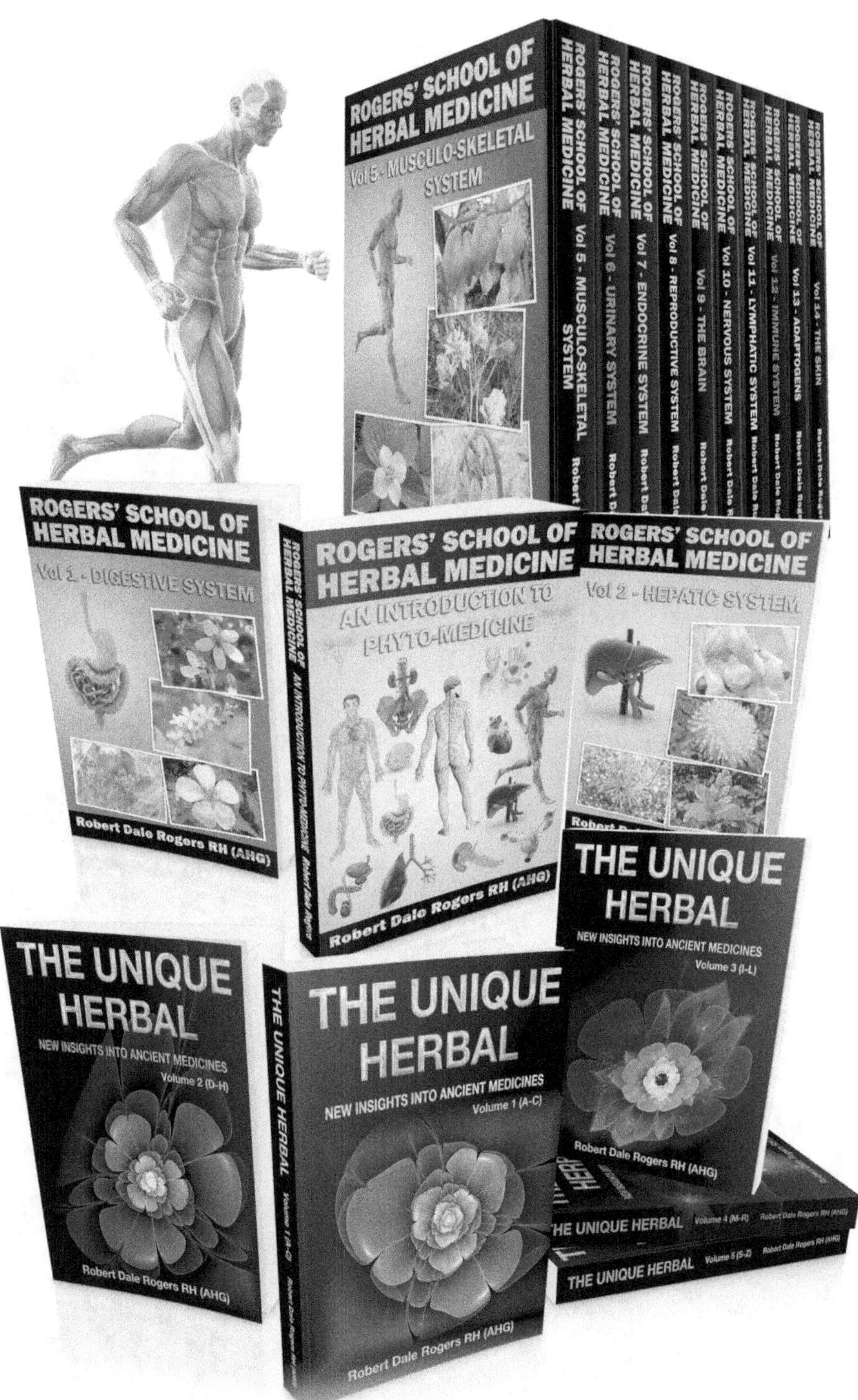
ROGERS' SCHOOL OF HERBAL MEDICINE
Vol 5 - MUSCULO-SKELETAL SYSTEM
ROGERS' SCHOOL OF HERBAL MEDICINE
Vol 5 - MUSCULO-SKELETAL SYSTEM
Vol 6 - URINARY SYSTEM
Vol 7 - ENDOCRINE SYSTEM
Vol 8 - REPRODUCTIVE SYSTEM
Vol 9 - THE BRAIN
Vol 10 - NERVOUS SYSTEM
Vol 11 - LYMPHATIC SYSTEM
Vol 12 - IMMUNE SYSTEM
Vol 13 - ADAPTOGENS
Vol 14 - THE SKIN
ROGERS' SCHOOL OF HERBAL MEDICINE
Vol 1 - DIGESTIVE SYSTEM
Robert Dale Rogers RH (AHG)
ROGERS' SCHOOL OF HERBAL MEDICINE
AN INTRODUCTION TO PHYTO-MEDICINE
Robert Dale Rogers RH (AHG)
ROGERS' SCHOOL OF HERBAL MEDICINE
Vol 2 - HEPATIC SYSTEM
Robert Dale Rogers RH (AHG)
THE UNIQUE HERBAL
NEW INSIGHTS INTO ANCIENT MEDICINES
Volume 3 (I-L)
Robert Dale Rogers RH (AHG)
THE UNIQUE HERBAL
NEW INSIGHTS INTO ANCIENT MEDICINES
Volume 2 (D-H)
Robert Dale Rogers RH (AHG)
THE UNIQUE HERBAL
NEW INSIGHTS INTO ANCIENT MEDICINES
Volume 1 (A-C)
Robert Dale Rogers RH (AHG)
THE UNIQUE HERBAL   Volume 4 (M-R)   Robert Dale Rogers RH (AHG)
THE UNIQUE HERBAL   Volume 5 (S-Z)   Robert Dale Rogers RH (AHG)

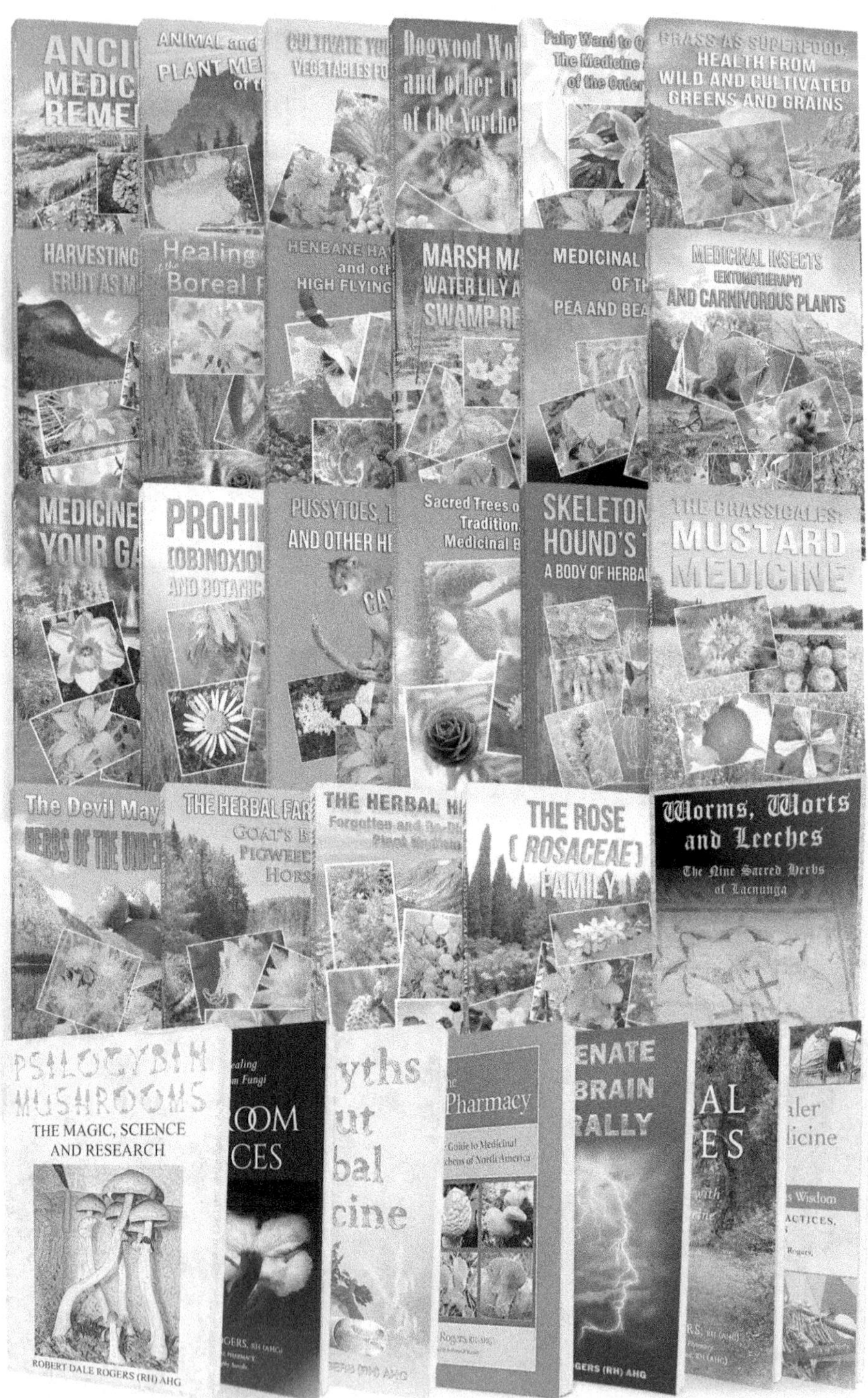